QUALITY
IMPROVEMENT

A GUIDE FOR INTEGRATION IN NURSING

D1536826

Anita Finkelman, MSN, RN

Visiting Lecturer, Nursing Department
Recanati School for Community Health Professions
Faculty of the Health Sciences
Ben-Gurion University of the Negev
Beersheba, Israel

JONES & BARTLETT
LEARNING

World Headquarters
Jones & Bartlett Learning
5 Wall Street
Burlington, MA 01803
978-443-5000
info@jblearning.com
www.jblearning.com

Jones & Bartlett Learning books and products are available through most bookstores and online booksellers. To contact Jones & Bartlett Learning directly, call 800-832-0034, fax 978-443-8000, or visit our website, www.jblearning.com.

Substantial discounts on bulk quantities of Jones & Bartlett Learning publications are available to corporations, professional associations, and other qualified organizations. For details and specific discount information, contact the special sales department at Jones & Bartlett Learning via the above contact information or send an email to specialsales@jblearning.com.

12476-7

Production Credits

VP, Executive Publisher: David D. Cella
Executive Editor: Amanda Martin
Editorial Assistant: Emma Huggard
Director of Vendor Management: Amy Rose
Senior Marketing Manager: Jennifer Scherzay
Product Fulfillment Manager: Wendy Kilborn

Composition and Project Management: S4Carlisle Publishing Services
Cover Design: Scott Moden
Rights & Media Specialist: Wes DeShano
Media Development Editor: Troy Liston
Cover Image: © adistock/Shutterstock
Printing and Binding: McNaughton & Gunn
Cover Printing: McNaughton & Gunn

Library of Congress Cataloging-in-Publication Data
Names: Finkelman, Anita Ward, author.
Title: Quality improvement : a guide for integration in nursing / Anita Finkelman.
Description: Burlington, MA : Jones & Bartlett Learning, [2018] | Includes bibliographical references and index.
Identifiers: LCCN 2016051851 | ISBN 9781284105544
Subjects: | MESH: Quality Improvement | Nursing Process | Integrative Medicine | United States
Classification: LCC RT41 | NLM WY 100 AA1 | DDC 610.73—dc23 LC record available at https://lccn.loc.gov/2016051851

6048

Printed in the United States of America
21 20 19 18   10 9 8 7 6 5 4 3 2

Contents

Acknowledgments

I thank my family, Fred, Shoshannah, and Deborah, for tolerating my long years of writing and supporting my efforts—being there when I was frustrated and also celebrating goals met. The Jones & Bartlett Learning team is always a joy to work with on projects, and I appreciate the support of Amanda Martin, Emma Huggard, and Jennifer Scherzay. My experiences in practice, administration, and education and all my students have given me opportunities to consider many aspects of nursing practice and education and the critical need for improvement.

Preface

Alice in Wonderland provides a window into a world that is confusing, often viewed as nonsensical, where language and terminology are not clear; where characters change forms and their identities are uncertain; and where time is not always based on reality. One of the main characters, the Red Queen, makes it clear that you cannot expect to improve if you allow the status quo to continue. Alice, the main character, struggles in this world to find her way, as if in a maze, not knowing where to go or what her destination may be. Alice is full of questions as she tries to make Wonderland clearer to herself and engage others in Wonderland. She does discover that to be shown something improves her understanding. "What is the use of a book," thought Alice, "without pictures and conversation." Alice also comments on change, "How puzzling all these changes are! I'm never sure what I'm going to be, from one minute to another."

Why have I chosen to use *Alice in Wonderland* to introduce this preface and also each section in the text? The world of health care and quality improvement is also confusing; language and terminology, roles and responsibilities, functions, quality improvement process and measurement, and many other elements are not always clear. Trying to understand the system and quality improvement takes effort and comes with frustration. You need to ask questions and seek out information, information that changes and expands your knowledge. Quality improvement itself is based on change—data and measurement. If we want to provide quality care, however, it is clear we cannot continue with the status quo. You will be entering a maze of information about quality improvement, which at times is confusing and at other times makes perfect sense. As a nurse, you must engage as Alice did in the journey to reach the goal.

As is typically the case when a nurse feels motivated to write a textbook, I was driven by the desire to provide resources for students to expand learning opportunities. This desire is influenced by my clinical and teaching experiences. Specifically, I sensed the need to help guide efforts toward quality improvement in nursing. As described in the text, the quality of health care in the United States has been the subject of intense scrutiny. For example, in May 2016, a study noted that if errors were considered in the listing of causes of death, they would be the third most common cause of death in the United States (Makary & Daniel, 2016). This statistic represents one example of many supporting the need for quality improvement.

In exploring the specifics of quality improvement, it is important to understand the national view of healthcare quality, which is fairly new and has been strongly influenced by the Institute of

Medicine's *Quality Chasm* reports. Quality improvement is related to change, but not all change is improvement. Knowledge is very important to improvement, but not all knowledge leads to improvement. We need more than knowledge about quality improvement; we must take actions and implement effective changes. The complexity of improvement is one of the difficulties we have in health care, and this complexity is compounded by both the complex healthcare system and the complexity of health problems and treatment for individual patients. None of these challenges, however, should be used as excuses to avoid what must be done: improve care daily, one patient at a time and throughout the system, whether that be within the healthcare delivery system, within an individual healthcare organization, or at the local, state, national, or even global level. To accomplish this goal requires a clear, effective framework that provides direction for planning and implementation of continuous quality improvement (CQI). Nurses must be prepared to participate in all settings and positions to engage in CQI, demonstrating leadership. As Kennedy (2016) states, "A Culture of Safety begins with us. We need to follow the evidence and own up to our role" (p. 7).

This text is divided into 3 sections and 12 chapters. Section I covers Chapters 1–4. This initial content focuses on healthcare quality perspectives. The chapters consider the attributes of quality care and factors that influence it, such as ethical and legal concerns, accreditation, standards, education, professional concerns, and change. Section II includes Chapters 5–10, focusing on planning and measurement to meet CQI outcomes. The final section, Section III, includes Chapters 11 and 12 and covers the last phase of the quality improvement process, preventing quality problems or responding to problems based on measurement. In conclusion, Chapter 12 discusses the need for nursing engagement and effective leadership in CQI.

Each chapter begins with Chapter Objectives, a Chapter Outline, and Key Terms relevant to chapter content. Following the chapter conclusions, the end of chapter content, Apply CQI, includes the following resources and activities for additional student learning:

- *Chapter Highlights* identifies some of the key points in the chapter content.
- *Critical Thinking and Clinical Reasoning and Judgment* provides opportunities for students to examine more of the content by completing individual and team activities, including written assignments, development of presentations and visuals, and discussion in class or online.
- *Connect to Current Information* identifies web links related to some of the chapter content—for example, government sites and healthcare profession organizations.
- *EBP, EBM, and Quality Improvement: Exemplar* provides a citation for a reference that explores evidence-based practice (EBP), evidence-based medicine (EBM), and quality improvement. It then poses questions about the reference to consider.
- *Evolving Case Study* is a case scenario focused on CQI with questions to consider.
- *References* identify references used to develop the chapter content.

Chapters include figures, exhibits, and tables to provide additional data and information supporting chapter content. Chapters also include Stop and Consider boxes, which highlight important thoughts relating to the content. As the student reads the chapter, he or she should stop and consider the statement in relation to the content and personal views. Finally, two appendices are included at the end of the text:

- Appendix A: Examples of Affordable Care Act of 2010 Provisions Related to Quality Care
- Appendix B: Examples of Major Healthcare Organizations and Agencies, Governmental and Nongovernmental, Related to Quality Improvement

References

Carroll, L. (1865). *Alice's Adventures in Wonderland*. London: Macmillan Publishing.
Carroll, L. (1872). *Through the Looking-Glass and What Alice Found There*. London: Macmillan Publishing.
Kennedy, M. (2016). A culture of safety starts with us. *American Journal of Nursing, 116*(5), 7.
Makary, M., & Daniel, M. (2016). Medical error—the third leading cause of death in the U.S. *BMJ*, (May 3). Retrieved from http://www.bmj.com/content/353/bmj.i2139/rr-40

Section I

Healthcare Quality Perspectives

"Begin at the beginning," the King said, very gravely, "and go on till you come to the end: then stop."

Lewis Carroll, *Alice's Adventures in Wonderland* (1865)

© Mopic/Shutterstock

The goal of the maze is to reach a state of quality care. To find your way out of the Continuous Quality Improvement Maze you first must begin to understand quality care and improvement: What is it? What is the status of quality care? What influences quality care—ethics, legal, accreditation, standards, education, professional concerns, and change

Healthcare Quality

CHAPTER OBJECTIVES

At the conclusion of this chapter, the learner will be able to:

- Examine the *Quality Chasm* reports and their impact on healthcare delivery.
- Analyze the current status of healthcare quality in the United States.
- Synthesize the key elements of the vision of healthcare quality.
- Examine the relationship between value and costs in healthcare delivery.
- Appraise the impact of the Affordable Care Act of 2010 on continuous quality improvement.
- Assess the National Quality Strategy and implications for nursing.
- Appraise the status of leadership, interprofessional teamwork, and nursing responsibility for continuous quality improvement.

OUTLINE

KEY TERMS

Continuous quality improvement (CQI)	Learning healthcare system	Pay for performance
Discrimination	Macrosystem	Process
Disparity	Macroview	Quality care
Diversity	Mesosystem	Quality gap
Error	Microsystem	Safety
Health literacy	Microview	Structure
Healthcare organizations (HCOs)	Outcome	System thinking

Introduction

As expressed by Nance (2008), the medical community has made great strides toward acknowledging and correcting the problem of medical injury in our society:

> We know how to prevent medical injuries. The Institute of Medicine [IOM] report that got so much attention also made a clear and unambiguous observation: It's not bad people, it's bad systems. Fix those systems! More than a half-century of thought, experimentation, and hard work in cognitive psychology, human factors engineering, and several high-hazard fields, most notably aviation, underlie that recommendation. System failures cause human failures. Fix systems if you want to stop medical mistakes and injuries. The efforts to fix systems have been enormous. Since the Institute of Medicine [IOM] report, there has been a steady crescendo of increasing development, testing, and implementation of new safe practices by hospitals throughout country. (p. vii)

As we learn more about **continuous quality improvement (CQI)**, we are better able to appreciate its complexity. Many **healthcare organizations (HCOs)** are trying out innovations and revising visions of how healthcare delivery should be viewed and the type of leadership required for integration and coordination of care so that care is patient centered (Bisognano & Kenney, 2012). The publication of *To Err Is Human* (IOM, 1999) and *Crossing the Quality Chasm* (IOM, 2001a) is sometimes described as the Big Bang in healthcare quality. In the words of Sollecito and Johnson (2013), "Suddenly, quality improvement was acknowledged to be a professional responsibility, a quality-of-care issue rather than a managerial tactic" (p. 25).

The content in this chapter reviews the overall view of healthcare quality—the CQI framework—and other background information needed to begin an examination of CQI. It echoes the sentiment of a question posed by Nash, Evans, and Bowman (2006): "After decades of research and numerous press reports indicating just how poor the quality of health care is in the United States, how can we continue denying that improving the quality of care is one of the most, if not the most, pressing public health issue today?" (p. 3).

Nurses have a responsibility to participate actively in improving care in their daily practice, whether that be in care delivery, management, education, or research, and should participate in healthcare policy-making at local, state, federal, and even global levels. This text supports the need for nursing engagement and leadership, but to achieve this objective requires knowledge and then application.

Healthcare Quality in the United States

The early reports from the National Academy of Medicine (NAM), then known as Institute of Medicine (IOM), describe **quality care** as "providing patients with appropriate services in a technically competent manner, with good communication, shared decision-making, and cultural sensitivity" (IOM, 2001a, p. 232). This definition emphasizes an active relationship with the patient and expectation of high performance on the part of the system and its providers.

Improving care has a long history, although major efforts toward this end were slow in arriving. Nursing was directly involved early on with the work of Florence Nightingale in the late 1800s and early 1900s. Nightingale began to examine the healthcare environment, collecting and analyzing data and recommending changes. Others also began to address health delivery problems, but how to systematically assess care and then determine solutions was an unknown area. Later in this text, models and theories about CQI and their influence on the development of effective methods to measure and improve care over time are discussed. It is critical for nurses to continue to develop their engagement in CQI and to participate in all aspects of CQI, including the development of measurement methods—monitoring, collecting and analyzing data, creating new solutions—to help prevent quality care problems. We have made progress, with acceleration in ideas, technology, and research, but from this expansion we have also learned we do not know enough. We now look at CQI from the system perspective, but each nurse must also consider the key concerns from an individual provider perspective: (1) How can I improve care for my patients? (2) How can I improve the system of care? Other industries have made great strides in addressing safety concerns, but health care has been much slower in developing improvement efforts.

Millenson (2006) aptly describes one of the key obstacles to the quality improvement initiative:

> Like the civil rights movement, the quality improvement movement cast doubts on deeply held traditional beliefs; in this case, those of the individual physician. While it might have been the individual doctor's "duty" to pursue process improvement and outcomes measurement, it was in his "interest," given traditional financial incentives. (p. 15)

This view of "duty" rather than "interest" did slow down CQI efforts; however, this trend has changed with the greater emphasis on the need for improvement. One might also consider how nurses responded, as nursing has also been slow to become more competent in CQI and assume greater leadership. Elements of CQI have been included in nursing standards for a long time, but until recently, these efforts had not been enough to move CQI toward center stage in nursing. Consider, for example, the publication of *The Future of Nursing* (IOM, 2010a) and its emphasis on nursing competency and leadership as a requirement for CQI.

The *Quality Chasm* Reports and the Healthcare Delivery System

As articulated by Gantz, Sorenson, and Howard (2003) over a decade ago, "The movement [quality improvement] now reaches beyond the walls of health care since *quality* is a part of everyday conversation not only among providers and payers but also consumers" (p. 324). This insight remains true today, and consumers are even more involved in commenting on health care. To appreciate the current views and status of U.S. health care, it is necessary to gain a historical perspective, particularly focusing on the 1990s to current date. Why is this background important? Healthcare delivery is influenced by healthcare policy, and so it is important to examine some of the policy issues—i.e., how they are identified and their impact. For nurses to assume greater leadership, they need this background information. The place to begin is with President W. Clinton's administration.

Presidents may form short-term commissions without approval of Congress to examine issues and problems. President W. Clinton established the President's Advisory Commission on Consumer Protection and Quality in the Healthcare Industry, which published a final report, *Quality First: Better Healthcare for All Americans* (1998). The report indicated that there was concern about healthcare quality, and we needed to know more about its status and how quality improvement is accomplished and maintained. The commission recommended that the NAM assume the responsibility for additional extensive examination.

First, a recent development involving some of the key players in the CQI effort should be pointed out:

> On March 15, 2016, the division of the National Academies of Sciences, Engineering, and Medicine (the Academies) that focuses on health and medicine was renamed the Health and Medicine Division (HMD) instead of using the name Institute of Medicine (IOM). This new name builds on the heritage of the IOM's work in medicine while emphasizing its increased focus on a wider range of health matters. (NAS/HMD, 2016)

When this organization is mentioned in this text, it will be referred to as NAS/HMD.

The NAS/HMD is a nonprofit agency that is located in Washington, DC. The organization is not connected to the government, but rather serves as an advisor to the government, policy makers, businesses, educators, and professionals. Since its work is highly respected, it has great influence. How does the NAS/HMD provide advice? Typically, it is asked to examine a specific problem by an external party such as Congress, the president, government agencies, professional organizations, and so on, as was the case with President Clinton's Advisory Commission on Consumer Protection and Quality in Healthcare. The NAS/HMD staff invites a panel of experts to examine the problem. The panel is provided with staff support. Often a panel will work for several years, examining information and data and asking for expert testimony. Then a report is published that provides information and recommendations. These recommendations may be ignored or may be used to initiate changes in policy, laws, regulations, education, and so on. The reports cover a broad range of topics, including health care. See the Connect to Current Information section at the end of the chapter for a link to the site, which provides free access to the reports.

Since 1999, the NAS/HMD has examined many issues and published reports related to healthcare quality, referred to as the *Quality Chasm* reports. Through this process of using multiple panels of experts representing a variety of professions, these reports describe the problems, define critical terms for consistency, develop aims or goals and a vision of a quality healthcare system, develop a framework for national monitoring, and address the issue of healthcare professions competencies that are needed to meet the goals and the vision. The following descriptions provide an overview of the critical reports in this series. These reports have had a major impact on how the United States views its healthcare system and provide important direction for planning and implementing national and state CQI initiatives and HCO quality improvement programs (Finkelman & Kenner, 2016).

To Err Is Human *(1999)*

As requested by President Clinton's commission, the NAS/HMD, then known as the IOM, began to examine health care, focusing on errors. This report did not just become a policy report that sat on a bookshelf; it was the report that opened Pandora's box. The media took note of this report and ran stories on the radio and television news, newspapers, and other print publications. Why was this topic so interesting? The report noted that approximately 44,000 to nearly 100,000 patients died annually in the United States due to errors. This information was overwhelming to consumers who trusted the healthcare delivery system. It came at a time when healthcare consumers had found their voice, mostly due to the experience of the managed care era when consumers became angry about the growing loss of choice in health care. At the time of the report, there was little systematic monitoring of healthcare data, meaning the description of death rates due to errors was probably not accurate; in all likelihood, the true rate was higher. The report's concern about errors was one aspect that was discussed, but also important was the recognition of the need for systematic monitoring.

Another issue that arose from this examination was the concern about the "blame culture," in which HCOs focus on blaming individual staff for errors and ignore the impact of system issues. This critical topic is discussed in further detail in other chapters. The report provided two important definitions: **Safety** is "freedom from accidental injury (IOM, 1999, p. 4). **Error** is the "failure of a planned action to be completed as intended or the use of a wrong plan to achieve an aim" (IOM, 1999, p. 4). Safety is a part of healthcare quality. It is not the only dimension of quality, but resolving errors is important in achieving a high-quality healthcare system (IOM, 2001a; Sadeghi, Barzi, Mikhail, & Shabot, 2013).

The report concluded with recommendations, particularly noting that improving patient safety requires a comprehensive approach. There is no one magic solution. The other critical conclusion was that the system must move away from the prevailing blame culture. It is important to realize that at the time of this report the United States really had no comprehensive view or model of quality care or any method for monitoring and evaluating care. We had some pieces to the puzzle, but no system.

Crossing the Quality Chasm *(2001)*

With the publication of *To Err Is Human*, it was recognized that we needed to know more about the healthcare delivery system and its quality. A second panel was formed to continue this examination, resulting in *Crossing the Quality Chasm* (IOM, 2001a). This report concluded that the U.S. healthcare delivery system was dysfunctional, with great variety in performance, fragmented and poorly organized, confusing, and complex. There was treatment overuse, underuse, and misuse, all of which have a major impact on quality. This situation is often referred to as a **quality gap**. These outcomes were disturbing. In addition, other aspects of concern were noted. Chronic disease was a growing problem, crossing the life span, with many people having more than one chronic disease. The system was not prepared to deliver quality care for this population. In addition, there was concern that there was a problem with disparities in health care, although there was limited understanding of this problem.

The report began the process of describing a vision of the U.S. healthcare delivery system focused on quality, and this helped to develop a structure for CQI. If the only *Quality Chasm* report had been the 1999 report, we would not be where we are today, making more and more efforts to improve care. *Crossing the Quality Chasm* examined health care with greater depth, which was needed to fully recognize that the system had serious problems and was very weak. However, even though the first two reports indicated there were many problems, it took more reports, examination, and work to drive the need for CQI and make it a priority (Bisognano & Kenney, 2012).

Envisioning the National Healthcare Quality Report *(2001)*

As was noted in the first two *Quality Chasm* reports, there was great need for systematic monitoring of healthcare quality so that we would better understand the status of quality care and then use this information to improve care. *Envisioning the National Healthcare Quality Report* describes an initial framework for a national healthcare quality monitoring report that would be completed annually. As expressed in this report (IOM, 2001b), "*The National Healthcare Quality Report (NHQR)* should serve as a yardstick or the barometer by which to gauge progress in improving the performance of the healthcare delivery system in consistently providing high-quality care" (p. 2). The framework for the annual report is influenced by the aims and the vision as well as other recommendations from *Quality Chasm* reports. The annual report makes data and analysis available to decision makers and the public. The original description of the framework has changed, but the core elements are the same. The Agency for Healthcare Research and Quality (AHRQ), which is an agency in the U.S. Department of Health and Human Services (HHS), is responsible for the annual *NHQR*, with the most current report accessible at the AHRQ website. A link is provided in the Connect to Current Information section at the end of the chapter.

Priority Areas for National Action *(2003)*

When the direction changed from developing a framework to routinely monitoring care quality, the question of what should be monitored arose. It was clear that not all aspects of care could or should be monitored. The *Priority Areas for National Action* report discusses the issue of prioritizing and identified the focus areas used in the first annual report (IOM, 2003a). As was expected, the focus areas have changed as certain areas have improved, reducing the need for monitoring, redefinition of areas, and new areas that need to be added.

Health Professions Education: A Bridge to Quality *(2003)*

After the NAS/HMD spent considerable time describing healthcare delivery problems and identifying aims, a vision, and setting up a system to monitor care, attention turned to the need for healthcare professionals to be prepared and competent to ensure that care is of the highest quality possible. This need impacts both staff education and academic education, as both settings prepare staff for professional roles such as physician, nurse, pharmacist, healthcare administrator, and many others. If the healthcare system is working toward improvement but the new healthcare professionals entering the system are not prepared in core areas, then improving care will be difficult.

The report's expert panel identified five healthcare professions core competencies that are necessary to reach an acceptable level of quality care (IOM, 2003b, p. 4).

1. Provide patient-centered care.
2. Work in interdisciplinary/interprofessional teams.
3. Employ evidence-based practice.
4. Apply quality improvement.
5. Utilize informatics.

The report recommended that all healthcare profession education programs adopt these core competencies. It is significant that the emphasis was not on a specific healthcare profession, but rather focused on all healthcare professions. These competencies should be common to all healthcare professions, although there are other specific competencies that also pertain to each profession. HCO staff who are not prepared in these areas need to be updated, as the competencies apply not only to students but also to staff. These competencies are directly related to healthcare problems and possible solutions. This text emphasizes these competencies for nurses because they are integral to understanding and application of CQI.

Nursing Reports

The NAS/HMD has had a major impact on nursing, as it has published several reports on nursing. The report *Nursing and Nursing Education: Public Policy and Private Action* (IOM, 1983) recommended that nursing have an active role at the National Institutes of Health (NIH), and as a result, Congress established the Center for Nursing Research at NIH in 1993. It is now called the National Institute for Nursing Research (NINR). The NINR has an impact on nursing and CQI. It provides greater nursing professional emphasis on research, which is necessary for evidence-based practice (EBP), a critical component of CQI and focus of one of the core competencies.

The second major report, *Keeping Patients Safe: Transforming the Work Environment for Nurses* (IOM, 2004a), emphasizes the need to transform the work environment for nurses, focusing on the 24/7 role of nurses in acute care and how their work impacts the quality of care. The report's recommendations focus on four areas: (1) adopting transformational leadership and evidence-based management, (2) maximizing the capability of the workforce, (3) designing work and workspaces to prevent and mitigate errors, and (4) creating and sustaining cultures of safety (IOM, 2004a, pp. 7–14). This examination of acute care nursing provides important information about the status of nursing in the healthcare system and what needs to improve. The report strongly supports the need for nurses to assume more active roles in CQI but concludes that nurses are not sufficiently prepared to do this. Nursing leadership is also emphasized in this report.

In 2010, a landmark report titled *The Future of Nursing: Leading Change, Advancing Health* was published, which continued the earlier work done by the NAS/HMD (IOM, 2010a). This report discusses changes needed in nursing degrees, the need to increase the number of BSN-prepared nurses and doctoral-prepared nurses, barriers to scope of practice, the need for lifelong learning, workforce issues, and other relevant professional concerns. *Keeping*

Patients Safe (IOM, 2004a) provides the critical groundwork for *The Future of Nursing* report. In many respects, *Keeping Patients Safe* discusses more significant information about nursing practice, such as the major role of nurses in the healthcare delivery system, the need for nurses to be leaders in CQI (although they are often not prepared to do so), staffing and staff schedules, the blame culture, work design and its impact on quality, the need for transformational leadership, the nursing shortage, risks of working long hours, and the need for greater use of surveillance or ongoing monitoring of patients. Although this report's content is significant for nursing, it received minimal attention when published compared to the attention given *The Future of Nursing*. The 2010 report and the progress report published in 2015 are discussed in more detail in other chapters in this text.

Public Health Reports

The *Quality Chasm* reports also examine public health. The two major public health reports are *The Future of the Public's Health in the 21st Century* (IOM, 2003c) and *Who Will Keep the Public Healthy?* (IOM, 2003d). Although we often think of the public health system as separate from the "healthcare delivery system," it should be an integral part of the entire healthcare delivery system. Today, there is much more focus given to the entire system and recognition that more needs to be done to provide care and meet health needs within the patient's community. Public/community health delivery also requires improvement, and in addition, there will be greater need for public health services and thus for public health professionals. The first report identifies aspects of public health that are important in reviewing: population health approach, public health infrastructure, partnerships, accountability, evidence, and communication. In addition to the five healthcare professions competencies identified in the report *Health Professions Education* (IOM, 2003b), the second public health report notes that effective public health requires that staff be competent in informatics, genomics, communication, culture, community-based participatory research, global health, policy and law, and public health ethics.

Impact of the Quality Chasm Reports

The *Quality Chasm* reports have had a major impact on U.S. views of quality care, influencing innovations to improve care and healthcare legislation, such as the Patient Protection and Affordable Care Act of 2010 (ACA). Staff may wonder why it is important to pay attention to this work on quality care and its numerous reports. The answer: It represents the leading source of critical examination of the healthcare delivery system and its outcomes. Its recommendations influence the creation of new legislation and regulations and impact government departments and agencies, such as the HHS, Centers for Medicare and Medicaid Services (CMS), Food and Drug Administration (FDA), Centers for Disease Control and Prevention (CDC), AHRQ, Occupational Safety and Health Administration (OSHA), National Institute for Occupational Health and Safety (NIOSH), and state and local departments and services.

The *Quality Chasm* reports have led to many changes in health care, but one of the most notable is that "suddenly, quality improvement was acknowledged to be a professional responsibility, a quality-of-care issue rather than a managerial tactic" (Sollecito & Johnson, 2013, p. 25). The responsibility for CQI has typically been more important to higher healthcare administration; however, now this responsibility has been expanded to include healthcare providers, who can make major changes in the quality of care on a daily basis.

The recommendations led to changes in HCOs and CQI-related organizations' requirements, such as those of The Joint Commission, which accredits most HCOs. Healthcare professional organizations and educational institutions also consider the *Quality Chasm* reports' recommendations relevant to their goals and use them in developing initiatives to improve care and healthcare professional education, such as the following examples, many of which are discussed in other sections of this text:

- The Joint Commission designation of annual safety goals, which are monitored by organizations accredited by The Joint Commission (the goals change annually depending on the need)
- The Joint Commission and World Health Organization (WHO) initiatives focusing on reducing errors globally
- The development of the Institute for Healthcare Improvement and resources about CQI for staff, education programs, and healthcare professions students
- Institute for Healthcare Improvement 5 Million Lives Campaign collaborating with The Joint Commission's High 5s Project
- CMS changes in reimbursement and development of the Hospital Acquired Complications initiative
- Development of increased interest in interprofessional collaborative teams leading to need to improve interprofessional education; publication of major reports on these topics jointly developed by an interprofessional group
- Development of web-based information and tools to improve care
- Establishment of the CMS Hospital Quality Initiative, providing comparison information on quality
- Publication of *The Future of Nursing: Leading Change, Advancing Health* (IOM, 2010a), a critical report influenced by the previous *Quality Chasm* reports on CQI and related nursing reports

- Publication of *Educating Nurses: A Call for Radical Transformation* (Benner, Sutphen, Leonard, & Day, 2010), a major report about a study that concludes there is need to improve nursing education
- Passage and implementation of the ACA, which is focused on healthcare delivery, access to care, and costs

The pressure to focus more on CQI has been influenced by the *Quality Chasm* reports, but also by initiatives that developed from these reports and other reports that followed (Draper, Felland, Liebhaber, & Melichar, 2008). Changes, such as the preceding examples, are ongoing. The Joint Commission changed its focus to requiring that their accredited HCOs report on core quality measures for accreditation, rather than using a broad-based approach that tries to assess all aspects of an HCO. Since insurers typically expect HCOs such as hospitals to be accredited, there is now increased HCO motivation to meet these requirements to ensure reimbursement of services. The Magnet Recognition Program® places greater emphasis on HCO nursing service responsibilities and leadership in HCO quality improvement, supporting the recognition of nurses meeting critical CQI responsibilities and the need for this leadership. These examples and others are discussed in more detail throughout this text, but they are mentioned here to illustrate the major impact of the *Quality Chasm* reports on health policy, healthcare delivery, nursing practice, and healthcare profession education. In 2014, The U.S. Senate Committee on Health, Education, Labor, and Pensions held meetings on healthcare quality and discussed the recommendations from the *Quality Chasm* reports, their outcomes, and the current quality status. **Exhibit 1-1** provides excerpts of this discussion, illustrating how important this topic is in the United States and the concern about the need for improvement.

Since the first report in the *Quality Chasm* series was published in 1999 there have been many other reports that expanded on the topic and also focused on more specific issues related to quality care and to specialty care such as emergency care, oncology, women's health, pediatrics, pain management, chronic disease, genomics, EBP, and others. All reports are available through the NAS/HMD website, listed in the Connect to Current Information section at the end of chapter.

Reports on Diversity and Disparities in Health Care

With the extensive examination of the healthcare system, the early *Quality Chasm* reports noted that there was most likely a serious problem with disparities in health care, which is also related to efforts to improve public/community health (IOM, 2001a). This led to additional reports on this problem and to the development of a *National Healthcare Disparities Report* (*NHDR*) that would be available with the *NHQR* and also administered by the AHRQ. In 2010, the NAS/HMD was asked to

Exhibit 1-1 Excerpts from Expert Testimony, U.S. Senate Committee on Health, Education, Labor, and Pensions (HELP), Subcommittee on Primary Health and Aging. Patient Safety Hearing. (July 17, 2014)

Peter Pronovost, MD, PhD, FCCM: Medicine today has preventable harm as the third leading cause of death. We do not Bates, and I used published literature to estimate that over 220,000 preventable deaths occur from health care; that is over 600 deaths daily, which is far more than from mining or faulty automobiles yet receiving far less attention. This estimate is conservative and does not include more than 120,000 deaths from teamwork failures, 80,000 deaths from misdiagnosis, or thousands of deaths from sepsis. Medicine today squanders a third of every dollar spent on therapies that do not get patients well, that result from treating preventable complications, and that result from administrative inefficiencies and fraud. This is about $9000 per U.S. household, (Fineberg, 2012) money that could be better spent on preschool education and STEM, on innovation, and on securing a better tomorrow for all Americans. Medicine today invests heavily in information technology. The Federal government and health care organizations have spent hundreds of billions of dollars on health information technology with little to show for it. The promised improvements in safety have not been realized and productivity has decreased rather than increased.

Ashish Jha, MD, MPH: So here we are, 15 years after *To Err is Human* and it is critical to ask a simple question: how much progress have we made? First, I want to start off with some good news. We have dramatically increased our awareness of patient safety issues and changed how we think about medical errors. In the past, medical errors were thought to be the result of individuals behaving badly. We blamed the doctor who ordered the wrong treatment, the pharmacist who dispensed the wrong dose, or the nurse who gave the medication to the wrong patient. This idea that adverse events were due to bad people led to a "deny and defend" culture among healthcare professionals and prevented progress on patient safety. Today, we know better. We know that medical errors are largely the result of bad systems of care delivery, not individual providers.

Four years ago, the New England Journal of Medicine published a terrific study from North Carolina hospitals that found that between 2002 and 2007, there had been little or no progress in reducing harm from unsafe medical care (Landrigan, Parry, Bones, Hackbarth, Goldman, & Sharek, 2010). A recent study led by Dr. John James found that between 200,000 and 400,000 Americans die each year from unsafe medical care, which makes it the third leading killer in the U.S., behind only heart disease and cancer (James, 2013). Finally, in an eye-opening November 2011 report on adverse events in hospitals, the Office of the Inspector General (OIG) in the Department of Health and Human Services found that 13.5 percent of Medicare patients suffered an injury in the hospital that prolonged their stay or caused permanent harm or death. An additional 13.5 percent of Medicare patients suffered temporary harm such as an allergic reaction or hypoglycemia. Together, the data suggest that more than one in four hospitalized Medicare beneficiaries suffers some sort of injury during their inpatient stay, much higher than previous rates. The OIG report also found that unsafe care contributes to 180,000 deaths of Medicare beneficiaries each year, and that Medicare pays at least $4.4 billion to treat these injuries (HHS, 2010)

Despite all the focus on patient safety, it seems we have not made much progress at all. The news is not all bad, of course -- and there are areas where we have made meaningful gains. The area of safety that has seen the biggest improvement is healthcare associated infections.

While much attention in patient safety has been paid to acute hospitals, we have generally paid far less attention to what happens when patients are discharged. In a different report, the OIG at HHS found that 22 percent of Medicare beneficiaries in skilled nursing facilities (SNF) suffered a medical injury that prolonged their stay or caused permanent harm or death. An additional 11 percent suffered temporary medical injury. All told, OIG estimates that adverse events cost Medicare roughly $2.8 billion per year, and about half of these events are preventable. The OIG report is particularly alarming given that about 20 percent of hospitalized Medicare patients go to a SNF after discharge (HHS, 2014). We need a renewed call to improve patient safety as a national priority.

The strategy for improvement has to focus on three main areas: metrics, accountability, and incentives. Getting the metrics right may be the most important. The fundamental problem is that most healthcare organizations don't track the safety of their care. In addition, I believe that health information technology has a critical role to play in improving patient safety. But metrics and reporting alone will not be enough. We also need to make safe care part of the business of providing healthcare. And this requires incentives.

Tejal Gandhi, MD, MPH, CPPS: I would like to talk to you today about ambulatory patient safety and the priorities and challenges that we currently face. Much of the effort of the patient safety movement over the past 15 years, since the Institute of Medicine report To Err is Human (http://www .nap.edu/catalog.php?record_id=9728), has focused on improving patient safety in the hospital setting. However, it is important to remember that most care is given outside of hospitals, and there are numerous safety issues that exist in other health settings that are quite different from those we face in hospitals (Gandhi, 2010). The setting that we know the most about, in terms of ambulatory safety issues, is primary care. I will touch on 3 areas in particular--medication safety, missed and delayed diagnoses, and transitions of care. Studies have shown that medication errors are common in primary care, and that adverse drug events, or injuries due to drugs, occur in up to 25% of patients within 30 days of being prescribed a drug (http://www.ncbi.nlm.nih.gov/pubmed/12700376). In addition, a key medication safety issue in ambulatory care, that is not an issue in hospitals, is nonadherence. Missed and delayed diagnosis is a key issue as well-- this is the most common type of outpatient malpractice claim (usually missed and delayed diagnosis of cancer in primary care). Lastly, we know that patients are vulnerable during transitions in care. These transitions occur all the time in health care--hospital to home, nursing home to emergency department, rehabilitation center to visiting nurse. Transitions are high-risk times, when key pieces of information (such as medication changes, pending test results, additional workups that need to happen) can be lost. For example, one study found that after hospital discharge, within 3 to 5 days, one-third of patients were taking their medications differently than how they were prescribed at discharge (Schnipper, et al., 2006). A major theme throughout ambulatory safety is patient engagement--partnering with patients to achieve safer care.

Joanne Disch, PhD, RN, FAAN: The estimate by James (2013) that possibly 400,000 PDs occur each year is more accurate than the previous Institute of Medicine (IOM) projection of 98,000/year (*To Err Is* Human, 1999). However, I would respectfully suggest that the title of this hearing understates the problem – and the title of the hearing should be changed to 'More than 1000 preventable deaths - and 10,000 preventable serious complications a day - is too many. . ."

This morning, I will highlight some of the key factors influencing patient safety, and make three recommendations which I know, from my 46 years as a nurse, make a difference: (1) assuring an adequate and appropriately educated supply of registered nurses at the bedside; (2) actively engaging patients and families as partners in their care; and (3) moving hospitals and other healthcare settings to embrace a safety culture and become high reliability organizations. My comments focus on the hospital setting since that is where we have the most data, although the principles apply to other settings.

Nurses are the cornerstones of the American health care system. Registered nurses form the largest element (2.6 million), with more than half (58%) working in medical and surgical hospitals (BLS, 2013). They provide care

24/7 and are on the 'ground floor' of care delivery. They are the eyes and ears of patients and their families, as well as physicians and other HCPs who are interacting with the patient intermittently. The nurse's role is to assess the patient's condition and response to treatment; perform indicated treatments; prevent complications; assist the patient and family in adjusting to the treatment or impact of chronic illness; and create a safe environment within which health, healing or a peaceful death can occur. It is the nurse who sees a skin breakdown that will lead to a bedsore; it is the nurse who notices the older woman's unsteady gait and puts in place strategies to prevent a fall; it is the nurse who notices that the dose of the drug ordered is not relieving the pain and who initiates a conversation with the physician to get the order changed. Individuals who have been hospitalized, or have had a family member hospitalized, understand the essential role of the nurse. Actually, nursing care is the reason for hospitalization . . . and it is the nurse who is the 'last line of defense' against error.

Data from U.S. Senate Committee on Health, Education, Labor, & Pensions. (2014). Subcommittee hearing: More than 1,000 preventable deaths a day is too many: The need to improve patient safety. Retrieved from http://www.help.senate.gov/hearings /more-than-1-000-preventable-deaths-a-day-is-too-many-the-need-to-improve-patient -safety. Testimony examples are excerpted from longer transcripts available at the URL.

Other references noted in comments from the congressional testimony:

Bureau of Labor Statistics (BLS). (2013). Employment projections 2012–2022. Retrieved from http://www.bls.gov/news.release/ecopro.t08.htm

Fineberg H. (2012) Shattuck lecture. A successful and sustainable health system--how to get there from here. *New England Journal of Medicine, 366*, 1020–1027.

Gandhi, T. (2010). Patient safety beyond the hospital. *New England Journal of Medicine, 363*, 1001–1003

Landrigan C., Parry G., Bones C., Hackbarth A., Goldmann D., Sharek P. (2010). Temporal trends in rates of patient harm resulting from medical care. *New England Journal of Medicine, 363* (22) 2010, 2124–2134.

James J. (2013). A new, evidence-based estimate of patient harms associated with hospital care. *J Patient Saf. 9*(3): 122–128.

Schnipper, J. et al. (2006). Role of pharmacist counseling in preventing adverse drug events after hospitalization. *Archives of Internal Medicine, 166* (5), 565–571.

U.S. Department of Health and Human Services: Office of Inspector General (HHS). (November 2010) Adverse events in hospitals: National incidence among Medicare beneficiaries. Washington, D.C.: Author.

U.S. Department of Health and Human Services: Office of Inspector General (HHS). (February 2014) Adverse events in skilled nursing facilities. Washington, D.C.: Author review the AHRQ monitoring system, and this led to the following improvement recommendations (IOM, 2010b, p. xi):

- Track national priorities for quality improvement and high-impact measurement areas to inform collective action across federal and other public and private sector healthcare delivery programs.
- Conceptually and operationally link quality improvement and disparities elimination in the *NHQR* and *NHDR*.
- Highlight quality achievement by presenting best-in-class benchmarks: Move from only presenting historical trend data to also extrapolating rates of change to indicate when gaps might be closed at the existing pace; present an assessment of the effect on population health of bridging quality and equity gaps.
- Analyze and present data in meaningful ways that identify for Congress, states, and others the results of and prospects for evidence-based policies and interventions
- Support broader and sustained dissemination of report content.

Unequal Treatment *(2003)*

Unequal Treatment (IOM, 2003e) examined healthcare disparities and noted that bias, prejudice, and stereotyping may result in disparities, and the healthcare delivery system had a healthcare disparities problem. This problem is found consistently across a variety of healthcare settings and diagnoses. **Disparities** is defined as "racial or ethnic differences in the quality of healthcare that are not due to access-related factors or clinical needs, preferences, and appropriateness of intervention" (IOM, 2003e, pp. 3–4). Any **diversity** characteristic could be applied to this definition—for example, gender, religion, ethnicity, and so on. Among the goals of Healthy People 2020, a federal initiative, are to "achieve health equity, eliminate disparities, and improve the health of all groups" (HHS, ODPHP, 2010). This objective relates to conclusions and recommendations in the *Quality Chasm* reports on quality and disparities. There was concern that discrimination existed in the healthcare system. The goal is to reduce **discrimination**, defined as "differences in care that result from bias, prejudices, stereotyping, and uncertainty in clinical communication and decision-making" (IOM, 2002, p. 4).

Health Literacy *(2004)*

Health Literacy expanded the discussion about diversity to include **health literacy**, defined as "the degree to which individuals have the capacity to obtain, process, and understand basic information and services needed to make appropriate decisions regarding their health" (IOM, 2004b, p. 2). Health literacy has a major impact on quality care and the health of individuals and communities. For example, if a patient or family cannot understand medication directions, then an error may occur or the patient may not take medication as prescribed, influencing health outcomes. Healthcare providers need to recognize that understanding may be more than just the ability to read. Vulnerable populations are at greater risk for health literacy problems. The AHRQ announced in 2011 that low health literacy in older Americans is linked to poorer health status and a higher risk of death, more emergency room visits, and more hospitalizations (HHS, AHRQ, 2011). Today, efforts are being made to address this problem, but much more needs to be done. This topic is discussed in other chapters, as it is highly relevant to meeting CQI outcomes and nursing care.

Guidance for the National Healthcare Disparities Report *(2002)*

Due to the recognition of a major problem in healthcare disparities, it was recommended that in addition to annual monitoring of healthcare quality there is need to also annually monitor healthcare disparities. *Guidance for the National Healthcare Disparities Report* describes how disparities should be monitored and how to best integrate this information with quality monitoring (IOM, 2002). Both are administered by the AHRQ and found on the same website. If healthcare disparities are to be reduced, it is critical that there be a comprehensive review of the status and need to monitor change over time. Developing interventions to improve has become an important goal for HCOs and healthcare professions. Other content in this text elaborates on healthcare diversity and the problem of disparities.

In addition to reviewing these important reports, it is necessary to consider diversity in healthcare professions. In the Sullivan Commission on Diversity in the Healthcare Workforce report, it is noted that the United States needs greater workforce diversity to better meet the needs of a growing diverse patient population and reduce healthcare disparities (Sullivan, 2004). Since the publication of this report, there has been greater emphasis on increasing the number of minorities in all healthcare professions. In nursing, funding has been granted to assist in examining diversity in the profession and to support programs in nursing schools to increase faculty and student diversity, although the lack of diversity continues to be a concern.

Healthy People 2020

The Healthy People 2020 initiative focuses on community and public health. This initiative is now in its third 10-year cycle. The HHS Office of Disease Prevention and Health Promotion (2010) describes the Healthy People initiative as follows:

> *Healthy People* is used as a tool for strategic management by the federal government, states, communities, and many other public- and private-sector partners. Its comprehensive set of objectives and targets is used to measure

progress for health issues in specific populations, and serves as (1) a foundation for prevention and wellness activities across various sectors and within the federal government, and (2) a model for measurement at the state and local levels. (p. 1)

The Healthy People vision is a society in which all people live long, healthy lives, and this initiative aims to (Healthy People, 2015):

1. Attain high quality, longer lives free of preventable disease, disability, injury, and premature death.
2. Achieve health equity, eliminate disparities, and improve the health of all groups.
3. Create a social and physical environment that promotes good health for all.
4. Promote quality of life, healthy development, and healthy behaviors across life stages.

These goals are directly related to the work of the NAS/HMD, and there has been collaboration between the NAS/HMD and the Healthy People initiative. At the request of Healthy People, NAS/HMD participated in a review of Healthy People and provided comments about the revision of its leading indicators (IOM, 2011a). This collaboration demonstrates how NAS/HMD is integrated throughout many aspects of healthcare policy and initiatives that address improving health and healthcare delivery. **Figure 1-1** describes the key aspects of the current Healthy People cycle. Further information can be accessed through the Healthy People website, listed in the Connect to Current Information section at end of the chapter.

Stop and Consider #1
Up until 1999, we had limited in depth knowledge of healthcare quality.

Status of Healthcare Quality

As we get into a more detailed examination of CQI and how nurses can be involved in the effort, it is important to review the current status of healthcare quality and disparities. We now know we have annual reports on quality and disparities to help us monitor and analyze the status, and the current reports are accessible through the AHRQ website. Where do we stand, and what should concern us?

Since the publication of the 1999 *Quality Chasm* report, additional concerns have been identified and discussed:

For more than a decade, reports of the Institute of Medicine (IOM) have focused attention on a persistent set of problems within the American healthcare system that urgently need to be addressed, including poor quality;

Healthy People 2020

A society in which all people live long, healthy lives

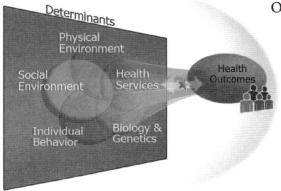

Overarching Goals:

- Attain high quality, longer lives free of preventable disease, disability, injury, and premature death.
- Achieve health equity, eliminate disparities, and improve the health of all groups
- Create social and physical environments that promote good health for all.
- Promote quality of life, healthy development and healthy behaviors across all life stages.

Figure 1-1 Healthy People 2020

Reproduced from Healthy People 2020. (2016). Framework. Retrieved from http://www.healthypeople.gov.

lax safety; high cost; questionable value; and the misdistribution of care based on income, race, and ethnicity. Each report has called for substantive transformation of the nation's healthcare system. Many have pointed out a disturbing paradox: the coexistence of overtreatment and undertreatment. The committee that authored this report found a similar situation: learning and adoption that are maddeningly slow—as with hand washing—coexisting with overly rapid adoption of some new techniques, devices, and drugs, with harmful results. Exemplary efforts under way across the nation are working on these problems . . . . But the pace of change is too slow, and adoption is too spotty; the system is not evolving quickly enough. (IOM, 2012, p. xi)

Based on comments like this and others, much work still must be done. Despite reports, initiatives, and work done by the government, HCOs, and healthcare providers, the United States continues to have quality care problems. In 2016, a study noted that if healthcare errors were considered a disease, errors would be the third-leading cause of death in the United States (Makary & Daniel, 2016). This is a significant statement, particularly if you consider this study alongside the 1999 report *To Err Is Human* (IOM, 1999), which identified a high rate of errors many years ago.

Also in 2016, it was revealed that the National Institutes of Health Clinical Center has had major quality problems, so much so that its leadership would be replaced (Bernstein & McGinley, 2016). The Clinical Center serves as a hospital for clinical trials and is the largest hospital of its kind in the world. It has a long history of providing care that is needed and exemplary; however, an independent review board "concluded that patient safety had become 'subservient to research demands'" (Sun, 2016). The review also noted that when compared to other hospitals, the center had no adequate systems for staff to report problems, such as near misses and errors, anonymously and supervisors did not address problems. This conclusion demonstrates grave problems and indicates that even with all the discussion about CQI and in a hospital that is so well known, there are HCOs providing care in an environment in which CQI is not a priority.

Since 1999, the healthcare community has recognized some elements of CQI that are important determinants of whether quality care is provided. Examples include movement toward a patient-centered system, greater engagement of patients and families, health informatics that continues to develop and provide tools that can be used while providing care, monitoring of care, CQI measurement, and more. As a result of the *Quality Chasm* reports, there is now greater recognition for more national approaches; many of the current initiatives are discussed in this text. We know we need leadership that guides CQI and staff engaged in the process. But despite all of these insights, much more needs to be learned about CQI and how to achieve it. CQI is not something that really has an end point, which is why quality improvement is referred to as *continuous* quality improvement.

Quality Care

As noted in *To Err Is Human*, an organized process was begun to examine the U.S. healthcare system. After several expert panels and published reports, it was clear that the system had major problems; however, there have been efforts made to improve since 2004 by more effective implementation of CQI (IOM, 2001a). There has also been some effort to include CQI content in nursing programs, although more is required. Monitoring is now done on an annual basis, with some of the resulting information available to the public and healthcare providers on the Internet.

In addition, the federal government has assumed a major role in monitoring and developing solutions to improve care as well as funding initiatives to improve care. The HHS is the major federal agency responsible for protecting the health of all Americans and providing essential health services. The department has a number of agencies that assist in meeting HHS goals, particularly to better ensure quality care (HHS, 2016a):

- *Centers for Medicare and Medicaid Services (CMS).* Manages all aspects of the Medicare Program and the Medicaid Program. Medicaid is a shared program, functioning at both the federal and the state levels, and Medicare is a federal program.
- *Agency for Healthcare Research and Quality (AHRQ).* Focuses on improving the quality, safety, efficiency, and effectiveness of health care for all Americans. As one of twelve agencies within the HHS, the AHRQ supports research and programs that help consumers, healthcare professionals, and

HCOs make more informed decisions and improve the quality of healthcare services and outcomes.

- *Centers for Disease Control and Prevention (CDC).* Collaborates to create the expertise, information, and tools that people and communities need to protect their health through health promotion, prevention of disease, injury and disability, and preparedness for new health threats; also offers information and resources about workplace safety, although the primary responsibility for this charge rests with the U.S. Department of Labor.
- *Food and Drug Administration (FDA).* Ensures safe use of food, drugs, and medical devices and equipment.
- *Indian Health Service (IHS).* Focuses on providing quality care to Native Americans and Alaskan Native populations.
- *Substance Abuse and Mental Health Services Administration (SAMSA).* Focuses on quality care for substance abuse and mental health needs.
- *Health Resources and Services Administration (HRSA).* Serves as the primary federal agency for improving access to healthcare services for people who are uninsured, isolated, or medically vulnerable, including people living with HIV/AIDS, pregnant women, and mothers and children. HRSA provides leadership and financial support to healthcare providers in every state and U.S. territory. The agency trains health professionals and improves systems of care in rural communities. HRSA oversees organ, bone marrow, and cord blood donation. It supports programs that prepare against bioterrorism, compensates individuals harmed by vaccination, and maintains databases that protect against healthcare malpractice and healthcare waste, fraud, and abuse.
- *National Institutes of Health (NIH).* Seeks fundamental knowledge about the nature and behavior of living systems and the application of that knowledge to enhance health, lengthen life, and reduce the burdens of illness and disability. NIH includes the National Institute of Nursing Research (NINR).

These federal government agencies are not new, but today they have been influenced by the *Quality Chasm* reports and recommendations, leading to an increase in their CQI activities.

The National Quality Forum (NQF), a public–private partnership established in 1999, is now an important organization leading healthcare performance improvement and advising policy makers. Its three-part mission is to improve the quality of American health care by helping set national priorities and goals for quality improvement, to endorse national consensus standards for measuring and publicly reporting on performance, and to promote the attainment of national goals through education and outreach programs (NQF, 2016). The NQF is particularly recognized for establishing NQF-endorsed measures, now considered by many to be the gold standard in measurement, providing advice about CQI measurement to government agencies and others (Burstin, Leatherman, & Goldmann, 2016). Additional information about its measures is found in the chapters of this text relating to measurement and on the NQF website.

A major source of data about the status of health care is the *National Quality and Disparities Report* (HHS, AHRQ, 2015b). As mentioned earlier, the *Quality Chasm* reports recommended annual monitoring of quality care and also disparities. It is a reporting system that is congressionally mandated and has provided reports since 2003. In 2014, the *NHQR* and *NHDR* reports were combined and are now referred to as one report, *QDR*. The new version combines both the quality and the disparities data and also includes data from the National Quality Strategy (NQS) priorities. Examples of improvement have been noted in a recent report: "hospital care was safer in 2013 than in 2010, with 17 percent fewer harms to patients and an estimated 1.3 million fewer hospital-acquired conditions, 50,000 fewer deaths, and $12 billion in cost savings over three years (2011, 2012, and 2013)" (Kronick, 2015). Adverse events were still a major problem, with 121 adverse events per 1,000 hospitalizations. Tracking quality care is improving, although screening still remains a problem. These reports are typically not focused on the current year because it takes time to collect the data and complete analysis. More detailed and comprehensive current *QDR* data are available at the AHRQ website, which is identified in the Connect to Current Information section at the end of the chapter. The work is not completed; it is ongoing to ensure that there is a health system that meets the NQS priorities of patient safety, person-centered care, care coordination, effective treatment, healthy living, and affordable care.

Disparities

Healthcare disparities, a component of healthcare quality, continue to be of concern throughout the United States, supported by data from the *National Healthcare Quality and Disparities Reports*. It is important, however, to ask whether the implementation of the ACA has made a difference in decreasing disparities. According to the report, the ACA has made a difference; for example, "The uninsurance rate dropped from 40.3 percent to 33.2 percent for Hispanics, and the rate declined from 14.0 percent to 11.1 percent for whites" (HHS, AHRQ, 2016). These figures demonstrate that there is some decrease in uninsurance rates due to implementation of the ACA, but some people have complained of experiencing increased costs. Due to the reimbursement changes, more people, both adults and children, receive care.

Global Healthcare Quality

Quality healthcare is not just a U.S. concern. There is global interest in quality care and initiatives to improve health in many countries. For example, a 2014 issue of the *International Journal for Quality in Health* focused on hospital quality improvement. The WHO has long worked to improve health and healthcare delivery, particularly in developing countries, although their work applies to all countries. The WHO website devotes space to patient safety (WHO, 2015), accessible through the link in the Connect to Current Information section at the end of the chapter. One of the WHO's initiatives is to apply a surgical unit–based safety program. It provides resources for healthcare provider training about safety and quality, change implementation (e.g., use of checklists, hand hygiene, reduction of bloodstream infections), and patient engagement. These global initiatives reflect the same concerns that are important in U.S. healthcare quality.

Interconnection is a key characteristic of the world today. Informatics allows greater communication and sharing of information, which can improve the quality of care. For example, healthcare providers and researchers can easily share information and collaborate. Problems such as natural or man-made disasters, epidemics, refugee health and social concerns, poor nutrition, impact of war and injuries to civilians, and other problems require that countries work together to ensure greater health and safety for all. Medical technology and healthcare informatics are developed in many countries and then used globally, improving care in more than one country and thereby demonstrating greater collaboration. While modern transportation allows people to travel anywhere, it should be noted that travel does present some risks, such as sharing infectious diseases, which is a particular problem in areas of the world that do not have effective control of diseases.

Stop and Consider #2

Healthcare quality in the United States falls below many countries.

The Vision of Healthcare Quality

In the words of Cosgrove (2013), "Quality is elusive. Not only achieving it. But defining it. Measuring it. Planning it and improving it" (p. ix). The healthcare system has focused sporadically on different aspects of CQI but has now moved to a major emphasis on CQI (Hall, Moore, & Barnsteiner, 2008). From the mid-1970s to today, The Joint Commission and regulatory agencies have agreed that quality care is an important issue. Managed care concerns were the focus from 1980 to 2000. Quality assurance programs were focused on from 1980 through 2008; however, this term is not used today. EBP and health informatics became important in 1990 and continue to expand in all types of HCOs. Quality improvement moved into focus in the mid-1990s, with changes in terminology from quality assurance to quality assessment, quality improvement, and finally CQI. Around 2000, patient safety became more of a concern and is considered to be a dimension of quality care.

Before this text moves into the specifics of quality improvement, it is important to describe the national view of healthcare quality, which is fairly new and has been strongly influenced by the *Quality Chasm* reports and the extensive work done to develop these reports. Quality improvement is related to change, but not all change is improvement. Knowledge is very important to improvement, but not all knowledge leads to improvement. We need more than knowledge about quality improvement; we must take actions and implement effective changes. The complexity of improvement is one of the difficulties we have in health care, and this complexity is compounded by both the complex healthcare system and the complexity of health problems and treatment for individual patients. None of these challenges, however, should be used as excuses to avoid what must be done: improve care daily, one patient at a time and throughout the system, whether the focus may be at the level of the collective HCO system, the individual HCO level, or the local, state, national, or even global level. To accomplish this goal requires a clear, effective framework that provides direction for planning and implementing CQI.

Vision

Crossing the Quality Chasm (IOM, 2001a) not only extended the examination of the healthcare delivery quality problem, but it also supported steps toward developing a more systematic view of quality care and improvement strategies. **Exhibit 1-2** describes the vision. Included in this vision is the development of a future vision, which is referred to as "new," rules for redesigning the system and improving care that are intended as improvements to current rules (IOM, 2001a, pp. 61–62). The rules are described as follows (Reproduced with permission from Health IT and patient safety: Building safer systems for better care, pp. 39-40, 2012 by the National Academy of Sciences, Courtesy of the National Academies Press, Washington, D.C.):

1. *Care based on continuous health relationships.* Patients should receive care whenever they need it and in many forms, not just face-to-face visits. For example, access to care may also be provided over the Internet, by telephone, through telehealth, and by other means.
2. *Customization based on patient needs and values.* The system of care should be designed to meet the most common types of needs, but it should also be capable of responding to individual patient choices and preferences.
3. *The patient as the source of control.* Patients should be given the necessary information and opportunity to exercise the degree of control they choose over healthcare decisions that affect them. The health system should be able to accommodate differences in patient preferences and encourage decision-making.
4. *Shared knowledge and the free flow of information.* Patients should have unfettered access to their own medical information and to clinical knowledge. Clinicians and patients should communicate effectively and share information.
5. *Evidence-based decision-making.* Patients should receive care based on the best available scientific knowledge. Care should not vary illogically from clinician to clinician or from place to place.

Exhibit 1-2   Rules for the 21st-Century Healthcare System

Current Approach (Old Rule)

Care is based primarily on visits.
Professional autonomy drives variability.
Professionals control care.
Information is a record.
Decision making is an individual responsibility.
Do no harm is an individual responsibility.
Secrecy is necessary.
The system reacts to needs.
Cost reduction is sought.
Preference is given to professional roles over the system.

New Rule

Care is based on continuous healing relationships.
Care is customized according to patient needs and values.
The patient is the source of control.
Knowledge is shared and information flows freely.
Decision making is evidence based.
Safety is a system property.
Transparency is necessary.
Needs are anticipated.
Waste is continuously decreased.
Cooperation among clinicians is a priority.

Reproduced with permission from Institute of Medicine. (2001). Crossing the quality chasm: A new health system for the 21st century. Washington, DC: The National Academies Press. Courtesy of the National Academies Press, Washington, DC.

---

6. *Safety as a system property.* Patients should be safe from injury caused by the care system. Reducing risk and ensuring safety require greater attention to systems that help prevent and mitigate errors.
7. *The need for transparency.* The healthcare system should make information available to patients and their families so that they can make informed decisions when selecting a health plan, hospital, or clinical practice or when choosing among alternative treatments. This information should include a description of the system's performance in achieving measures relating to quality, EBP, and patient satisfaction.

8. *Anticipation of needs.* The health system should anticipate patient needs, rather than simply react to events.

9. *Continuous decrease in waste.* The health system should not waste resources or patient time.

10. *Cooperation among clinicians.* Clinicians and institutions should actively collaborate and communicate to ensure an appropriate exchange of information and coordination of care.

These rules should not be viewed as a list of choices, but rather a package that is needed to improve care (IOM, 2001a). This perspective crosses all types of healthcare settings and applies to all healthcare professions. Since the publication of these rules, much has been done to address them, but much more is still required. Content in this text relates to all of these rules, and CQI models embed many, if not all, of these rules in their approaches. One can also see how they are related to the six aims or goals identified in the following section and can then compare them with the five healthcare professions core competencies. The work done in the *Quality Chasm* reports connected the elements discussed so that in the end there would be a complete picture.

Aims

Crossing the Quality Chasm also developed six aims or goals. Clear direction and leadership are needed to improve health care, and these aims provide that direction. The six aims or goals identified to guide this process are described as follows (IOM, 2001a, pp. 39–40):

1. *Safe.* Avoiding injuries to patients from the care that is intended to help them

2. *Timely.* Reducing waits and sometimes harmful delays for both patients who receive and those who give care

3. *Effective.* Providing services based on scientific knowledge to all patients who could benefit from those services and refraining from providing services not likely to benefit the patient

4. *Efficient.* Avoiding waste of equipment, supplies, ideas, and energy

5. *Equitable.* Providing care that does not vary in quality because of personal characteristics such as gender, ethnicity, geographic location, and socioeconomic status

6. *Patient-centered.* Providing care that is respectful of and responsive to individual patient preferences, needs, and values, ensuring that patient values guide all clinical decisions

Some organizations refer to the aims as STEEEP. Each one of the aims is now important in healthcare delivery and in CQI. These aims are emphasized in this text and should be integrated into nursing education and nursing practice.

Framework for Monitoring Quality

As mentioned earlier, monitoring care is required to effectively improve care, and the AHRQ now monitors care annually. Federal legislation mandates this monitoring. In 2014, substantial changes were made in this monitoring and annual reporting. As noted earlier, the *QDR* has expanded to include more on performance (assess performance; identify areas that are improving and need improvement), disparities data, and the tracking progress of NQS priorities. Electronic access to this report has also been expanded. As described by the HHS (2016):

> The *QDR* provides a comprehensive overview of the quality of health care received by the general U.S. population and disparities in care experienced by different racial, ethnic, and socioeconomic groups. The report is based on more than 250 measures of quality and disparities covering a broad array of health care services and settings.

The current *QDR* is not the same as the original reports, but the original reports provided the base for this monitoring and allowed experimentation and adaptation to improve the monitoring and methods for reporting results. Integrated in the *QDR* framework and monitoring are the quality improvement elements mentioned previously, aims, definitions, vision, and so on. There is greater integration today of multiple views of CQI, but there is also still some confusion and need for more organized approaches, as will be noted in other chapters.

System Approach

With greater interest in viewing health care as a system comes greater emphasis on understanding the healthcare system in order to improve it. In addition, with efforts to establish a patient-centered approach to care, understanding how the patient views the healthcare system is also important.

Macroviews and Microviews of Healthcare Quality

There are two important approaches to viewing the overall picture of healthcare quality—the macroview and the microview. The **macroview** of healthcare quality focuses on the broader issues from a local, state, federal, or even global perspective. At this broad level, there is much interaction not only between people and healthcare providers, but also between services and funding. This funding may be provided by local, state, or federal sources, but federal sources provide a lot of the funding for healthcare services and research. The national reports on healthcare quality and disparities are examples of the macroview of CQI. The **microview** of healthcare quality focuses on the healthcare provider, which can be an HCO or individual healthcare provider such as a physician, nurse, or pharmacist. The macroview provides many of the standards that are used to assess care as well as regulate care, whereas the microview implements and ensures that these standards are met and, if not, makes changes to improve care at the patient care level.

Health care today is complex, and so it is not always easy to separate these perspectives. For example, when people travel, they interact with healthcare delivery systems nationally or globally. Both views must use the same terminology and measurement, share information, apply a similar understanding of the roles of all providers, collaborate, and provide patient-centered care. Such a system, however, has not yet been realized.

Macrosystem, Mesosystem, and Microsystem

Within the microview of the healthcare delivery system is the **macrosystem**. An example of the macrosystem is the HCO (e.g., a hospital or a medical corporation with multiple hospitals). Within the macrosystem are the mesosystems and the microsystems (Nelson et al., 2008). If the macrosystem is a large multistate corporation, then the mesosystem might be individual HCOs within the system such as a hospital or a home health agency that is part of the healthcare system. Within one HCO, the **mesosystems** are departments, clinical centers, or services. Regardless of the type of organizational structure, drilling down to the microsystem level is critical in improving care. It is at this level that most nurses practice, and they have the most to offer in improving care. **Microsystems** are the clinical units, the smallest unit of the system, and it is here that the patient has the most influence.

Nurses work within all of these systems and need to understand them and how they impact nurses and nursing practice—structures, processes, and outcomes. Healthcare systems are neither simple nor stagnant; they change, requiring adaptation. **System thinking**, seeing the whole, how its parts interrelate, and how these parts all impact workflow, is important for success. This type of thinking is an integral part of effective CQI, allowing us to prevent, identify, and lessen the harm of errors; use problem solving and critical thinking along with clinical reasoning and judgment to make sound decisions based on best evidence; plan and use effective timelines; use interprofessional teams; and evaluate to determine outcomes. As stated by Fallon, Begun, and Riley (2013), "Systems thinking encourages consideration of unintended consequences of an intervention. Unintended consequences are results that are different from the outcomes expected as a result of a purposeful action" (p. 220). When nurses focus only on what they are doing each day, their views and options are limited and improved care will not occur.

Need for Definitions

Definitions are important in CQI. If the CQI process is undertaken with unclear definitions or if staff involved in any step of the process use different definitions, then data and outcomes will be negatively impacted. For example, if two people are measuring the length of the same room and each person is using a different definition for a foot, then it will not be possible to compare the results. While this logic may seem rather obvious, in healthcare quality there has been limited consensus on definitions of critical terms. The *Quality Chasm* reports build on one another, defining terms and then using them consistently across the reports. Defining key terms, such as quality, safety, and error, was a critical part of developing a clear framework, and the effort to standardize terminology remains crucial to the CQI process; indeed, it is embraced by this text.

The definition of quality care used in the *Quality Chasm* reports and mentioned earlier in this chapter (IOM, 2001a) supports earlier work by Donabedian (1980). Donabedian described quality care as having three elements: structure, processes, and outcomes. As the topic of CQI is examined in this text, it is important to keep this definition in mind along with the three elements of quality. When **structure** is examined, the focus is on how the organization's elements are put together and how this coming together of parts impacts quality. This view recognizes that an organization is a system that has parts, and a thorough understanding of it considers both the whole and the parts. When **process** is reviewed, the focus is on how the parts of the system function independently and interact. **Outcomes** are critical; considering them turns the focus to results. Historically, healthcare professionals had problems agreeing on a universally accepted definition of quality care. The *Quality Chasm* reports' definition, noted in this chapter, was used as the guide in developing a vision, goals, a proposed framework to monitor care, and recommendations. It has been used by many of the major CQI initiatives that followed.

CQI is defined as "a structured organizational process for involving personnel in planning and executing a continuous flow of improvements to provide quality healthcare that meets or exceeds expectations and usually involves a common set of characteristics" such as staff education, CQI teams, inclusion of CQI in HCO planning, and commitment and engagement to CQI (Sollecito & Johnson, 2013, pp. 4–5). Quality improvement has also been influenced by approaches and methods found in other businesses—for example, safety in the aviation industry. Key strategies to achieve improved quality include the following (Draper et al., 2008, p. 3):

- Having supportive hospital leadership and keeping them actively engaged in the work
- Setting expectations for all staff—not just nurses—that quality is a shared responsibility
- Holding staff accountable for individual roles
- Inspiring and using physicians and nurses to champion efforts
- Providing ongoing, visible, and useful feedback to engage staff effectively
- Applying the most current and rigorous techniques of the scientific method and statistical process control

Today, CQI is the most common approach used to improve care that supports the definition of quality care found in this chapter. As the topic of CQI is further examined in this text, there will be continued discussion of what it means and how it is implemented to achieve positive outcomes.

Stop and Consider #3

The most accepted view of healthcare quality is the application of STEEEP.

Value and Cost

Although some may find this claim difficult to accept, cost and quality are connected. The U.S. healthcare system is the most expensive healthcare system in the world, and yet it does not have the best quality. In one study that examined costs associated with harm while hospitalized, results noted that there were increased total costs, variable costs, and length of stay, and these factors had a negative impact on the long-term hospital finances. This problem will increase as healthcare delivery focuses more on value and performance rather than focusing just on volume (Adler et al., 2015). However, increasing cost does not necessarily mean better care. We must get much better at providing efficient *and* effective care. The report *Best Care at Lower Cost: The Path to Continuously Learning Health Care in America* presents

> a vision of what is possible if the nation applies the resources and tools at hand by marshaling science, information technology, incentives, and care culture to transform the effectiveness and efficiency of care—to produce high-quality health care that continuously learns to be better. (IOM, 2012, p. ix)

The report recognizes that there is a connection between cost and quality, and it needs to be addressed. **Figure 1-2** describes missed opportunities in reducing waste and harm. These missed opportunities act as barriers to best care at lower cost and are discussed throughout this text.

To achieve the goal of best care at lower cost, the healthcare system needs to manage the ever-increasing complexity and reduce ever-increasing costs (IOM, 2012). Discussed in this text, other reports emphasize the complexity and rapidly expanding knowledge (science and research) within the healthcare system; such reports focus on EBP, clinical guidelines, and comparative research (IOM, 2011b, 2011c, 2011d). In general, the U.S. healthcare system needs to improve care while reducing expenses and waste, consider the cost of care, and determine if the cost is reasonable, such as the extremely high costs of some medications and treatments (Rockoff & Silverman, 2015).

Addressing the key concerns found in Figure 1-2, *Best Care at Lower Cost* concludes with the overall recommendation of achieving a learning healthcare

Figure 1-2 Schematic of the Healthcare System
Reproduced from Institute of Medicine. (2012). Best care at lower cost: The path to continuously learning health care in America. Washington, DC: The National Academies Press. Courtesy of the National Academies Press, Washington, DC.

system. What is meant by the learning healthcare system discussed in this critical report? A **learning healthcare system**

> links personal and population data to researchers and practitioners, dramatically enhancing the knowledge base on effectiveness of interventions and providing real-time guidance for superior care in treating and preventing illness. A healthcare system that gains from continuous learning is a system that can provide Americans with superior care at lower cost. (IOM, 2012, p. ix)

As we discuss CQI throughout this text, there will be themes, and the descriptors in this recommendation represent one of them.

Examples of some of the CDC data on U.S. healthcare expenditures include the following (HHS, CDC, 2016): National health expenditures for 2013 were $2.9 trillion and for 2014 were $3.0 trillion. Percentage of health expenditures for hospital care with comparison of change from 2013 and 2014 was 32.1% (32.1%); nursing home and continuing care retirement, 5.3% (5.1%); physician and clinical services, 20.1% (19.1%); and prescriptions, 9.3% (9.8%). Current CDC data are found at the CDC website.

Data comparing the United States with other countries indicate that the United States spends more on health care. According to the World Bank (2015),

> total health expenditure [or the total percentage of the gross domestic product relating to health care] is the sum of public and private health expenditure. It covers the provision of health services (preventive and curative), family planning activities, nutrition activities, and emergency aid designated for health but does not include provision of water and sanitation.

The rates for the United States for 2011, 2012, and 2013 were 17.1%, 17.0%, and 17.1%, respectively. These rates are higher than those found in the United Kingdom, France, or Germany.

When comparing measures of access, equity, quality, efficiency, and healthy lives, the United States ranks last in a 2013 list of 11 countries (Australia, Canada, France, Germany, Netherlands, New Zealand, Norway, Sweden, Switzerland,

United Kingdom, United States) (Commonwealth Fund, 2014). In this ranking, the United States has the highest cost and poorest performance. This finding occurs despite the implementation of many ACA provisions, though the United States is still in the early stages of the ACA's implementation. It is hoped the ACA will have greater impact on improving access and care and reducing costs in the years to come. It is also important to note that many of the countries in the ranking have universal healthcare coverage, which the United States does not have. Detailed findings about the U.S. healthcare rankings include the following (Commonwealth Fund, 2014):

- *Healthy lives.* The United States ranks last in infant mortality rankings and in deaths that were potentially preventable with timely access to effective health care; it ranks second to last in healthy life expectancy, at age 60 years.
- *Access to care.* People in the United States have the hardest time affording the health care they need. The United States ranks last in every measure of cost-related access. More than one-third (37%) of U.S. adults reported forgoing a recommended test, treatment, or follow-up care because of cost.
- *Healthcare quality.* The United States ranks in the middle for two of four measures of quality—effective care (3rd out of 11 countries) and patient-centered care (4th out of 11 countries); however, it does not perform as well providing safe or coordinated care.
- *Healthcare efficiency.* The United States ranks last due to low marks on the time and dollars spent dealing with insurance administration, lack of communication among healthcare providers, and duplicative medical testing. Forty percent of U.S. adults who visited an emergency room reported they could have been treated by a regular doctor had one been available. This is more than double the rate of patients in the United Kingdom.
- *Equity of healthcare.* The United States ranks last in this category. About 4 out of 10 (39%) adults with below-average incomes in the United States reported a medical problem but did not visit a doctor in the past year because of costs, compared with less than 1 out of 10 in the United Kingdom, Sweden, Canada, and Norway. There were also large discrepancies between the length of time in the United States that lower-income adults waited for specialists, emergency care, and after-hours care compared with higher-income adults.

We have better data now than we did in 1999 when the NAS/HMD began to examine care and published the first *Quality Chasm* report, *To Err Is Human*; however, current data do not demonstrate enough improvement. The reasons for providing these examples in this chapter is to present you with a better picture of how cost and quality are connected. An important change related to the cost of care and how it relates to quality is the amplified emphasis on **pay for performance**. This emphasis can be positive, as it may stimulate improvement, but it can also be problematic if providers are focused on "how they appear" rather than actually providing quality care. For example, an opinion column published in the *New York Times*, written by a surgeon, noted that there are problems with using quality report cards when reported information may be used to penalize physicians, and this may then influence physicians to be too cautious (Jauhar, 2015; McCabe, Joynt, Welt, & Resnic, 2013). As stated by Jauhar (2015), "Surgical report cards are a classic example of how a well-meaning program in medicine can have unintended consequences. . . . It would appear that doctors, not patients, are the ones focused on doctors' grades—and their focus is distorted and blurry at best" (p. A27).

The *QDR* examines not only quality but also some measures of affordability of care, although few of its measures are used for this concern. The 2014 report, reflecting on 2013 data, indicates some problems with affordability. It worsened over time from 2002 to 2010, particularly for (1) people who indicated a financial or insurance reason for not having a usual source of care and (2) people unable to get or delayed in getting needed medical care, dental care, or prescription medicines due to financial or insurance reasons (HHS, AHRQ, 2015b). The affordable care measures include access to care problems due to healthcare costs and inefficient care due to use of services associated with more harm than benefits. The ACA has already had some impact on decreasing these problems.

The NQS cost of care priority focuses on providing affordable care or reducing the cost of quality health care for individuals, families, employers, and government. This priority is associated with paying, rewarding, and incentivizing providers to deliver high-quality, patient-centered care. The focus needs to move from volume to value in the purchase of health care or quality. Value-based purchasing is also a provision included in the ACA. How does the legislation support this change? First, it supports the NQS as the national framework for healthcare quality. In addition, it recommends the use of standardized quality measures, advocates for investment in CQI programs, recommends increased connection between quality performance and payment for Medicare payment, and encourages greater alignment between private and public purchasing of care. There are challenges to measurement that need to be considered; for example, measures need to be accurate and reliable and should not set up a scenario where the provider and others view the measures as the end point and thus limit the understanding of quality care. Healthcare measurement at this point is weak. Measurement is an important topic discussed in this text.

Stop and Consider #4

Value and cost in health care are not the same.

Healthcare Reform and Quality Improvement: Affordable Care Act of 2010

The ACA, often referred to as healthcare reform, primarily focuses on reimbursement with its provisions to reduce the number of uninsured and underinsured. It does not establish a universal health system for the United States. The United States is unusual in that most developing countries have universal healthcare coverage; however, to date, there has been insufficient political support in the United States for this type of coverage. The ACA continues to be a point of political contention. In 2012 and again in 2014, the Supreme Court upheld the law, although it did give more flexibility to states regarding use of Medicaid. It also was an issue in the 2016 presidential race. In 2014, the number of uninsured U.S. citizens was 32 million, a decrease of nearly of 9 million since 2013. In early 2016, the number was 20 million, or 9.1% of the overall population, with an estimated 20 million people gaining insurance coverage since the passage of the ACA in 2010 (HHS, 2016b). There were also major changes in increased enrollment of critical groups: young adults, racial minority groups, and ethnic groups. Because the implementation of the ACA spans several years, data on the insured and uninsured will change.

The law has also had an impact on nursing education and practice and areas that are related to CQI. Examples of these provisions include the following:

- Funding—grants and loans for students and faculty
- Education and training funds focused on geriatrics
- Primary care: advanced practice traineeships
- Funding for nurse-managed clinics
- Health prevention and public health
- Increased workforce diversity
- Community-based transition programs
- Establishment of the Patient-Centered Outcomes Research Institute
- Efforts toward nondiscrimination in health care
- Continued support for the Preventive Services Task Force
- Creation of the National Health Care Workforce Commission

This text does not focus on the ACA, but rather discusses how it impacts, or might impact, quality improvement.

Integration of Quality Improvement in Healthcare Reform

A major goal of the ACA is to expand coverage to millions of uninsured Americans (Majerol, Newkirk, & Garfield, 2015). The legislation does recognize that to focus solely on cost and reimbursement is not helpful, as the U.S. healthcare system needs to also improve healthcare delivery. Access to care may be a barrier to achieving positive health outcomes; for example, postponing care or not getting it at all, not taking medications regularly due to cost, and so on, lead to poor health outcomes, and in this respect, reimbursement and costs impact the quality of care that people receive. This concern led to the addition of provisions to the ACA relating to quality improvement. Appendix A identifies some of these provisions.

CQI has been greatly affected by other recent national legislation, such as the Health Insurance Portability and Accountability Act (HIPAA) of 1996, the American Recovery and Reinvestment Act (ARRA) of 2009, and the Health Information Technology for Economic and Clinical Health (HITECH) Act, which requires the establishment of a National Coordinator for Health Information Technology in HHS (Fallon et al., 2013). ARRA provides funding to assist physicians in adopting electronic records. As of 2015, to avoid Medicare payment penalties, physicians who care for Medicare patients must use electronic records. HITECH also requires that physicians document clinical quality measures. The ACA requires greater reporting of measures to ensure quality and establishes the NQS. States have also moved to more direct monitoring of healthcare quality by requiring reporting for serious adverse events.

As discussed in this chapter, the *Quality Chasm* reports brought the problem of healthcare disparities to the forefront (IOM, 2001a, 2002, 2003e, 2004b). The ACA is not developed to specifically address the problem of disparities; however, it is now recognized that it is difficult to resolve issues of reimbursement, cost, access, and quality without consideration of disparities. For example, health literacy is discussed in the ACA as a provision "to communicate health and healthcare information clearly; promote prevention; be patient-centered and create medical or health homes; assure equity and cultural competence; and deliver high-quality care" (Somers & Mahadevan, 2010, p. 4).

Current Status of the Implications of the Affordable Care Act and Quality Health Care

Since 1999, we have been able to get a better picture of the healthcare delivery system with the annual *QDR*. In 2014, the journal *Patient Safety and Quality Healthcare*, which began publishing in 2004, devoted its August issue to the future, asking patient safety experts to look 5 years into the future and describe the status of healthcare quality. Generally, the comments predicted modest improvement focused on continuing progress with current changes in the CQI process. Carr (2014) reports the following expert opinion:

> Former hospital CEO Paul Levy predicted that healthcare will continue to be "'islands of excellence surrounded by a sea of mediocrity" because medical education is largely unchanged and hospital leaders are focused more on market concentration and the bottom line than on safety and quality.

Other experts share this view, as Carr (2014) further elucidates:

Jim Conway, adjunct lecturer at the Harvard School of Public Health, . . . reminds us that there is no end to that journey and expects that "sustainability" will be a new challenge, especially for organizations that engage in isolated, limited improvement projects. Sustainability comes from system-wide commitment to continual improvement. Organizations that work to embody the principles of high reliability know that sustaining the gains they have made means never taking those gains for granted or believing that past or even performance offers protection from future hazards.

Why do problems persist despite some improvement? The work described in the *Quality Chasm* reports clarified many of the problems, but Fineberg, who led the IOM (now known as the NAS/HMD) for many years, identifies some of the critical inefficiencies that also continue to cause current problems in the healthcare system (Fineberg, 2012, p. 1023):

- Less emphasis on patient outcomes in the payment system
- Reward for inefficiency such as complications and readmissions
- Indifference of providers to reduce costs; lack of personal and professional concern about this problem
- Failure to take full advantage of professional skills of nurses
- Lack of uniform systems and processes to ensure safe and high-quality care
- Problems with patient flow, use of services, overcrowding (such as in emergency departments delaying treatment and admissions)
- Insufficient involvement of patients in decision-making
- Insufficient attention to prevention, disparities, primary care, health literacy, population health, and long-term results
- Fragmented and uncoordinated delivery, without continuity of care
- Lack of information on resource costs, performance, comparative effectiveness, quality of care, and health outcomes
- Scientific uncertainty about effectiveness and cost
- Cultural predisposition to believe that more care is better
- Administrative complexity related to multiple insurers
- Fraud and a problematic malpractice system

There are other issues, but the issues listed here summarize the key points.

Stop and Consider #5

The ACA is not legislation that supports universal health coverage in the United States, and its major focus is not on quality care but rather reimbursement.

An Important Step Toward Improvement: National Quality Strategy

As discussed throughout this chapter, the *Quality Chasm* reports and similar initiatives focused the U.S. healthcare system on CQI. There was a great need to identify the problems and examine approaches to addressing them. Laying the groundwork and then recommending annual monitoring of healthcare quality and disparities were major steps toward a healthcare environment that commits to quality at its core. There was, however, still a need to have a clearer overall national perspective of CQI. The *Quality Chasm* reports and other sources such as the Institute for Healthcare Improvement provided initial ideas for a framework.

One of the ACA provisions related to quality improvement is the establishment of the National Quality Strategy (NQS), which addresses the need for a national quality improvement framework and adds an additional focus on population health and reduction in healthcare disparities (Burstin et al., 2016; HHS, AHRQ, 2015c). Since the publication of the first *Quality Chasm* report in 1999, it took 12 years for the federal government to develop this national framework for healthcare quality. A variety of theories and models supporting improvement had an impact on the NQS. There is additional information about quality improvement theories and models in other chapters of this text. It is important in this chapter, which focuses on the introduction of CQI, to recognize the importance of the NQS and understand its framework and implications of its use.

Development and Purpose of the National Quality Strategy

The NQS is now an important part of the national initiative to improve care. As required by the ACA, the development of the NQS framework was led by the AHRQ. To ensure a collaborative effort, the AHRQ included feedback from over 300 stakeholders representing the federal government, especially the HHS; the states; the private sector; and multi-stakeholder groups such as healthcare professional organizations and the recommendations found in the *Quality Chasm* series. An evidence-based approach was used to develop the NQS.

In a 2011 press release, the HHS commented that the NQS was a groundbreaking initiative supporting an approach that quality care can be measured and improved at multiple levels—namely at the level of the community, practice settings, and individual physicians (HHS, 2011). A critical problem noted was there were too many measures and no control or evaluation of them. This problem has led to redundancies and some overlap in measurement, which impacts the value of results. More systematic methods are needed to measure care quality and maintain the CQI process. Patient-centered care needs to be at the core of the NQS, as it is now considered the core concern in care delivery. The major purpose of the NQS is to provide a national approach to measure quality and ensure higher-quality care for all.

National Quality Strategy Design

The NQS consists of three aims, six priority strategies for improvement, and levers. The NQS is also working toward greater measure alignment across the HHS to establish core sets of measures that would be useful and meaningful for different groups of stakeholders. This effort is motivated by the concern about the proliferation of measures.

Aims

The three NQS aims are based on the Triple Aim framework and incorporate elements of STEEEP. It is recommended that HCOs adopt all of the aims. The Triple Aim is discussed in other sections of this text, but it is important to introduce it at the beginning of the discussion about quality improvement due to its influence on the NQS (HHS, AHRQ, 2015a):

1. *Better Care.* Improve the overall quality, by making health care more patient-centered, reliable, accessible, and safe.
2. *Healthy People in Healthy Communities.* Improve the health of the U.S. population by supporting proven interventions to address behavioral, social, and environmental determinants of health in addition to delivering higher-quality care.
3. *Affordable Care.* Reduce the cost of quality health care for individuals, families, employers, and government.

The second aim is important because it illustrates how various initiatives are connected to the NQS. An effective national view of quality requires collaborative initiatives and a consistent framework. Healthy People in Healthy Communities has been an important national healthcare initiative for many years, identifying and tracking objectives and measures/indicators for health improvement (Healthy People, 2015; HHS, CDC, 2015). With development of the NQS, these long-standing programs are brought into the overall national strategy.

Prioritizing Strategies

The aims connect to the six priorities and strategies, examining the most common health concerns. It is recommended that HCOs use the NQS priorities to guide efforts to improve health and healthcare quality. The six priorities are as follows (HHS, AHRQ, 2015a):

- Making care safer by reducing harm caused in the delivery of care
- Ensuring that each person and family is engaged as partners in their care
- Promoting effective communication and coordination of care

- Promoting the most effective prevention and treatment practices for leading causes of mortality
- Working with communities to promote wide use of best practices to enable healthy living
- Making quality care more affordable for individuals, families, employers, and government by developing and spreading new healthcare delivery models

Better Care

PRIORITIES

1. Making care safer
2. Ensuring that each person and family are engaged
3. Promoting effective communication and coordination of care
4. Promoting the most effective prevention and treatment practices
5. Working with communities to promote wide use of best practices to enable healthy living
6. Making quality care affordable

Healthy People/Healthy Communities   Affordable Care

Figure 1-3 National Quality Strategy Three Aims and Six Priorities.
Reproduced from Centers for Medicare and Medicaid Services, Center for Clinical Standards and Quality. (2015). 2015 national impact assessment of the Centers for Medicare & Medicaid Services (CMS) quality measures report. Retrieved from https://www.cms.gov/Medicare/Quality-Initiatives-Patient-Assessment-Instruments/QualityMeasures/Downloads/2015-National-Impact-Asessment-Report.pdf.

Levers

Nine levers are identified for the strategies. Each lever "represents a core business function, resource, and/or action that stakeholders can use to align to the strategy. In many cases, stakeholders may already be using these levers but have not connected these activities to NQS alignment" (HHS, AHRQ, 2015a). In addition to developing a national framework, the NQS also addresses the problem of too many measures and the negative impact that this has on CQI and healthcare providers. It results in confusion, lack of consistency, and disorganization. Given the description of a healthcare system that is dysfunctional having a CQI approach that is also confusing is not helpful. The levers are identified in **Figure 1-4**. The relationship between the aims and the levers is found in **Figure 1-5**. It is recommended that HCOs focus on at least one of the levers.

Federal healthcare programs now apply the NQS. It is recommended that other healthcare programs—both private and public—adopt the NQS; however, it is not required. The AHRQ provides tools and resources to support implementation of the NQS (HHS, AHRQ, 2015c). The NQS must provide an annual report to Congress, and the reports are posted on the AHRQ website. The 2015 congressional report states the following:

> Across the nation the National Strategy for Quality Improvement in Health Care (NQS) brings together federal agencies, healthcare payers, purchasers, providers, consumers, and other partners in pursuit of improved health and health care for all Americans. The NQS serves as a framework for aligning stakeholders across private and public sectors at the federal, state, and local levels. (HHS, 2015)

National Quality Strategy Levers			
Lever	**Icon**	**Definition**	**Example**
Payment		Reward and incentivize providers to deliver high-quality, patient-centered care.	Join a regional coalition of purchasers that are pursuing value-based purchasing.
Public Reporting		Compare treatment results, costs, and patient experience for consumers.	A regional collaborative may ask member hospitals and medical practices to align public reports to the National Quality Strategy aims or priorities.
Learning and Technical Assistance		Foster learning environments that offer training, resources, tools, and guidance to help organizations achieve quality improvement goals.	A Quality Improvement Organization may disseminate evidence-based best practices in quality improvement with physicians, hospitals, nursing homes, and home health agencies.
Certification, Accreditation, and Regulation		Adopt or adhere to approaches to meet safety and quality standards.	The National Quality Strategy aims and priorities may be incorporated into continuing education requirements or certification maintenance.
Consumer Incentives and Benefit Designs		Help consumers adopt healthy behaviors and make informed decisions.	Employers may implement workforce wellness programs that promote prevention and provide incentives for employees to improve their health.
Measurement and Feedback		Provide performance feedback to plans and providers to improve care.	A long-term care provider may implement a strategy that includes the use of Quality Assurance and Performance Improvement data to populate measurement dashboards for purposes of identifying and addressing areas requiring quality improvement.
Health Information Technology		Improve communication, transparency, and efficiency for better coordinated health and health care.	A hospital or medical practice may adopt an electronic health record system to improve communication and care coordination.
Workforce Development		Investing in people to prepare the next generation of health care professionals and support lifelong learning for providers.	A medical leadership institution may incorporate quality improvement principles in their training.
Innovation and Diffusion		Foster innovation in health care quality improvement, and facilitate rapid adoption within and across organizations and communities.	Center for Medicare & Medicaid Innovation tests various payment and service delivery models and shares successful models across the Nation.

Figure 1-4 National Quality Strategy Levers
Reproduced from U.S. Department of Health and Human Services. (2014). National Quality Strategy: Using levers to achieve improved health and health care. Retrieved from http://www.ahrq.gov /workingforquality/reports /nqsleverfactsheet.htm

Figure 1-5
Relationship of the
National Quality Strategy
Aims and the Levers
Reproduced from U.S. Department
of Health and Human Services.
(2016). National Quality Strategy:
Overview [PowerPoint presenta-
tion]. Retrieved from http://www
.ahrq.gov/workingforquality/nqs
/overview2016.pptx

How should the healthcare delivery system implement the NQS (HHS, AHRQ, 2015d)? It is hoped that HCOs are knowledgeable about the NQS and adopt its elements as recommended. Adopters should also include healthcare profession education programs such as all nursing degree programs, which should include this content and ensure that nursing students at all levels know about NQS and can apply it to their practice. The overall goal is an effective healthcare delivery system that is consistent and emphasizes CQI from the same perspective. The NQS website offers resources such as tools and reports for healthcare providers and policy makers. The Connect to Current Information section at the end of the chapter provides a link to this site.

Current Status of the National Quality Strategy

The NQS priorities are patient safety, person-centered care, care coordination, effective treatment, healthy living, and care affordability. As noted previously, they are monitored as part of the annual *QDR*. This information is then included in the annual NQS report to Congress (HHS, 2015; HHS, AHRQ, 2015b). Multiple healthcare organizations and government agencies participate in providing data for the report. **Figure 1-6** provides an overview of how the NQS works.

Stop and Consider #6
Up until the development of the National Quality Strategy, the United States had no clear national healthcare perspective.

Introduction to Leadership, Interprofessional Teamwork, and Nursing Responsibility for CQI

Leadership, including nursing leadership, is required in all phases of CQI. HCO leaders ensure that CQI is part of all aspects of the organization, including the mission, goals and objectives, organization, processes, policies and procedures,

Figure 1-6 National Quality Strategy: How It Works

Reproduced from U.S. Department of Health and Human Services (2016). National Quality Strategy: Overview [PowerPoint presentation]. Retrieved http://www.ahrq.gov/workingforquality/nqs/overview2016.pptx

position descriptions and performance appraisal, and all aspects of clinical practice. They must work to integrate standards, accreditation requirements, staff education, ethics, and legal requirements into the organization, as discussed in other sections of this text. Teamwork is critical to successful CQI, and leaders in the HCO must provide support to teams with resources, guidance, and staff education about teams. As articulated by Gantz and colleagues (2003), "Quality improvement and performance should be a way of life for best practices and high performers who seek to understand, change, improve, and enhance patient care outcomes" (p. 329).

Nurses usually think of nursing leaders as being in management or administration positions; however, every nurse needs to be a leader and develop leadership competencies (Finkelman, 2016). These competencies are needed as nurses provide care working with teams, advocating for patients, and engaging in CQI in direct care. Nurses also need these competencies when they participate in organizational activities such as committees, task forces, and other situations where professional issues are considered and nurses need to share the nursing perspective. *The Future of Nursing* report includes the following recommendation: "expand opportunities for nurses to lead and diffuse collaborative improvement efforts" (IOM, 2010a, p. S-9).

Responsibility for CQI is the core issue in this text. Every healthcare profession has the responsibility to (1) ensure that its educational programs prepare graduates who can apply quality improvement in their individual practice and participate in CQI programs within HCOs and (2) actively commit to improving care in all types of healthcare settings. These objectives are not simple to accomplish. CQI has not always been an important content topic in healthcare professions education, including nursing. It is mentioned, of course, but there is typically limited in-depth examination of quality care and methods to improve care—although this situation is slowly improving. One of the five healthcare professions core competencies is to apply quality improvement, and this core competency is tied to the other four core competencies, with all needed to effectively continuously improve care.

The *Quality Chasm* series has had an impact on the entire healthcare system. Not only has the recognition of CQI as a professional responsibility influenced how HCOs view quality care and how the government at local, state, and federal levels works toward improving care, but also now there is much more emphasis on the role of individual healthcare providers—and in this text, the focus is on nurses. CQI is not something that is just done by a single department in an HCO with staff occasionally hearing about it. It must be part of daily work and the provision of care, and it must impact all staff, both professional and nonprofessional. Each staff member must ask: How can I improve what I do?

Stop and Consider #7

Nursing needs to develop more leadership in quality improvement.

Conclusions

This chapter sets the stage for an in-depth examination of the healthcare system from the perspective of quality care and the roles and responsibilities of nurses in CQI. This is a complex area, involving many viewpoints and methods. Nurses should assume more CQI responsibilities at the point of care and within HCOs. This chapter provides background information and an overview of our current knowledge of CQI so that nurses will be well informed as they begin their journey toward competence in quality improvement. Fineberg frames this journey well with the following words:

> To achieve a successful and sustainable health system, we must be able and willing to try many different things. But therein lies a unifying idea: Do many things. No single stroke will solve this problem. A successful and sustainable health system will not be achieved by supporting prevention, it will not be achieved by championing competition, it will not be achieved by comparing the effectiveness of different practices, it will not be achieved by striking commercial influence from professional decision-making, it will not

be achieved by changing the way we pay doctors, and it will not be achieved by just reengineering the system. It requires all these changes and more. We need the cleverness of the fox and the persistence of the hedgehog. We must be willing to adopt many strategies and use them to reach one big goal. (p. 1026)

Apply CQI
Chapter Highlights

- Concern about the quality of health care in the United States has been particularly high since 1999 when a report (*To Err Is Human*) was published, followed by a number of other critical reports referred to as the *Quality Chasm* reports.
- The Institute of Medicine (IOM), whose name has been changed to the National Academy of Sciences, Health and Medicine Division (NAS/HMD), has a major role in examining healthcare quality through its review panels and published reports with recommendations.
- Five healthcare professions core competencies were identified by one of the major reports, *Health Professions Education* (2003), and apply to all healthcare professions.
- The *Quality Chasm* reports identified the need for national annual reports on healthcare quality and disparities that are now administered by the Agency for Healthcare Research and Quality (AHRQ) (through the *National Healthcare Quality and Disparities Report* [QDR]).
- Continuous quality improvement (CQI) is now a major concern of all healthcare organizations (HCOs) and professions, with emphasis on STEEEP.
- Based on data and reports that indicate certain populations do not receive equitable care, leading to healthcare disparities, diversity in health care and disparities are now integrated into the need for improvement.
- Healthy People 2020, a national health initiative, guides views of healthy individuals and communities.
- U.S. healthcare does not rate as high as it should when compared to other countries' healthcare systems.
- *The Quality* Chasm reports provide a vision of U.S. health care that is now incorporated into many quality improvement initiatives.
- Macro- and microviews of healthcare quality are integrated into CQI. The macrosystem, mesosystem, and microsystem should be understood for each HCO.
- Value and cost are related and have to be considered in CQI.
- The Patient Protection and Affordable Care Act of 2010 (ACA) is legislation that is primarily focused on reimbursement; however, it does include some provisions on quality improvement, recognizing that focusing solely on cost will limit our ability to reach improved care and health.

- The National Quality Strategy (NQS) is a significant national initiative assisting in developing and maintaining quality care within the healthcare delivery system.
- Every nurse needs to be a leader and assume an active role in CQI.

Critical Thinking and Clinical Reasoning and Judgment: Questions and Learning Activities

1. Select one of the *Quality Chasm* reports described in this chapter. Go to the author's website (https://www.nationalacademies.org/hmd/Reports.aspx) and find the report. Read the executive summary, and then in your own words describe why the report is important to healthcare delivery and to nursing.

2. Consider the following questions about the ACA: (1) Why does the ACA not establish universal health coverage? (2) Why would one describe the ACA as mostly focused on reimbursement of care? (3) Review the examples of quality improvement provisions in this chapter and in Appendix A. Select one and identify why the provision relates to nursing care.

3. Review this chapter's discussion of the NQS, and visit the AHRQ's website to further research the NQS. How is the NQS directly related to nursing care and the nursing profession? Identify the NQS elements that are based on important CQI elements discussed in this chapter. Discuss your views with your student team.

4. Why do you need to be actively engaged in CQI as a student and then as a practicing nurse?

Connect to Current Information

- National Academy of Sciences/Health and Medicine Division
  https://www.nationalacademies.org/hmd/
- U.S. Department of Health and Human Services
  http://www.hhs.gov
- Agency for Healthcare Research and Quality
  http://www.ahrq.gov
- Healthy People 2020
  http://www.healthypeople.gov
- National Healthcare Quality and Disparities Reports (current annual reports)
  http://nhqrnet.ahrq.gov/inhqrdr/
- National Quality Strategy
  http://www.ahrq.gov/workingforquality/
- World Health Organization
  http://www.who.int/en/
- National Quality Forum
  http://www.qualityforum.org/Home.aspx

EBP, EBM, and Quality Improvement: Exemplar

Ricciardi, R., Moy, E., & Wilson, N. (2016). Finding the true north. Lessons from the National Healthcare Quality and Disparities Report. *Journal of Nursing Care Quality, 31*(1), 9–12.

This article offers a commentary about the *National Healthcare Quality and Disparities Report (QDR)* and its impact on quality care.

Questions to Consider

1. How does the article describe the *QDR* and its relevance?
2. Why is the NQS included in the discussion?
3. What example is described to support the impact that nurses can have on quality care?

Evolving Case Study

Your hospital has recently revised its CQI vision and aims based on work done in the *Quality Chasm* series and the NQS recommendations. As nurse manager for an emergency department (ED), you need to take this information and make it "real" for staff in the ED. The medical director and you will present this information to the staff, but you need to figure out how it applies to daily work and engage staff. You both agree that the staff will not appreciate the "words" on the paper unless you can attach their meaning to their work in the ED.

Case Questions

1. What information would you use as your base about the vision and the aims?
2. How would you then apply this information to the ED and the work done by staff?
3. You suspect you will be asked how the ACA impacts this approach. What information should you prepare on this topic?

References

Adler, L., Yi, D., Li, M., McBroom, B., Hauck, L., Sammer, C., ... Classen, D. (2015). Impact of inpatient harms on hospital finances and patient clinical outcomes. *Journal of Patient Safety.* doi: 10.1097/PTS.0000000000000171

Benner, P., Sutphen, M., Leonard, V., & Day, L. (2010). *Educating nurses: A call for radical transformation.* San Francisco, CA: Jossey-Bass.

Bernstein, L., & McGinley, L. (2016, April 21). NIH hospital needs sweeping reform to better protect patient safety, panel says. *The Washington Post.* Retrieved from https://www.washingtonpost.com/national/health-science/nih-hospital-needs-sweeping-reform-to-better-protect-patient-safety-panel-says/2016/04/21/52c1cb00-080d-11e6-b283-e79d81c63c1b_story.html?tid=a_inl

Bisognano, M., & Kenney, C. (2012). *Pursuing the triple aim.* San Francisco, CA: Jossey-Bass.

Burstin, H., Leatherman, S., & Goldmann, D. (2016). The evolution of healthcare quality measurement in the United States. *Journal of Internal Medicine, 279,* 154–159.

Carr, S. (2014). Looking to the future of patient safety. *Patient Safety and Healthcare Quality*. Retrieved from http://www.psqh.com/july-august-2014/looking-to-the-future-of-patient-safety

Commonwealth Fund. (2014). U.S. health system ranks last among eleven countries on measures of access, equity, quality, efficiency, and healthy lives. Retrieved from http://www.commonwealthfund.org/publications/press-releases/2014/jun/us-health-system-ranks-last

Cosgrove, D. (2013). Foreword. In S. Sadeghi, A. Barzi, O. Mikhail, & M. Shabot (Eds.), *Integrating quality and strategy in health care organizations*. Burlington, MA: Jones & Bartlett Learning.

Donabedian, A. (1980). *Explorations in quality assessment and monitoring, volume 1: The definitions of quality and approaches to its assessment*. Ann Arbor, MI: Health Administration Press.

Draper, D., Felland, L., Liebhaber, A., & Melichar, L. (2008). The role of nurses in hospital quality improvement. Center for Studying Health System Change. *Research Brief, March*(3), 1–8.

Fallon, L., Begun, J., & Riley, W. (2013). *Managing health organizations for quality performance*. Burlington, MA: Jones & Bartlett Learning.

Fineberg, H. (2012). A successful and sustainable health system—How to get there from here. *New England Journal of Medicine, 366*(11), 1020–1027.

Finkelman, A. (2016). *Leadership and management for nurses. Core competencies for quality care* (3rd ed.). Upper Saddle River, NJ: Pearson Education.

Finkelman, A., & Kenner, C. (2016). *Professional nursing concepts. Competencies for quality leadership* (3rd ed.). Burlington, MA: Jones & Bartlett Learning.

Gantz, N., Sorenson, L., & Howard, R. (2003). A collaborative perspective on nursing leadership in quality improvement. *Nursing Administrative Quarterly, 27*(4), 324–329.

Hall, L., Moore, S., & Barnsteiner, J. (2008). Quality and nursing: Moving from a concept to a core competency. *Urological Nursing, 28*(6), 417–425.

Healthy People. (2015). Healthy people 2020. Retrieved from http://www.healthypeople.gov

Institute of Medicine (IOM). (1983). *Nursing and nursing education: Public policy and private action*. Washington, DC: The National Academies Press.

Institute of Medicine (IOM). (1999). *To err is human*. Washington, DC: The National Academies Press.

Institute of Medicine (IOM). (2001a). *Crossing the quality chasm*. Washington, DC: The National Academies Press.

Institute of Medicine (IOM). (2001b). *Envisioning the national healthcare quality report*. Washington, DC: The National Academies Press.

Institute of Medicine (IOM). (2002). *Guidance for the national health care disparities report*. Washington, DC: The National Academies Press.

Institute of Medicine (IOM). (2003a). *Priority areas for national action*. Washington, DC: The National Academies Press.

Institute of Medicine (IOM). (2003b). *Health professions education: A bridge to quality*. Washington, DC: The National Academies Press.

Institute of Medicine (IOM). (2003c). *The future of the public's health in the 21st century*. Washington, DC: The National Academies Press

Institute of Medicine (IOM). (2003d). *Who will keep the public healthy?* Washington, DC: The National Academies Press.

Institute of Medicine (IOM). (2003e). *Unequal treatment*. Washington, DC: The National Academies Press.

Institute of Medicine (IOM). (2004a). *Keeping patients safe. Transforming the work environment of nurses*. Washington, DC: The National Academies Press.

Institute of Medicine (IOM). (2004b). *Health literacy. A prescription to end confusion*. Washington, DC: The National Academies Press.

Institute of Medicine (IOM). (2010a). *The future of nursing. Leading change, advancing health*. Washington, DC: The National Academies Press.

Institute of Medicine (IOM). (2010b). *Future directions for the national healthcare quality and disparities reports*. Washington, DC: The National Academies Press.

Institute of Medicine (IOM). (2011a). *Leading health indicators for Healthy People 2020: Letter report.* Washington, DC: The National Academies Press.

Institute of Medicine (IOM). (2011b). *Learning what works: Infrastructure required for effectiveness research: Workshop summary.* Washington, DC: The National Academies Press.

Institute of Medicine (IOM). (2011c). *Finding what works in health care: Standards for systematic reviews.* Washington, DC: The National Academies Press.

Institute of Medicine (IOM). (2011d). *Clinical practice guidelines we can trust.* Washington, DC: The National Academies Press.

Institute of Medicine (IOM). (2012). *Best care at lower cost: The path to continuously learning health care in American.* Washington, DC: The National Academies Press.

Jauhar, S. (2015, July 22). Giving doctors grades. *New York Times*, p. A27.

Kronick, R. (2015). New AHRQ report shows patient safety and access improvements, but disparities remain. Retrieved from http://www.ahrq.gov/news/blog/ahrqviews/042015.html

Majerol, M., Newkirk, V., & Garfield, R. (2015). The uninsured: A primer—Key facts about health insurance and the uninsured in America. The Henry J. Kaiser Family Foundation. Retrieved from http://kff.org/uninsured/report/the-uninsured-a-primer/

Makary, M., & Daniel, M. (2016). Medical error: The third leading cause of death in the U.S. *BMJ*, May 3. Retrieved from http://www.bmj.com/content/353/bmj.i2139/rr-40

McCabe, J., Joynt, K., Welt, F., & Resnic, F. (2013). Impact of public reporting and outlier status identification on percutaneous coronary intervention case selection in Massachusetts. *JACC Cardiovascular Interventions, 6*(6), 625–630.

Millenson, M. (2006). Duty versus interest. The history of quality health care. In D. Nash & N. Goldfarb (Eds.), *Closing the quality chasm* (pp. 15–29). Sudbury, MA: Jones & Bartlett Publishers.

Nance, J. (2008). *Why hospitals should fly? The ultimate flight plan to patient safety and quality care.* Bozeman, MT: Second River Healthcare Press.

Nash, D., Evans, A., & Bowman, K. (2006). An overview of quality in the healthcare system. In D. Nash & N. Goldfarb (Eds.), *The quality solution: The stakeholders guide to improving health care* (pp. 3–14). Sudbury, MA: Jones & Bartlett Publishers.

National Academies of Science, Engineering, and Medicine (NAS), Health and Medicine Division (HMD). (2016). About our web address and division name. Retrieved from https://www.nationalacademies.org/hmd/About-HMD/Division-Name.aspx

National Quality Forum (NQF). (2016). About NQF. Retrieved from http://www.qualityforum.org/Home.aspx

Nelson, E., Godfrey, M. M., Batalden, P. B., Berry, S. A., Bothe, A. E., Jr., McKinley, K. E., . . . Nolan, T. W. (2008). Clinical microsystems: Part 1. The building blocks of health systems. *The Joint Commission Journal of Quality and Patient Care, 34*(7), 367–378.

President's Advisory Commission on Consumer Protection and Quality in the Health Care Industry. (1998). *Quality first: Better health care for all Americans.* Retrieved from http://www.hcqualitycommission.gov

Rockoff, J., & Silverman, E. (2015, April 26). Pharmaceutical companies buy rivals' drugs and then jack up the prices. *The Wall Street Journal.* Retrieved from http://www.wsj.com/articles/pharmaceutical-companies-buy-rivals-drugs-then-jack-up-the-prices-1430096431#:HilJLi6HwyKdqA

Sadeghi, S., Barzi, A., Mikhail, O., & Shabot, M. (2013). *Integrating quality and strategy in health care organizations.* Burlington, MA: Jones & Bartlett Learning.

Sollecito, W., & Johnson, J. (2013). The global evolution of continuous quality improvement: From Japanese manufacturing to global health services. In W. Sollecito & J. Johnson (Eds.), *McLaughlin and Kaluzny's continuous quality improvement in healthcare* (4th ed., pp. 1–48). Burlington, MA: Jones & Bartlett Learning.

Somers, S., & Mahadevan, R. (2010). *Health literacy implications of the affordable care act.* Hamilton, NJ: Center for Health Care Strategies.

Sullivan, L. (2004). *Missing persons. Minorities in health professions.* Washington, DC: Sullivan Commission on Diversity in the Healthcare Workforce. Retrieved from http://www.aacn.nche.edu/media-relations/SullivanReport.pdf

Sun, L. (2016, May 10). Exclusive: Patient safety issues prompt leadership shake-up at NIN hospital. *The Washington Post.* Retrieved from https://www.washingtonpost.com/national/health-science/exclusive-patient-safety-issues-prompt-leadership-shake-up-at-nih-hospital/2016/05/10/ad1f71f6-0ffb-11e6-8967-7ac733c56f12_story.html

U.S. Department of Health and Human Services (HHS). (2011, March 21). Press release: National quality strategy will promote better health, quality care for Americans. Retrieved from http://www.business-wire.com/news/home/20110321006087/en/National-Quality-Strategy-Promote-Health-Quality-Care

U.S. Department of Health and Human Services (HHS). (2015). *2015 annual progress report to congress: National strategy for quality improvement in health care.* Retrieved from http://www.ahrq.gov/workingforquality/reports/annual-reports/nqs2015annlrpt.htm

U.S. Department of Health and Human Services (HHS). (2016a). HHS family of agencies. Retrieved from http://www.hhs.gov/about/agencies/index.html

U.S. Department of Health and Human Services (HHS). (2016b). 20 million people have gained health insurance coverage because of the Affordable Care Act, new estimates show. Retrieved from http://www.hhs.gov/about/news/2016/03/03/20-million-people-have-gained-health-insurance-coverage-because-affordable-care-act-new-estimates

U.S. Department of Health and Human Services (HHS), Agency for Healthcare Research and Quality (AHRQ). (2011). Low health literacy linked to higher risk of death and more emergency room visits and hospitalizations. Retrieved from http://archive.ahrq.gov/news/newsroom/press-releases/2011/lowhlit.html

U.S. Department of Health and Human Services (HHS), Agency for Healthcare Research and Quality (AHRQ). (2015a). About the National Quality Strategy. Retrieved from http://www.ahrq.gov/workingforquality/about.htm

U.S. Department of Health and Human Services (HHS), Agency for Healthcare Research and Quality (AHRQ). (2015b). *National healthcare quality and disparities report: Chartbook on care affordability.* Retrieved from http://www.ahrq.gov/research/findings/nhqrdr/2014chartbooks/careafford/careafford-care.html

U.S. Department of Health and Human Services (HHS), Agency for Healthcare Research and Quality (AHRQ). (2015c). NQS tools. Retrieved from http://www.ahrq.gov/workingforquality/toolkit.htm

U.S. Department of Health and Human Services (HHS), Agency for Healthcare Research and Quality (AHRQ). (2015d). Three tips for facilitating the quality improvement process. Retrieved from http://www.ahrq.gov/cahps/quality-improvement/improvement-guide/4-approach-qi-process/index.html

U.S. Department of Health and Human Services (HHS), Agency for Healthcare Research and Quality (AHRQ). (2016). National Healthcare Quality Disparities Reports. Retrieved from http://nhqrnet.ahrq.gov/inhqrdr/

U.S. Department of Health and Human Services (HHS), Centers for Disease Control and Prevention (CDC). (2015). Healthy communities program. Retrieved from https://www.cdc.gov/nccdphp/dch/programs/healthycommunitiesprogram/

U.S. Department of Health and Human Services (HHS), Centers for Disease Control and Prevention (CDC). (2016). Health expenditures. Retrieved from http://www.cdc.gov/nchs/fastats/health-expenditures.htm

U.S. Department of Health and Human Services (HHS), Office of Disease Prevention and Health Promotion (ODPHP). (2010). *Healthy people 2020.* ODPHP Publication No. B0132. Retrieved from https://www.healthypeople.gov/sites/default/files/HP2020_brochure_with_LHI_508_FNL.pdf

World Bank. (2015). Health expenditure total. Retrieved from http://data.worldbank.org/indicator/SH.XPD.TOTL.ZS/

World Health Organization (WHO). (2015). Patient safety. Retrieved from http://www.who.int/patientsafety/en/

CHAPTER 2

Quality Improvement: Ethics, Standards, Regulatory, Accreditation, and Legal Issues

CHAPTER OBJECTIVES

At the conclusion of this chapter, the learner will be able to:

- Analyze ethical issues in healthcare delivery and nursing implications.
- Apply standards to the continuous quality improvement process.
- Illustrate the implications of regulations to continuous quality improvement.
- Examine accreditation and its importance to quality health care.
- Examine legal issues that relate to quality health care.

OUTLINE

KEY TERMS

Accreditation	Ethics	Scope of practice
Autonomy	Fraud	Self-determination
Beneficence	Justice	Self-regulation
Certification	Malpractice	Standard
Code of ethics	Negligence	Veracity
Collaboration	Nursing regulation	
Ethical dilemma	Reasonably prudent nurse	

Introduction

Moving beyond the previous chapter's overview of the history, key players, and current initiatives of the continuous quality improvement (CQI) movement, this chapter will consider the ethics, standards, regulations, accreditation process, and legal issues related to CQI. These issues apply to all healthcare settings and to all healthcare professionals and staff and can affect CQI by acting as barriers and also as support for positive CQI outcomes.

Ethical Concerns

Finkelman and Kenner (2016) frame the discussion of **ethics** by comparing ethics to a related concept, *morals*: "Ethics refers to a standardized code or guide to behaviors. Morals are learned through growth and development, whereas ethics typically is learned through a more organized system, such as standardized ethics code developed by a professional group" (p. 174). Ethical standards, often presented as a **code of ethics**, guide behaviors. These standards are part of quality care and should not be ignored. Since there is greater concern today about ethical behavior, or the rightness and wrongness of the behavior of organizations and individual staff, healthcare organizations (HCOs) are emphasizing ethics more. For example, the American Nurses Association (ANA) designated 2015 as the year of ethics, recognizing its importance to the profession (ANA, 2015a). The following are four major principles of ethics (see **Figure 2-1**). The principles are

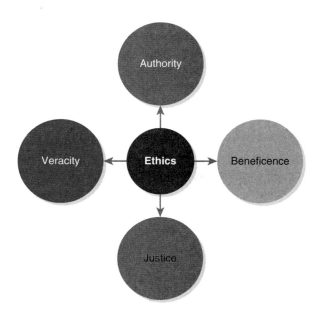

FIGURE 2-1 Critical Ethical Principles.

part of nursing professional ethics (ANA, 2015a; Finkelman & Kenner, 2016, p. 175; Koloroutis & Thorstenson, 1999).

1. **Autonomy**. *Patients have the right to determine their own rights.* This principle applies to CQI when you consider issues such as patient-centered care, patient decision-making, and privacy and confidentiality.
2. **Beneficence**. *Nurses should not inflict harm and should safeguard the patient.* This principle applies to CQI when you consider prevention of errors, quality monitoring, analysis of quality care concerns such as errors and failure to meet outcomes, and development and evaluation of solutions to problems.
3. **Justice**. *Patients should be treated fairly.* This principle applies to CQI when you consider patient equality, health literacy, and methods to reduce healthcare disparities.
4. **Veracity**. *Patients should be told the truth.* This principle applies to CQI when staff communicate clear information about patient care, obtain patient consent, report concerns about care delivery, and disclose errors to patients.

Nursing's Social Policy Statement: The Essence of the Profession

Nursing's Social Policy Statement (ANA, 2015b) describes the scope of nursing practice and how the nursing profession relates to the public for which it is accountable. Nursing is directly related to a number of social concerns, one of which specifically addresses the need for quality healthcare delivery and outcomes. Social responsibility requires nurses to assist with social concerns, providing nurses with the authority to do this; however, nurses need to be competent and follow a code of ethics. They are accountable for the care they provide based on their scope of practice. Professional collaboration, which is directly related to the need for teamwork, is required to meet the goal of effective nursing practice. The ANA (2015b) defines **collaboration** as follows:

> A professional healthcare partnership grounded in reciprocal and respectful recognition and acceptance: each partner's unique expertise, power, and sphere of influence and responsibilities; the commonality of goals; the mutual safeguarding the legitimate interest of each party; and the advantage of such a relationship. (ANA, 2015b, p. 86; nursing scope and standards of practice)

Guide to the Code of Ethics for Nurses: Interpretation and Application

The primary source for a code of ethics for nurses was developed by the ANA "as a guide for carrying out nursing responsibilities in a manner consistent with quality in nursing and the ethical obligations of the profession" (Fowler, 2016, p. xix). Provision 3 in the ANA Code focuses on issues related to CQI:

> Protection of the rights of privacy and confidentiality, protection of human participants in research, performance standards and review mechanisms,

professional responsibility in promoting a culture of safety, protection of patient health and safety by acting on questionable practice, and patient protection and impaired practice. (ANA, 2015b)

Many of the code's other provisions are indirectly related to CQI.

Fraud and Healthcare Quality

When fraud occurs there are both ethical and legal issues. Fraud and abuse in health care are not rare. **Fraud** is intentional deception for one's own gain, and it is a criminal act. Abuse and fraud are similar acts, but with abuse, it is often difficult to prove intention.

Healthcare fraud and abuse have increased over the years. In some instances, HCOs and individuals that work for HCOs have committed fraud or deliberately deceived another person or organization for personal gain. In other instances, patients, such as those undergoing psychiatric treatment, have been abused, as described in this section. Nurses have been involved in these problems. Health care is a business, a very large industry, and it provides many opportunities for fraud, particularly related to reimbursement. Healthcare fraud and abuse impact healthcare quality and also drain from money that could be used to provide and improve care.

The most common fraud example is deceiving reimbursement sources such as the federal government, particularly the Medicare and Medicaid programs, although fraud also occurs with other types of reimbursement/insurers. In 2013, the federal government recovered more than $4.2 billion due to fraud in federal healthcare programs, such as Medicare and Medicaid (HHS, DOJ, 2013). It is important that this money was recovered; even though this instance does not represent all the money that was lost, it represents a poor statement about ethics and legal concerns. For example, this fraud was related to billing for "phantom patients" (patients who did not exist), billing for medical goods or services that were not provided, billing for more hours than there are in a day, and double-billing for healthcare goods and services provided (HHS, 2014). In 2015, more than 240 individuals (doctors, nurses, and other licensed professionals) were arrested in one week for alleged participation in Medicare fraud involving $712 million in false billings (FBI, 2015).

There have been major fraud issues with Medicare that led the Centers for Medicare and Medicaid (CMS) to create a website focused on fraud called Stop Medicare Fraud. Because Medicare fraud exhausts healthcare resources and thereby contributes to rising healthcare expenses, it impacts all Americans. Identifying and preventing such corruption can improve the quality of health care and help make it more affordable for families, businesses, and the federal government (HHS, 2015a). The CMS offers the following examples of healthcare fraud (HHS, 2015a):

- A healthcare provider bills Medicare for services patients never received.
- A supplier bills Medicare for equipment patients never received.

- Someone uses another person's Medicare card to get medical care, supplies, or equipment.
- Someone bills Medicare for home medical equipment after it has been returned.
- A company offers a Medicare drug plan that has not been approved by Medicare.
- A company uses false information to mislead potential Medicare beneficiaries into joining a Medicare plan.

The CMS website encourages Medicare beneficiaries to report problems and ask questions they may have about billing and other issues so that potential problems can be investigated. The Connect to Current Information section at the end of the chapter provides a link to this site.

Healthcare fraud does not just happen in Medicare and Medicaid and may be associated with CQI directly by using a cover-up. An example occurred in 2016 at an academic medical center (Beckers Hospital Review, 2016). What is notable about this case is a nurse served as a whistleblower. This is a person who reports on an employer or others who could retaliate (Westrick, 2014). The whistleblower laws protect the whistleblower from retaliation when these lawsuits are initiated. The nurse filed a whistleblower civil lawsuit that led to an investigation of the number of patients, estimated at 100, who experienced infections after bronchoscopy. The way the medical center decided to deal with the increase in infections was to just stop checking the bronchoscopes routinely. In doing this they of course did not identify any problems. The nurse asked that this not be done and recommended the hospital use an external agency to investigate the quality problem, but this had no affect. This case is significant as it includes a cover-up to make CQI look better and includes a healthcare professional who asks for help outside the organization and then files a lawsuit. This takes great strength to make this type of stand against care that is not only of poor quality but when healthcare professionals purposely take actions to appear as if care has not problems. Nurses and others do encounter this type of situation in their work places and must decide how to address it.

One of the major fraud and abuse episodes occurred in the 1980s and 1990s. During this period there were large national psychiatric service corporations, which were investor-owned or for-profit. Many new hospitals were built, and there was a great deal of merging of corporations. The following types of fraud and abuse are now known to have occurred (U.S. House of Representatives, 1992, 1994; U.S. Senate, 1992):

- HCOs documented admissions when the patients were never actually admitted.
- Parents were told that their children were seriously ill and needed admission when this was not the case.

- Patients were given medications they did not need, or there was documentation indicating patients received large amounts of medications that were never actually given; in either case, the hospitals billed for the medications.
- Patients were charged for medications and other treatment they never received.
- Patients were restrained unnecessarily and for long periods.
- Patients were denied their rights.
- Patients were subjected to verbal abuse.

When these problems were finally identified on a national level, there were extensive congressional reviews that detailed a lack of professional and business ethics in healthcare delivery (U.S. House of Representatives, 1992, 1994; U.S. Senate, 1992). Some states, such as Texas, had worse problems than others. Senator Moncrief commented in Congress that "in Texas, we have uncovered some of the most elaborate, aggressive, creative, deceptive, immoral, and illegal schemes being used to fill empty hospital beds with insured and paying patients" (U.S. House of Representatives, 1992, p. 7). Hospital administration, physicians, nurses, and others were involved in these activities, although some physicians and nurses did report the activities to the authorities, such as the state board of nursing (Mohr, 1996, 1997). However, some of them experienced negative results for stepping up to report unethical and illegal activities; for example, some of these employees reported being blacklisted so that it was difficult to get a new job, being the victims of false claims to licensing boards about use of drugs, being subjected to verbal abuse, and receiving other threats.

As an example of the complexity of CQI, in 2014, a major healthcare fraud concern was identified in the Veterans Health Administration (VA) hospitals and their services. This healthcare system identified measures/indicators to determine quality status outcomes and in many cases assess performance of providers and administrators. Some of these measures/indicators were connected to wait times for initial appointments. Some hospitals were involved in elaborate schemes to demonstrate they met the measures/indicators; these schemes included changing or falsifying documentation. All of this fraud had a direct impact on the quality of care received; access was delayed, and in some cases care was never received. This is a clear example of the relationship between ethics and legal issues and quality care. In this case, the focus on CQI outcomes incentivized staff to do the wrong thing, to make the wrong decisions to meet the outcomes. Such behavior is always a risk when outcomes are set and then used to assess performance of individuals and organizations. With the increasing use of this method in CQI, it has become even more important for healthcare professionals to understand ethics and apply ethical principles, recognizing the need to maintain ethics in decisions and practice.

Even in 2016, problems continued in some VA medical centers; for example, care and misconduct allegations at a Cincinnati, Ohio, VA hospital prompted a recent Inspector General investigation and in Long Island, New York, VA hospital (Krause, 2016; Rebello & Santora, 2016).

The website for the Office of Inspector General of the U.S. Department of Health and Human Services (HHS) provides information about CMS current fraud cases. The following are specific examples of legal cases listed for January, February, and early March 2016 (HHS, OIG, 2016).

- Former owner and operator of California Medical Equipment Supply Company sentenced for roles in $1.5 million Medicare fraud scheme. (January 2016)
- Federal jury convicts physician in Medicare fraud scheme. (January 2016)
- Physician assistant sentenced to 14 months in prison for accepting illegal kickbacks. (January 2016)
- Owner and manager of three home health agencies convicted in $57 million healthcare fraud scheme. (January 2016)
- Physician pleads guilty for role in $20 million healthcare fraud scheme. (February 2016)
- Individual sentenced to more than 14 years in prison for multimillion-dollar healthcare fraud and money laundering scheme. (March 2016)
- Physician convicted in hospital kickback scheme. (March 2016)
- Former fugitive pleads guilty in multimillion-dollar healthcare fraud scheme. (March 2016)
- Physician pleads guilty for role in $20 million healthcare fraud scheme. (February 2016)

This list of examples indicates that fraud persists and is a major problem with implications for how it hurts others and the cost involved. The list covers only a short period of time and represents fraud that took place only in the CMS program. In addition, the list indicates that participants in fraud cover many types of healthcare professionals and others involved in the healthcare industry and a variety of types of HCOs and HCO-related businesses. Because this problem has increased and drains resources, it is addressed in the Affordable Care Act of 2010 (ACA) by increasing penalties, expanding screening for fraud, and improving coordination of information across states. The HHS Healthcare Fraud Prevention and Enforcement Action Team (HEAT) is an example of the government's efforts to decrease healthcare fraud. HEAT brings together multiple stakeholders to prevent waste, fraud, and abuse in Medicare and Medicaid (HHS, 2015b). Its mission statement includes the importance of preventing fraud, as it impacts quality care. HHS works closely with the Department of Justice in this initiative.

The federal government has increased monitoring and enforcement of laws to prevent fraud. Who has been involved in the fraud? Physicians, nurses, pharmacists, healthcare administrators, and other healthcare providers have been involved in fraud cases. Every staff member has an obligation to follow the four ethical principles and to report concerns to organization administration or, if necessary, to legal authorities.

With the increased number of ethical and legal concerns in health care, such as the healthcare fraud examples discussed in this chapter, HCOs have become more interested in organizational ethics. We see this now in many industries, but what does it mean? The organizations develop organization compliance committees with the goal of ensuring ethical business practices. These committees establish standards; provide staff education on ethics; develop systems for staff to report ethical and legal concerns, including policies, procedures, and staff education; and develop audits and monitor outcomes. Staff need to understand how the organization's mission, vision, and goals relate to a code of conduct and its relationship to the HCO's compliance program.

When the program is developed, a critical element is implementation of a method for staff to anonymously report ethical concerns. Staff must feel that their identity will be protected and that reporting concerns will not lead to any personal negative result. In the psychiatric care fraud and abuse examples, nurses had limited confidential methods to report their concerns, and those who stepped forward met with negative consequences. This type of culture does not lead to an effective compliance program. The need for HCO monitoring of ethical concerns has become so important that in 1996 the Health Care Compliance Association (HCCA) was established and then expanded over the years as need increased (HCCA, 2015). Staff can now complete certification requirements in healthcare compliance to more effectively assist HCOs in their compliance efforts.

Ethical Leadership

Leaders need to apply ethical principles in their decision-making and ensure that staff apply these principles in their work settings. All types of healthcare providers and HCOs need to ensure that there is a process for measuring quality and that strategies are used to improve care (Baily, Bottrell, Lynn, & Jennings, 2006; Jennings, Baily, Bottrell, & Lynn, 2007; White & O'Sullivan, 2012). There is greater emphasis today on pushing CQI down to the bedside level or the direct care level. This means that CQI is no longer just the responsibility of management and CQI programs/departments within HCOs; it is also the responsibility of each staff member. Healthcare leaders need to communicate to staff that attending to CQI efforts is an expectation and directly connected to the organization's ethics.

Ethical decision-making is connected to decisions nurses make about CQI. Typically, this process occurs when there is an ethical dilemma. When **ethical dilemmas** occur, significant emotions are often involved, making it even more difficult to resolve them. Using facts is an important part of describing and understanding an ethical dilemma. This process needs to include patient, family, and staff perspectives. In the end, choices must be made, and none of the options are ideal (an ethical dilemma). There is no "magic" answer to an ethical dilemma.

Stop and Consider #1

Nurses have been involved in healthcare fraud.

Standards and Quality Improvement

Standards and regulations impact practice, management, and CQI in health care and relate to individual professions, to HCOs, and to the government (local, state, and national). A **standard** is an "authoritative statement defined and promoted by a profession by which the quality of practice, service, or education can be evaluated" (ANA, 2015b, p. 146). Standards are viewed as the minimum, not maximum, expectation. They should be met, but they are not the end point in improvement. Nursing standards of practice include both standards of care that guide the provision of care and standards of professional performance describing the competent level of professional practice (ANA, 2015b). Standards are an important part of CQI in that individual healthcare professions have standards that guide practice, states and the federal government have standards that must be applied by law and regulations to HCOs, healthcare professionals must commit to state scope of practice and meet licensure requirements, and accrediting organizations establish standards required for accreditation of HCOs and also healthcare profession education programs. Individual HCOs also have standards.

Individual Professional Standards

Nursing regulation, as defined by the National Council for State Boards of Nursing (2007), "exists to protect the health, safety, and welfare of the public in their receipt of nursing services—and much more." **Self-regulation** is an important aspect of a profession. Nurses are expected to maintain their competence, often through required continuing education for licensure and/or certification. Even if this is not required, it is expected as part of self-regulation; as nurses practice, they should participate in peer review within their HCOs. ANA's *Nursing: Scope and Standards of Practice* emphasizes the

> essential role of the nurse in care coordination, promoting wellness, providing individualized care in nurse-managed health centers, and participation in

medical homes. It identifies these and other nursing services as vital to the effort—to alleviate the financial and social costs of treating preventable and chronic diseases. (ANA, 2015b, p. 26)

Healthcare professional organizations develop standards for their members. For example, the ANA standards *Nursing: Scope and Standards of Practice* (ANA, 2015b) are the major standards for nursing. The ANA also has developed standards focused on specific practice areas such as nursing administration, staff education, gerontology, informatics, and other areas. Other healthcare professions, such as medicine, respiratory therapy, occupational health, social work, laboratory services, radiology, and so on, have similar types of standards. The main goal for these standards is to ensure quality care and provide a description of the professional responsibility to reach the profession's goal.

Typically, specialty groups within a profession also have standards. Examples of nursing specialty organizations include the Association of Occupational Health Nurses, American Association of Nurse Anesthetists, Association of Perioperative Registered Nurses, National Association of Neonatal Nurses, Infusion Nurses Society, and others. Nurses who work in these specialty areas are expected to follow these specialty standards. HCOs need to be aware of them and ensure that they are integrated into HCO standards and requirements. Standards change periodically due to changes in the healthcare knowledge, research, and delivery needs, and changes within the health professions. Nurses and HCOs need to be aware of changes. Ideally, they will participate in the development of changes in standards and apply them. The *Quality Chasm* five healthcare professions core competencies are now integrated into some healthcare professions education requirements, including nursing, although more needs to be done to implement this recommendation.

Healthcare Organization Standards

HCOs also establish standards that apply to their staff and work processes within the organization. It is important that HCOs remain aware of other standards to avoid conflicts. For example, is the HCO requiring staff to practice in a certain way that is not acceptable with the staff members' professional standards or other relevant standards? Such conflicts are not acceptable.

Stop and Consider #2

Standards are described as minimum standards.

Government Standards, Legislation, and Regulations

Government at the local, state, and federal levels has many standards that are integrated into laws and regulations. HCOs and healthcare professionals are required to follow all relevant standards. The HHS is particularly tasked with healthcare delivery on the federal level, and it has many agencies that do this work for the department. The department is directly impacted by the National Academies Health and Medicine Division (NAS/HMD) and its *Quality Series* reports and subsequent reports and often turns to this source to request in-depth examination of problems and provide external advice.

Government Standards

State and federal governments establish standards in laws and related regulations that must be met. Many of these standards are more than a guide; they are legal requirements. An example is the Emergency Medical Treatment and Active Labor Act of 1986 (EMATALA), which establishes the standard that all patients who require emergency treatment or who are in labor must be provided care regardless of ability to pay. This act establishes a level of care that is enforced by penalty of the law. An emergency department must monitor this activity in its CQI program. Now, in some situations it is difficult to determine what is an emergency, but emergency departments have no choice but to make every effort to meet this standard.

Legislation and Regulation

State laws and regulations have a major impact on how nursing is practiced within a state, which in turn impacts the status of healthcare delivery. Some federal laws also impact practice and decisions made. The American Nurses Association describes the Model of Professional Nursing Practice Regulation as a guide for the profession. Nursing practice integrates scope of practice, standards, ethics, specialty certification, nurse practice acts, rules and regulations, healthcare organization policies and procedures, and individual self-determination in care delivery. Quality, safety, and evidence are critical supporting elements of that practice (Styles, Bickford, & White, 2008, cited in ANA, 2015). The guiding principles of nursing regulation are: Protection of the public, competence of all practitioners regulated by the board of nursing, due process and ethical decision-making, shared accountability, strategic collaboration, evidence-based regulation, response to the marketplace and healthcare environment, and globalization of nursing (NCSBN, 2007).

Self-determination is a very important part of this model. During practice, each nurse must determine if there is a match with the scope of practice, clinical setting in which care is provided and the patient, individual skills and competencies, and the healthcare team's competencies. Individual judgment is part of this process. **Scope of practice** is "the description of the *who*, *what*, *where*, *when*, and *how* of nursing practice that addresses the range of nursing practice activities common to all registered nurses" (ANA, 2015b, p. 67). The ANA *Standards of Practice* and the *Code of Ethics* influence the scope of practice as designated by each state's Nurse Practice Act. All of which impact evidence-based practice and quality.

State Boards of Nursing and Nurse Practice Acts

State boards of nursing are responsible for ensuring that each state's Nurse Practice Act is followed in order to demonstrate effective practice and quality care for patients, the state's citizens. Each state has its own practice act, which is a law with regulations. The state boards also evaluate schools of nursing within the state to ensure they meet the requirements established by the state board, and these requirements are influenced by standards. The National Council for State Boards of Nursing (NCSBN) is an independent, nonprofit organization that provides counsel to state boards of nursing but cannot tell individual state boards what they must do. The NCSBN is also responsible for the nursing licensure exams (NCSBN, 2015a). The purpose of the state boards and the NCSBN is to address issues related to public health, safety, and welfare. The NCSBN description of the Transition to Practice and its relationship to CQI are discussed in this text.

The NCSBN is also involved in health policy—providing information, lobbying, and so on—with all levels of government. For example, the NCSBN is involved on policies related to interstate practice and telehealth, both of which have implications for CQI. In 2015, the NCSBN held a conference, Leadership and Public Policy, to examine these issues and their relationship to nursing. Other activities related to CQI are improving simulation education for nurses and research about workforce needs. The NCSBN publishes a journal, *Journal of Nursing Regulation*, to expand information about regulation and the profession. It also develops reports and books, such as *Nursing Pathways for Patient Safety* (Benner, Malloch, & Sheets, 2010).

The NCSBN is involved in helping state boards of nursing with their professional discipline activities. It is not possible to eliminate risk in nursing practice, and state boards of nursing know this but are mandated by their state Nurse Practice Act to protect the public. The NCSBN (2015b) summarizes its role in nursing discipline as follows:

> While the vast majority of nurses are competent and caring individuals who provide care according to the standard, violations of the Nurse Practice Act do

happen. When violations occur, the board of nursing takes formal action if it finds sufficient basis that the nurse violated the act or regulations. Currently, the rate of discipline on a license is less than 1 percent.

Professional Licensure

Professional licensure is administered at the state level through each state's board of nursing, but the licensure exam is offered on a national basis, administered through the NCSBN. The purpose of professional licensure is to ensure that all registered nurses and licensed practical nurses meet required standards to enter nursing practice at the *minimum* level of competence. The overall goal is to better ensure patients receive quality care. Renewal of licensure is required for practice, but there is no testing done. Many states require that licensed professionals in their states complete a certain number of continuing education credits; however, there is no current method to determine if this requirement makes any difference in practice and quality of care.

Certification

Certification is available for many nursing specialties. Through standardized examination, nurses are able to demonstrate expertise in a specialty area and validate knowledge for certification as determined by the American Nurses Credentialing Center (ANCC), although this is not the only provider of certification (ANCC, 2015). The goal is the same as for licensure—to ensure excellence in practice and thus impact the quality of care. To apply for certification, all eligibility requirements must be met, which may include practice requirements. Exams, portfolios, and continuing education are methods used to establish certification.

Stop and Consider #3
After the entry level exam (NCLEX), there are no more required testing for registered nurses.

Accreditation

Thus far, this chapter has discussed individual professional responsibilities and methods to ensure that individual healthcare providers meet certain standards. Attention to the individual provider, however, is not enough, as HCOs have critical responsibilities in working to improve care. **Accreditation** is a method used to assess organizations and determine if they meet *minimum* established standards.

The Joint Commission: Purpose and Description of Accreditation Process

The Joint Commission is an independent, not-for-profit organization that accredits and certifies HCOs and healthcare programs. The Joint Commission (2015a) vision is that "all people always experience the safest, highest quality, best value health care across all settings." This vision correlates with the NAS/HMD work, the Triple Aim (better care, healthy people/healthy communities, affordable care), and the National Quality Strategy. Most hospitals are accredited by this organization. Although it is a voluntary process, this accreditation has implications for marketing, for receipt of federal funds such as Medicare payment, and for insurers. Healthcare profession student clinical experiences must be offered in accredited HCOs. Accreditation focuses on hospitals, ambulatory health care, behavioral health care, critical access hospitals, home care, laboratory services, and nursing care centers.

Although accreditation is typically associated with HCOs in the United States, The Joint Commission also accredits HCOs in other countries. As is the case with other types of accreditation organizations, The Joint Commission has established *minimum* standards, which it periodically reviews and updates. HCOs that apply for accreditation or renewal of accreditation use these standards also as guidelines as they prepare to ensure that they can gain accreditation during the official process. Standards vary depending on the type of HCO. Examples of standard topics for one type of HCO, the hospital, include the following: the environment of care, human resources, infection prevention and control, information management, leadership, life safety, medical staff, medication management, National Patient Safety Goals, provision of care, treatment and services, record of care, rights and responsibilities of the individual, transplant safety, and waived testing (The Joint Commission, 2015b).

The Joint Commission has developed a measurement system with measure sets focused on specific medical problems—for example, acute myocardial infarction, pneumonia, heart failure, and so on. This measurement system includes a review of medical records documentation. This approach provides an assessment of quality; however, it does not require a review of all HCO activities.

The Joint Commission provides resources to both healthcare providers and the consumer/patient. Its website includes information about important content for healthcare providers, particularly focused on quality care such as the listing of the current National Patient Safety Goals, sentinel event alerts, staff training, and so on. From The Joint Commission website, consumers/patients can link to Quality Check to search for information about specific HCOs—information on measures that best indicate the status of quality care in a Joint Commission–accredited HCO. These measures are based solely on the perspective of The Joint Commission (The Joint Commission, 2015c). Consumers/patients can also report a safety or other type of concern about a Joint Commission–accredited HCO to the website link for this purpose. Additional information about The Joint Commission and its CQI activities and resources is found in other chapters. The Connect to Current Information section at the end of the chapter provides a link to its site.

Nursing and The Joint Commission Accreditation

Nurses in all types of HCOs accredited by The Joint Commission are involved in all phases of the accreditation process. Nurses in leadership and management positions must be actively engaged in all steps within the HCO—planning, implementation, and evaluating the process at the conclusion. Clinical nursing staff are also involved, and now, compared to the past, all staff, clinical and nonclinical, are more involved in the actual survey visit. Surveyors speak with them and engage them in the on-site process. Nurses need to also participate in CQI, which is part of accreditation; however, CQI should not be dependent on accreditation. CQI does not end when accreditation is received, not to be revisited until the accreditation period concludes and a renewal is needed.

The accreditation process, as described by The Joint Commission (2015d), is "data-driven, patient-centered, and focused on evaluating actual care processes. The objectives of the survey are not only to evaluate the organization, but to provide education and "good practice" guidance that will help staff continually improve the organization's performance." Preparing for accreditation and the survey visit is part of the process. All levels of staff participate in the preparation and the visit. HCOs conduct self-assessments to prepare for an accreditation survey visit. The preparation includes the following:

1. Planning, which requires time and input from relevant stakeholders
2. Offering effective staff education about accreditation
3. Implementing an effective plan for the accreditation process
4. Providing ongoing evaluation of the implemented plan

The danger is always that the HCO does all the work for accreditation and then takes a long break until accreditation time comes around again. This is not the intent of accreditation and in the end harms the HCO.

Examples of Other Accrediting Organizations

The following examples illustrate that accreditation is relevant to a variety of HCOs and associated organizations and processes, including nursing education programs. Other healthcare profession programs such as medicine, pharmacy, and physical therapy also go through accreditation processes for their specific professional education programs based on their professional standards.

Community Health Accreditation Partner

The Community Health Accreditation Partner (CHAP) has existed for more than 50 years (CHAP, 2015). It provides accreditation to community-based HCOs and related businesses. These HCOs include hospice, private duty agencies, home medical equipment businesses, home health, infusion therapy nursing, pharmacy, and public health. As is typical for most accreditation processes, the CHAP process includes a self-study and site visit. The review includes all aspects of the organization and its services.

Accreditation Commission for Health Care

The Accreditation Commission for Health Care (ACHC) is an accreditation program that focuses on accreditation of hospice; home health; durable equipment, prosthetics, orthotics, and supplies (DMEPOS); pharmacy; private duty services; sleep lab/center; and behavioral health. Quality improvement is an important component of ACHC accreditation (ACHC, 2015). The CMS recognizes this accreditation for home health, hospice, and DMEPOS. This accreditation applies a process similar to the process used for other accrediting organizations.

Utilization Review Accreditation Commission

The Utilization Review Accreditation Commission (URAC) is an independent, nonprofit organization that provides accreditation for health insurance plans (URAC, 2015). The goal is to promote CQI through its accreditation education and measurement programs—for example, by using benchmarking to compare insurance plan outcomes.

Accreditation of Nursing Education Programs

Nursing academic programs also undergo an accreditation process. There are two organizations that accredit schools of nursing: the Commission on Collegiate Nursing Education (CCNE), which is associated with the American Association of Colleges of Nursing, and the Commission for Nursing Education Accreditation (CNEA), which is associated with the National League for Nursing. Both accreditation programs use similar processes based on their own required standards, self-study, and survey or site visit.

Nursing academic programs choose which accreditation they wish to obtain; however, the type of degree programs offered by the school of nursing may impact their choice of accreditation organization. The CCNE accredits collegiate professional education (baccalaureate and graduate nursing programs, including the doctor of nursing practice [DNP] degree but excluding PhD programs) and post-baccalaureate nurse residency programs (CCNE, 2015). Programs that may be accredited by CNEA are practical (vocational), diploma, associate degree, baccalaureate, master's, and DNP programs that prepare advanced practice nurses, nurse executives, and nurse educators (CNEA, 2015).

The purpose of academic accreditation is to ensure that the nursing programs meet standards related to students, organization, curriculum, faculty, and program assessment to ensure that students get effective education and meet requirements to practice as designated by the school's state Nurse Practice Act and its scope of nursing practice and other role requirements. The process supports self-assessment and growth and improvement.

Stop and Consider #4
Healthcare organization accreditation is not required but is common.

Legal Issues

Legal issues are connected with ethics, standards, and regulation. HCOs retain attorneys to assist with legal concerns and risk factors related to potential legal problems. These attorneys work with HCO staff on risk management and quality care to prevent legal problems and to resolve them when they occur. All nurses need to understand negligence and malpractice and how their practice can be at risk. Disclosure of errors is an important topic and part of patient-centered care today. This topic is discussed further in other chapters of this text.

Negligence and Malpractice

Standards serve another function, which is also related to quality care. They are used by state boards of nursing and by the legal system to address nursing actions in licensure concerns and in legal cases, such as determining nursing negligence and malpractice. The nurse is expected to practice as a **reasonably prudent nurse**. *Reasonably prudent* means a nurse who has similar education and experience and average intelligence, judgment, foresight, and skill would respond like other similar nurses to the same situation, case, facts, or emergency using the standard of care, and particularly should follow professional standards (Westrick, 2014). Standards are used as a guide for expected care, although other sources are also used in legal cases, such as clinical guidelines, expert testimony, and other documents that might clarify practice expectations. **Negligence** is "failure to exercise reasonable care, or the degree of care that a reasonably prudent person would exercise under the same or similar circumstances" (Westrick, 2014, p. 369). Negligence may be intentional or unintentional. **Malpractice** is similar to negligence but more specific. It is "professional negligence committed by a person in his or her professionally licensed capacity" (Westrick, 2014, p. 369). Specific legal requirements must be met for negligence: There must be (1) duty to the patient, (2) proximate cause, and (3) damages or injury.

Nurses are sued, and when this occurs, it is important to consider the nurse's practice and whether or not expected standards were followed. Nurses may also be sued as individual healthcare providers in lawsuits against an HCO, the nurse's employer. In these cases, it is recommended that the nurse consult an attorney that represents the nurse, not the HCO. Many nurses carry professional insurance, and in this case, the insurer may require that when the nurse is involved in a potential lawsuit the nurse take certain steps and use an attorney recommended by the insurer. Negligence and malpractice and situations in which nurses are identified as having practice problems by their board of nursing are directly related to quality care; something may have been done or not done that impacted practice and patient outcomes, and standards may not have been met.

Guide to Nurses' Responses to Legal Problems Related to Errors

Nurses need to know the legal requirements within their state and federal requirements. They must follow the state Nurse Practice Act and report practice that does not meet the standards. This is part of professional responsibility. Complaints to a board of nursing typically focus on nursing practice that is unsafe; incompetent; unethical and affected by alcohol, drugs, or other chemicals or by a physical or mental condition; and/or in violation of a nursing or nursing-related law or rule (NCSBN, 2015c). Each board of nursing describes its procedure for reporting concerns to the board. The NCSBN (2015c) states the following:

> A nurse's practice and behavior is expected to be safe, competent, ethical, and in compliance with applicable laws and rules. Any person who has knowledge of conduct by a licensed nurse that may violate a nursing law or rule or related state or federal law may report the alleged violation to the state board of nursing where the situation occurred.

Stop and Consider #5
Nurses are sued for malpractice.

Conclusions

CQI does not stand alone. It is influenced by critical aspects of healthcare delivery, particularly ethics, standards, legislation and regulation, accreditation, and legal concerns. Nurses are expected to understand all of these aspects as members of a profession, and they need to participate actively in following requirements to improve care. The profession has specific methods and organizations, such as professional organizations and state boards of nursing, that focus on all of these concerns. All of these methods relate to CQI—ensuring quality care for patients.

Apply CQI

Chapter Highlights

- Ethical concerns are present every day in all healthcare settings and relate to all healthcare professionals.
- Professional codes of ethics are related to CQI.
- Healthcare fraud causes the nation to lose money that could have been used on healthcare delivery and impacts quality; the problem is increasing.
- Ethical leadership should be part of each HCO, but it requires effort to achieve.
- Individual professional standards, HCO standards, and government standards all have an impact on how we practice and on CQI.
- Regulations and legislation may indirectly or directly impact CQI. The Emergency Medical Treatment and Active Labor Act of 1986 is an example of specialty legislation that impacts CQI. The Affordable Care Act includes provisions related to CQI, fraud, and other issues that impact CQI.
- Accreditation of HCOs and health profession education programs are important parts of ensuring CQI. Practice is based on standards; educational programs follow standards to meet consistent education requirements, and both HCOs and educational programs include CQI in their ongoing activities.
- Negligence and malpractice are related to the quality of practice and related outcomes.

Critical Thinking and Clinical Reasoning and Judgment: Discussion Questions and Learning Activities

1. Why is professional ethics part of a discussion about quality improvement? Provide three examples to support your answer.
2. You are part of a standards committee at your HCO. The committee is working on its annual review of standards. What internal and external information should be reviewed?
3. Several classmates should ask about accreditation at the HCOs where the students are performing clinical rotations. Before interviewing,

work together to prepare a list of key questions. After the interview, summarize the interview information and discuss how it relates to quality improvement.

Connect to Current Information

- Stop Medicare Fraud
  https://www.stopmedicarefraud.gov
- The Joint Commission
  http://www.jointcommission.org
- American Association of Colleges of Nursing (accreditation page)
  http://www.aacn.nche.edu/ccne-accreditation
- Accreditation Commission for Education in Nursing
  http://www.acenursing.org
- American Nurses Credentialing Center
  http://www.nursecredentialing.org/certification.aspx
- ANA's *Guide to the Code of Ethics for Nurses: Application and Interpretation*
  http://www.nursesbooks.org/ebooks/download/CodeofEthics.pdf

EBP, EBM, and Quality Improvement: Exemplar

Benton, D., Péez-Raya, F., Gonzáles-Jurado, M., & Rodríguez-López, M. (2015). Keeping pace with an ever-changing world: A policy imperative. *Journal of Nursing Regulation, 6*(1), 20–24.

This article examines change and how it impacts healthcare regulation.

Questions to Consider:

1. What healthcare global initiatives are discussed in this article?
2. What changes are discussed?
3. How might these comments relate to the nursing profession and CQI?

Evolving Case Study

As a member of the staff development department, you and others in the department are beginning preparations for an upcoming Joint Commission survey—a process that takes many months. There are five staff members, including the director; however, three of you have not been through an accreditation survey as a staff educator. Since the last survey, the hospital has added 40 beds, there is a shortage of registered nurses in two medical units and one surgical unit, and there has been an increase in CQI activities and an increase in CQI program staff. There are still concerns about quality care problems that have not improved, such as medication errors.

Case Questions:

1. What would you include in the plan to prepare for The Joint Commission process? Your plan should identify a timeline.
2. What are the differences in the accreditation role of staff educators, administration/management, clinical staff, and nonclinical staff?
3. As part of your preparation of staff and expansion of accreditation content in staff orientation, how would you include accreditation, standards, regulation, and ethical and legal issues in the orientation discussion? What teaching–learning methods might you use?

References

Accreditation Commission for Health Care (ACHC). (2015). ACHC: For providers. By providers. Retrieved from http://www.achc.org/about-achc

American Nurses Association (ANA). (2015b). *Nursing: Scope and standards of practice.* Silver Spring, MD: Author.

American Nurses Association (ANA). (2016). Guide to nursing's social policy statement: understanding the Profession from social contract to social covenant. Silver Spring, MD: Author.

American Nurses Association (ANA). (2011, March 3). ANA, CMA, and ONA activities in the IOM recommendations. Retrieved from http://www.nursingworld.org/MainMenuCategories/ThePracticeofProfessionalNursing/workforce/IOM-Future-of-Nursing-Report-1/ANA-Activities-from-IOM-Future-of-Nursing-Report.pdf9

American Nurses Association (ANA). (2015a). *Code of ethics with interpretative statements* (3rd ed.). Silver Spring, MD: Author.

American Nurses Credentialing Center (ANCC). (2015). About ANCC. Retrieved from http://www.nursecredentialing.org/About-ANCC

Baily, M., Bottrell, M., Lynn, J., & Jennings, B. (2006). *The ethics of using QI methods to improve healthcare quality and safety.* New York, NY: The Hastings Center.

Beckers Hospital Review. (2016). UC health nurse sues health system for covering up scope-related outbreak. Retrieved from http://www.beckershospitalreview.com/quality/uc-health-nurse-sues-health-system-for-covering-up-scope-related-outbreak.html

Benner, P., Malloch, K., & Sheets, V. (Eds.). (2010). *Nursing pathways for patient safety.* St. Louis, MO: Mosby.

Community Health Accreditation Partner (CHAP). (2015). About CHAP. Retrieved from http://www.chapinc.org/

Commission on Collegiate Nursing Education (CCNE). (2015). CCNE accreditation. Retrieved from http://www.aacn.nche.edu/ccne-accreditation

Commission for Nursing Education Accreditation (CNEA). (2015). Overview: National League for Nursing Commission for Nursing Education Accreditation. Retrieved from http://www.nln.org/accreditation-services

Federal Bureau of Investigation (FBI). (2015, June 18). Healthcare fraud takedown. Retrieved from https://www.fbi.gov/news/stories/2015/june/health-care-fraud-takedown/health-care-fraud-takedown

Finkelman, A., & Kenner, C. (2016). *Professional nursing concepts: Competencies for quality leadership* (3rd ed.). Burlington, MA: Jones & Bartlett Learning.

Health Care Compliance Association (HCCA). (2015). About the Health Care Compliance Association. Retrieved from http://www.hcca-info.org/AboutHCCA/AboutHCCA.aspx

Jennings, B., Baily, M., Bottrell, M., & Lynn, J. (2007). *Healthcare quality improvement: Ethical and regulatory issues*. Garrison, NY: The Hastings Center.

Koloroutis, M., & Thorstenson, T. (1999). An ethics framework for organizational change. *Nursing Administrative Quarterly, 23*(2), 9–18.

Krause, B. (2016, February 15). Cincinnati VA at center of misconduct investigation. Retrieved from http://www.disabledveterans.org/2016/02/15/cincinnati-va-at-center-of-misconduct-investigation/

Mohr, K. (1996). Dirty hands: The underside of marketplace healthcare. *Advances in Nursing Science, 19*(1), 28–37.

Mohr, K. (1997). Outcomes of corporate greed. *Image: Journal of Nursing Scholarship, 29*(1), 39–45.

National Council State Boards of Nursing (NCSBN). (2007). *Guiding principles for nursing regulation*. Retrieved from https://www.ncsbn.org/3933.htm

National Council State Boards of Nursing (NCSBN). (2015a). National council state boards of nursing. Retrieved from https://www.ncsbn.org/index.htm

National Council State Boards of Nursing (NCSBN). (2015b). Discipline. Retrieved from https://www.ncsbn.org/discipline.htm

National Council State Boards of Nursing (NCSBN). (2015c). Filing a complaint. Retrieved from https://ncsbn.org/filing-a-complaint.htm

Rebelo, K., & Santora, M. (2016, September 19). Deaths, fraud allegations, and an inquiry into a Long Island VA hospital. Retrieved from http://www.nytimes.com/2016/09/20/nyregion/inquiry-into-northport-va-hospital-long-island.html?_r=

Styles, M., Schuman, M., Bickford, C., & White, K. (2008). *Specialization and Credentialing in Nursing Revisited: Understand the Issues, Advancing the Profession*. Found in American *Nurses Association. (2015). Nursing: Scope and Standards of Practice*. Silver Spring, MD: Author. Retrieved from http://www.nursingworld.org/modelofpracticeregulation

The Joint Commission. (2015a). The Joint Commission. Retrieved from http://www.jointcommission.org/

The Joint Commission. (2015b). Standards interpretation. Retrieved from http://www.jointcommission.org/standards_information/jcfaq.aspx

The Joint Commission. (2015c). About Quality Check. Retrieved from http://qualitycheck.org/help_qc_facts.aspx

The Joint Commission. (2015d). Facts about the on-site survey process. Retrieved from http://www.jointcommission.org/facts_about_the_on-site_survey_process/

U.S. Department of Health and Human Services (HHS). (2014). Common Medicaid rip-offs and tips to prevent fraud. Retrieved from http://www.cms.gov/Medicare-Medicaid-Coordination/Fraud-Prevention/FraudAbuseforConsumers/Ripoffs_and_Tips.html

U.S. Department of Health and Human Services (HHS). (2015a). Stop Medicare Fraud. About fraud. Retrieved from http://www.stopmedicarefraud.gov/aboutfraud/index.html

U.S. Department of Health and Human Services (HHS). (2015b). HEAT task force. Retrieved from https://www.stopmedicarefraud.gov/aboutfraud/heattaskforce/index.html

U. S. Department of Health and Human Service (HHS), Department of Justice (DOJ) Healthcare Fraud and Abuse Control Program. (2013). Departments of Justice and Health and Human Services announce record-breaking recoveries resulting from efforts to combat healthcare fraud. Retrieved from http://www.hhs.gov/news/press/2013pres/02/20130211a.html

U. S. Department of Health and Human Services (HHS), Office of the Inspector General (OIG). (2016). Medicare fraud strike force. Retrieved from http://oig.hhs.gov/fraud/strike-force/

U.S. House of Representatives. (1992, April 28). The profits of misery: How inpatient psychiatric treatment bilks the system and betrays our trust. Hearing before the Select Committee on Children, Youth and Families, One Hundred Second Congress, Second Session. Washington, DC: U.S. Government Printing Office.

U.S. House of Representatives. (1994, July 19). Deceit that sickens America: Health care fraud and its innocent victims. Hearings before the Subcommittee on Crime and Criminal Justice of the Committee on the Judiciary House of Representatives, One Hundred and Third Congress, One Hundred Congress, Second Session. Washington, DC: U.S. Government Printing Office.

U.S. Senate. (1992, July 28). Hearing before the Committee on the Judiciary United States Senate, Senate Bill 2652, One Hundred Second Congress, Second Session. Washington, DC: U.S. Government Printing Office.

Utilization Review Accreditation Commission (URAC). (2015). About URAC. Retrieved from https://www.urac.org/about-urac/about-urac/

Westrick, S. (2014). *Essentials of nursing law and ethics* (2nd ed.). Burlington, MA: Jones & Bartlett Learning.

White, K., & O'Sullivan, A. (Eds.). (2012). *The essential guide to nursing practice. Applying ANA's scope and standards in practice and education.* Silver Spring, MD: American Nurses Association.

CHAPTER 3

Healthcare Professions Core Competencies to Improve Care

CHAPTER OBJECTIVES

At the conclusion of this chapter, the learner will be able to:

- Analyze the five healthcare professions core competencies and implications for continuous quality improvement (CQI) and nursing.
- Compare the five healthcare professions core competencies with the Quality and Safety Education for Nurses competencies.
- Discuss the implications of education to healthcare CQI.

OUTLINE

KEY TERMS

Comparative effectiveness research	Evidence-based practice (EBP)	Point-of-care learning
Competency	Interprofessional education	Systematic review
Continuing education	Learning health system	Workplace learning
Evidence-based management (EBM)	Lifelong learning	

Introduction

Today, it is clearly recognized that in order for health care to improve in the United States, there must be improvement and ongoing changes in healthcare education in academic healthcare professional programs, staff education in the workplace, and professional continuing education. This chapter offers a description of relevant competencies that are important to improving practice and care outcomes, along with discussion of important strategies needed to improve care through more competent staff practice that are supported by accreditation of education programs, education standards, innovative education approaches such as simulation, staff education, interprofessional education, and improvement in continuing education for healthcare professionals. The goal is to establish a learning healthcare system that, in the words of the Institute of Medicine (IOM) (2007), is

> designed to generate and apply the best evidence for the collaborative healthcare choices of each patient and provider; to drive the process of discovery as a natural outgrowth of patient care; and to ensure innovation, quality, safety and value in health care. Advances in computing, information science, and connectivity can improve patient–clinician communication, point-of-care guidance, the capture of experience, population surveillance, planning and evaluation, and the generation of real-time knowledge—features of a continuously learning health care system. (p. 37)

Health Professions: A Bridge to Quality

The publication of *Health Professions: A Bridge to Quality* (IOM, 2003a) as part of the *Quality Chasm* reports was an important step in the development of the reports on quality care. The *Quality Chasm* reports published prior to this report primarily focused on understanding the status of care and healthcare delivery problems; describing a vision, aims, and framework for quality care; and offering recommendations for measuring and tracking progress. The piece that was missing in the process is greater understanding of the input in the continuous quality improvement (CQI) process (Finkelman & Kenner, 2012). The *Health Professions* report discussed this concern, and the connection of this report to previous reports is described in **Figure 3-1**.

One can spend a lot of effort trying to improve care during the care process and within healthcare organizations (HCOs), but something is missing from this effort. Are healthcare professions ready to provide quality care and work to ensure that there is CQI? This CQI agenda is really the critical topic of this text. If HCOs work to improve but the staff and new graduates from the various healthcare professions are not prepared in understanding and applying CQI every day in care settings, can we really ever reach the aims of safe, effective, safe, timely, effective, efficient, equitable, and patient-centered (STEEEP) care (IOM, 2001)?

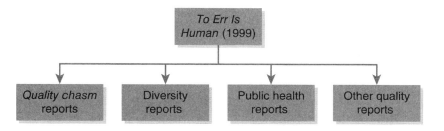

Figure 3-1 Development of the Health Professions Education Report by the Institute of Medicine.
Data from Finkelman, A. & Kenner, C. (2012). *Teaching IOM: Implications of the Institute of Medicine Reports for Nursing Education* (3rd ed.). Silver Spring, MD: American Nurses Association.

Figure 3-2 The Five Healthcare Professions Core Competencies.
Data from Institute of Medicine. (2003). *Health professions education: A bridge to quality.* Washington, DC: National Academies Press.

The first step was to identify the core competencies, and the approach taken was highly significant. Rather than identify core competencies for specific healthcare professions, the decision was made to identify core competencies for all healthcare professions—the same competencies to ensure a base of functioning in the healthcare delivery system. This approach had never been tried before. A **competency** is "an expected and measurable level of nursing performance that integrates knowledge, skills, abilities, and judgment based on established scientific knowledge and expectations for nursing practice" (ANA, 2015, p. 64). The five competencies are based on this definition. These core competencies are highlighted in **Figure 3-2** and discussed in the following sections. Healthcare professions meeting these competencies then act as a bridge to quality.

Provide Patient-Centered Care: Application to Nursing and CQI

The core competency to provide patient-centered care is described by the IOM (2003a) as follows:

Identify, respect, and care about patients' differences, values, preferences, and expressed needs; relieve pain and suffering; coordinate continuous care; listen to,

Figure 3-3 Providing Patient-Centered Care: Key Elements.

clearly inform, communicate with, and educate patients; share decision making and management; and continuously advocate disease prevention wellness, and promotion of healthy lifestyles, including a focus on population health. (p. 4)

Figure 3-3 highlights key elements of this competency.

The focus on the patient in health care has had a fluctuating history. Some healthcare professions, such as nursing, have historically put patients at the center of care. With the increasing concern about the quality of care and the work done by the National Academy of Sciences Health and Medicine Division (NAS/HMD), this focus has increased. Now, the term "patient-centered" care is commonly used, and when appropriate, this concept has been expanded to "family-centered" care.

As discussed in this text, this competency supports greater patient participation in CQI; for example, patients are encouraged to comment on care concerns (e.g., ask questions about their medications, note staff not washing their hands, and so on) and are asked to complete evaluation surveys. The focus of care is the patient, and this approach should improve care when nurses do the following:

- Recognize the importance of patient- and family-centered care and encourage them to actively participate in decisions.
- Understand the patient's and the family's journey—that is, their experiences with the healthcare system, both current and past.
- Incorporate elements of patient- and family-centered care in their daily work.
- Consider how they can improve the implementation of effective patient- and family-centered care.

Cosgrove (2012) explains the ideal approach to patient-centered care as follows:

> Patient-centered care requires shared decisions and open communication with patients. This type of decision-making requires listening to the patient and assists staff when they need to discuss benefits and risks with patients about their care so that the patient is prepared to participate actively in decision-making. The discussion should be based on evidence of best practice. (p. 18)

Healthy People 2020, as discussed in other chapters, is a national initiative to improve the health of U.S. citizens that also has an impact on quality of care. This initiative is also patient-centered, connecting it with the *Quality Chasm* recommendations. Its vision supports a society in which all people live long, healthy lives by focusing on four goals: healthcare quality, equity of health care, a healthy social and physical environment, and healthy development and behaviors across the life span (Healthy People, 2015). The patient is the center of each of the goals. Additional content about patient-centered care is found throughout this text.

Work on Interdisciplinary [Interprofessional] Teams: Application to Nursing and CQI

The core competency of interdisciplinary or interprofessional teams is described as "cooperate, collaborate, communicate, and integrate care in teams to ensure that care is continuous and reliable" (IOM, 2003a, p. 4). **Figure 3-4** highlights key elements of this competency.

Figure 3-4 Working Interprofessional Teams: Key Elements.

Teams are used in all HCOs, both teams composed of the same type of staff (intraprofessional), such as a nursing team, and teams that are interprofessional, representing multiple professions. All staff need to understand how teams are structured and function in order to participate effectively in the team environment. Organizations have their own cultures, and this culture impacts how the organization is structured and functions. The team approach to CQI is a key topic of this text.

Employ Evidence-Based Practice: Application to Nursing and CQI

The core competency of employ evidence-based practice (EBP) is described as "integrate best research with clinical expertise and patient values for optimum care, and participate in learning and research activities to the extent feasible" (IOM, 2003a, p. 4). **Figure 3-5** highlights key elements of this competency.

Evidence-Based Practice

What is **evidence-based practice (EBP)**? EBP is making clinical decisions using the best evidence possible. There are four types of evidence used in EBP (Melnyk & Fineout-Overholt, 2010): (1) evidence from research, (2) evidence from the patient's history and assessment, (3) clinical expertise, and (4) patient values and preferences. It is accepted that EBP has a positive impact on "constraining health costs, reducing geographic variation in the use of healthcare services, improving quality, supporting consumer-directed healthcare, and improving health coverage decisions" (IOM, 2008, p. 3).

Figure 3-5 Employ Evidence-Based Practice: Key Elements.

EBP is now an integral part of undergraduate and graduate nursing education. It took time for this to happen and pressure from HCOs, as they needed new graduates with at least baseline EBP knowledge. The process of recognizing and determining how to add this content so that this competency could be met varied. Some nursing programs dealt with this new need by eliminating research courses, adding EBP courses, combining research and EBP into one course, and/or adding EBP student projects. Most nursing education programs did not consider evidence-based management (EBM) content, but it too is important to include in leadership and management content, as well as CQI content (Kovner & Rundall, 2009). The IOM (2008) describes the need for continued efforts toward EBP as follows:

> The nation's capacity has fallen far short of its need for producing reliable and practical information about the care that works best. Medical-care decision-making is now strained, at both the level of the individual patient and the level of the population as a whole, by the growing number of diagnostic and therapeutic options for which there is insufficient evidence to make a clear choice. (p. 17)

Even though, EBP is now integrated in most HCOs, particularly hospitals, we still have much to do to ensure that best evidence is used, as articulated by the IOM (2011a):

> The demand for better evidence to guide healthcare decision-making is increasing rapidly for a variety of reasons, including the adverse consequences of care administered without adequate evidence, emerging insights into the proportion of healthcare interventions that are unnecessary, recognition of the frequency of medical errors, heightened public awareness and concern about the very high costs of medical care, the burden on employers and employees, and the growing proportion of health costs coming from out of pocket. (p. 1)

To support EBP improvement we need more nursing research to answer questions we have about best practice evidence, staff understanding of EBP, and effective methods to implement and maintain EBP.

Evidence-Based Management

Evidence should not be associated only with clinical care. It is very important to use evidence to support other decisions in health care, decisions typically made by managers. This is something that is usually not thought of in nursing curricula or by managers themselves. **Evidence-based management (EBM)** is the "systematic application of the best available evidence to the evaluation of managerial strategies for improving the performance of health services organizations" (Kovner & Rundall, 2009, p. 56). **Figure 3-6** provides an overview of the EBM steps.

```
┌─────────────────────────────────────┐
│      Formulating the Question        │
└─────────────────────────────────────┘
                  ↓
┌─────────────────────────────────────┐
│     Acquiring Research Evidence      │
└─────────────────────────────────────┘
                  ↓
┌─────────────────────────────────────┐
│    Assessing the Quality of Evidence │
└─────────────────────────────────────┘
                  ↓
┌─────────────────────────────────────┐
│       Presenting the Evidence        │
└─────────────────────────────────────┘
                  ↓
┌─────────────────────────────────────┐
│   Applying the Evidence to the Decision │
└─────────────────────────────────────┘
```

Figure 3-6 The Evidence-Based Management Process. Data from Kovner, A., Fine, D., & D'Aquila, R. (2009). *Evidence-based management in healthcare.* Chicago, IL: Health Administration Press.

HCO managers and leaders must be concerned with two aspects of the organization: Its functioning and its services (products). They are interconnected, although the latter focuses more on clinical care and EBP. EBM is concerned with management issues. How does the use of best evidence relate to management? For example, managers consider the effect of staffing levels on patient outcomes or evaluate a change in services that would impact CQI. An EBM approach provides evidence for making management decisions about these issues or problems, which in turn impact EBP. Decision-making is complex and requires a thoughtful process supported by best evidence, as described by the IOM (2008):

> The era of physician as sole healthcare decision maker is long past. In today's world, multiple people make healthcare decisions, individually or in collaboration, in multiple contexts for multiple purposes. The decision maker is likely to be the consumer choosing among health plans, patients or patients' caregivers making treatment choices, payers or employers making health coverage and reimbursement decisions, professional medical societies developing practice guidelines or clinical recommendations, regulatory agencies assessing new drugs or devices, or public programs developing population-based health interventions. Every decision maker needs credible, unbiased, and understandable evidence on the effectiveness of health interventions and services. (pp. 2–3)

Is manager and team leader decision-making the same as decision-making for clinicians (VA, 2015)? There are differences from a variety of perspectives. Clinicians may make more decisions than managers, but the decisions that managers make often involve and impact more people and costs and may require major changes in a unit, department, or HCO. Management decision-making often takes more time; for example, it can take weeks, months, or years to develop a plan and make long-range decisions, implement them, drive outcomes, and complete evaluation of outcomes. While clinical decisions tend to be more focused or specialized, management decisions are more heterogeneous.

There is great variety in management problems and approaches. Intuition is frequently used, with managers saying they had a gut feeling that some type of decision should be made. This approach is not EBM, although experience does help in making decisions and sometimes gut feelings are based on past experiences. Management decisions should involve multiple levels of staff, even though the manager may make the final decision. Reality has to be considered, such as the organizational hierarchy and its impact on decisions, but the manager should role model the importance of EBM and share information about factors that may impact decisions so that staff better understand the process and final decisions. Factors might be budget, changes in services or community health needs, staffing, staff and management changes, systemwide issues, policies and procedures, accreditation and government requirements, standards, and so on (VA, 2015). EBM may be used to get needed support for changes from higher levels of management and provider information for greater staff understanding—supporting decisions with objective evidence.

While clinical decision-making has been influenced more and more by EBP and staff are more prepared today to use EBP, managers still tend to follow trends or fads in management or use consultants to help them make decisions. According to the U.S. Department of Veterans Affairs (VA) (2009), "The leaders and managers of HCOs, while often strongly encouraging clinicians to adopt evidence-based practices, have been slow to apply the ideas to their own management." There needs to be more integration of EBM in healthcare decision-making about subjects such as planning, staffing, teams, budget, collaboration, coordination, communication, organization structure and function, and CQI.

Despite the common decision-making practices of managers, effective decisions should be based on solid evidence. HCOs are complex and demand clear decision-making. Patient care is the focus, and this makes use of careful decision-making even more important. As Walshe and Rundall (2001, p. 431) explain,

> Research evidence is more likely to be used in organizations that have a culture that values and encourages innovation, experimentation, data collection and analysis and the development of critical appraisal skills among managers. Organizations must cultivate what has been called a culture of learning through research.

The evidence that does exist is often not shared even within the same system. It must be noted that there is minimum evidence available related to best management practices, making it difficult for most managers to actively use EBM. However, this should not be viewed as a barrier to trying to use EBM. There are also potential barriers that make it difficult to effectively implement EBM, and understanding them helps managers as they make decisions and involve staff. Examples of the barriers such as workload and deadlines. The VA (2009) describes this problem as follows:

> Without a system in place to cope with heavy workloads, the pressure to meet deadlines restricts the time managers have to consider their decision-making process or to examine research. Attitudes that focus on making speedy decisions can interfere with managers' acceptance of research. In addition, a belief system reinforced by years of experience that management is an intuitive process will restrict support for management research.

EBM is fairly new from a perspective of a structured approach to decision-making to ensure use of evidence. It would be incorrect to say that management decisions have not been based on evidence, as many decisions are. The difference in using EBM is it is a specific process that consciously recognizes the importance of research evidence as well as other forms of evidence for best management practice. Managers may know what would be the best approach to take, but there are factors within the organization that make it difficult to make the decisions and implement them (Pearlman, 2006). More needs to be done to limit this problem and use EBM in as many management decisions as possible, particularly CQI decisions. Examples of strategies to improve use of EBM include the following (Rundall, Martelli, McCurdy, Graetz, & Arrayo, 2009, p. 15):

- Ask what is the evidence when decisions are made.
- Brief managers routinely on recent management research related to the organization's operational and strategic concerns.
- Incorporate research assessments into due diligence reports.
- Train management team members in the steps of evidence-based decision-making—about the process and its application.
- Establish ties with academic institutions and research centers.

It is also important that staff be informed about EBM in the same manner that they are informed about EBP. Information is key when making any decision, and HCOs need to make sure information is available when needed, which typically today includes use of electronic communication methods. Effective HCOs recognize the need to develop a questioning culture, one that encourages and supports staff to ask questions and seek answers. The following are strategies that an organization might use to develop this type of culture (Kovner & Rundall, 2009, p. 69):

- Organize research rounds (e.g., presentations by experts, updates on research, management research journal clubs, and research seminars).
- Analyze the results of past operational and strategic decisions, including comparing the system's performance with findings from research about other organizations.

- Conduct staff development programs to enhance managers' abilities to find, assess, and apply research findings.
- Link compensation to metrics related to obtaining and using relevant evidence in decision-making and sharing evidence with key stakeholders.
- Develop guidelines for decision-making that require an assessment of research evidence.

Learning Health System

Other reports, such as *Learning What Works: Infrastructure Required for Effectiveness Research: Workshop Summary* (IOM, 2011a), provide further examination of EBP and application to the EBP competency for all healthcare professions. The goal is develop a **learning health system**. This is a system that applies evidence to the care process. Along with the use of EBP and EBM, there is need for greater **comparative effectiveness research** to provide healthcare providers with state-of-the-science information to make the best quality and cost decisions for patients. Comparing evidence should be an active part of this process. The federal government provides resources for this through various agency websites, such as the Agency for Healthcare Research and Quality (AHRQ) and the Centers for Medicare and Medicaid Services (CMS). Another report, *Finding What Works in Health Care: Standards for Systematic Reviews* (IOM, 2011b), adds to this expanding examination of what is needed to apply EBP and, in doing so, relates to the EBP competency. A **systematic review** is a summary of evidence focused on a specific clinical question and provides critical appraisal of the evidence to determine if bias exists. Experts who understand the systematic review appraisal process should be the source of these reviews. Ideally, when EBP decisions are made in practice, they are based on these reviews, although in nursing we have not reached the point of sufficient reviews, mostly due to the need for more research to use as evidence. Research is the highest level of evidence; however, other types of evidence are also important. *Finding What Works* focuses on setting standards for the expanding development of systematic reviews to better ensure that these reviews provide effective information for clinical application.

Accelerating Change and Transformation in Organizations and Networks (ACTION) is an initiative led by the AHRQ (HHS, AHRQ, 2015). This initiative supports delivery system research in clinical sites by partnering with the clinical sites and supporting their efforts to test interventions to improve care. The focus is on real-world concerns in healthcare delivery. ACTION is associated with the mission of AHRQ, which is "to *produce evidence* to make health care safer, higher quality, more accessible, equitable, and affordable, and to work with HHS and other partners *to make sure that the evidence is understood and used*" (HHS, AHRQ, 2015). Accelerating means pushing forward, and this effort is needed in all aspects of healthcare delivery and CQI. Effective change requires evidence.

Apply Quality Improvement: Application to Nursing and CQI

The core competency of apply quality improvement is described (IOM, 2003a) as follows:

> Identify errors and hazards in care; understand and implement basic safety design principles, such as standardization and simplification; continually understand and measure quality of care in terms of structure, process, and outcomes in relation to patient and community needs; and design and test interventions to change processes and systems of care, with objective of improving care. (p. 4)

Figure 3-7 highlights the key elements.

Performance accountability is a critical factor in health care today. As more has been learned about the quality of U.S. health care, there has been greater need to evaluate performance: individual provider performance, team performance, and HCO performance. This need is tied into CQI and the greater need to aggregate state and national performance. Many external organizations make demands on HCOs for performance data. Some of the organizations are The Joint Commission, which accredits most of the HCOs in the United States; the CMS, the federal agency that administers both Medicare and Medicaid and funds these services (although Medicaid is jointly funded by the states and the federal government); and other organizations and government agencies.

Nursing practice has long been involved in CQI; however, as noted in many sources, including *Keeping Patients Safe: Transforming the Work Environment for Nurses* (IOM, 2003b) and *The Future of Nursing: Leading Change, Advancing Health* (IOM, 2010), nursing is a critical component of health care, with nurses providing care that is integral to patient outcomes. Both reports, however, comment on the need for greater nursing leadership in CQI. To accomplish this goal, nurses must know

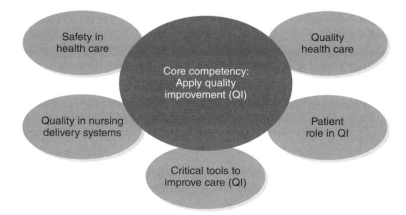

Figure 3-7 Apply Quality Improvement: Key Elements.

more about CQI and then apply this information. This text provides information to help nurses as they practice and improve care and meet this core competency.

Utilize Informatics: Application to Nursing and CQI

The core competency of utilize informatics is described as "communicate, manage knowledge, mitigate error, and support decision making using information technology" (IOM, 2003a, p. 4). **Figure 3-8** highlights key elements of this competency.

Since the publication of *Health Professions Education* (IOM, 2003a), there has been much more done to expand heath informatics technology (HIT) and develop resources for healthcare professions and HCOs, along with expanding medical technology used in care delivery. In a report on HIT, the issue of preparing staff to better utilize informatics is addressed. Staff who are not knowledgeable about HIT and do not apply their knowledge will not effectively use HIT and meet this core competency (IOM, 2012). It is a complex task to engage nursing staff in CQI, and to make this task easier, nurse managers need to depend on hiring new graduates who have a basic understanding of the CQI process and use of HIT in the process (Odell, 2011). HIT is discussed in more detail in other chapters in this text, notably its relationship to measurement and solutions to resolve problems and improve care.

Stop and Consider #1

The Institute of Medicine decided it is important for all healthcare professions to meet five core competencies.

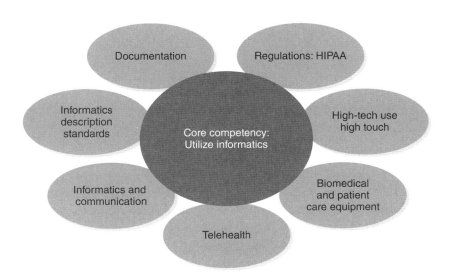

Figure 3-8 Utilize Informatics: Key Elements.

Quality and Safety Education for Nurses

The Quality and Safety Education for Nurses (QSEN) Institute provides a variety of competency-based resources to nurse educators (QSEN, 2014a). This initiative began in 2005 with a national study funded by the Robert Wood Johnson Foundation, focused on examining education on quality and safety for nursing students. The funding was initially provided to researchers at the University of North Carolina. The QSEN is now situated at the Frances Payne Bolton School of Nursing–Case Western Reserve University. The QSEN (2014b) seeks "to prepare nurses with the knowledge, skills, and attitudes necessary to continuously improve the quality and safety of the healthcare systems within which they work, based on the six quality and safety competencies" (QSEN, 2014b).

The multiphase project identified core knowledge, skills, and attitudes for pre-licensure students and then examined key content areas. In 2007, Phase II turned the focus to graduate education and also initiated pilots in 15 schools of nursing (QSEN, 2014c). In the first two phases of the project, QSEN faculty, experts from institutions across the nation, focused on defining the comprehensive set of quality and safety competencies for nursing and needed training (QSEN, 2014d). In Phase III, which began in 2009, the project joined with the American Association of Colleges of Nursing to increase faculty expertise and apply the QSEN competencies. Phase IV coincided with the publication of *The Future of Nursing* (IOM, 2010). The project continued with its work to prepare nurses to ensure high-quality, patient-centered care, supporting the recommendations found in *The Future of Nursing* report (QSEN, 2014e).

The QSEN competencies are focused on knowledge, skills, and attitudes (KSAs). *Knowledge* is the understanding of content required to meet the competencies—facts, concepts, and information and their relationships. *Skills* focus on psychomotor requirements or how something should be done to meet the competencies. *Attitudes* concern the affective, or emotions, responses, motivation, and perceptions. The QSEN competencies are based on the five healthcare professions core competencies, but they were adapted for this nursing initiative (IOM, 2003a). The QSEN competencies are the same for pre-licensure and graduate levels, but KSAs vary per competency.

In regard to integration of the QSEN into systemwide nursing education, Dolansky and Moore (2013) note the following:

> Many nurse educators report that the QSEN competencies are already integrated into their curriculum, but in our practice, we have noted that often this integration is at the individual level of care, rather than at the level of the system of care. The full effect of the QSEN competencies to improve the quality and safety of care can only be realized when nurses apply them at both the individual and system levels of care.

The following list provides a description of the QSEN competencies (QSEN, 2014f):

- *Patient-centered care KSAs.* Recognize the patient or designee as the source of control and full partner in providing compassionate and coordinated care based on respect for the patient's preferences, values, and needs.
- *Teamwork and collaboration KSAs.* Function effectively within nursing and interprofessional teams, fostering open communication, mutual respect, and shared decision-making to achieve quality patient care.
- *Evidence-based practice KSAs.* Integrate best current evidence with clinical expertise and patient/family preferences and values for delivery of optimal health care.
- *Quality improvement KSAs.* Use data to monitor the outcomes of care processes and use improvement methods to design and test changes to continuously improve quality and safety of healthcare systems.
- *Safety KSAs.* Minimize risk of harm to patients and providers through both system effectiveness and individual performance.
- *Informatics KSAs.* Use information and technology to communicate, manage information, mitigate error, and support decision-making.

The core KSAs for the competencies are found on the QSEN website; the Connect to Current Information section at the end of the chapter provides a link to this site. **Table 3-1** provides a brief comparison of the five interprofessional core healthcare professions competencies and the QSEN competencies for nurses.

TABLE 3–1 Comparing the Five Healthcare Professions Core Competencies and the QSEN Competencies for Nurses	
Healthcare Professions Core Competencies*	**QSEN Competencies for Nurses****
Provide patient-centered care.	Patient-centered care knowledge, skills, attitudes (KSAs)
Work on interdisciplinary [interprofessional] teams.	Teamwork and collaboration KSAs
Employ evidence-based practice.	Evidence-based practice KSAs
Apply quality improvement.	Quality improvement KSAs
—	Safety KSAs
Utilize informatics.	Informatics KSAs

Data from *Institute of Medicine (IOM). (2003). *Health professions education: A bridge to quality.* Washington, DC: The National Academies Press; **QSEN Institute. (2015). Definitions and pre-licensure KSAs. Retrieved from http://qsen.org /competencies/pre-licensure-ksas/; QSEN Institute. (2015). Definitions and graduate KSAs. Retrieved from http://qsen.org /competencies/graduate-ksas/

Stop and Consider #2

The accepted national five core healthcare professions core competencies are not identical to the QSEN core competencies.

Education to Improve Quality of Care

The *Health Professions* report (IOM, 2003a) concludes that competent healthcare staff are critical to healthcare improvement, but this requires healthcare profession education that supports inclusion of CQI in the curriculum and outcome-based education. There has been movement to increase content and learning experiences focused on CQI, although much more is needed (Finkelman & Kenner, 2012). The American Nurses Association (ANA) practice and professional standards and the *Nursing Professional Development: Scope and Standards of Practice* also support the need for staff education to improve care (ANA, NNSDO, 2010). In addition to the traditional teaching practices such as lectures, exams, and written assignments, other teaching–learning practices should be used—for example, grand rounds, root cause analysis assignments, use of structured communication methods in simulation and clinical settings, greater use of simulation that integrates CQI, interprofessional workshops on CQI, cases, web-based activities such as discussion, and team projects. Multiple methods should be used in academic nursing programs and in staff education.

Critical Nursing Documents and Initiatives Emphasizing CQI Through Education

Nursing professional organizations have long developed and published information about nursing practice and the healthcare delivery system. It is important to consider examples of some of these publications and initiatives that impact nursing practice and nursing education and their relationship to the five healthcare professions core competencies to improve practice.

The American Association of Colleges of Nursing and the National League for Nursing: Nursing Education Standards

The American Association of Colleges of Nursing (AACN) nursing education standard publications are *The Essentials of Baccalaureate Education for Professional Nursing Practice* (2008), *The Essentials of Master's Education in Nursing* (2011), and *The Essentials of Doctoral Education for Advanced Nursing Practice* (2006). All three of these documents comment on and/or integrate the healthcare professions core competencies. Nursing programs that follow AACN standards apply the relevant *Essentials* to their programs and are accredited by the AACN accrediting body, which impacts an education program's curriculum and expected competencies of graduates. The baccalaureate *Essentials* document specifically mentions many of the core competency concerns such as patient-centered care and quality care. One of the major goals for master's education is to lead change to improve quality outcomes, and the doctor of nursing practice (DNP) *Essentials* emphasize leadership, change, and quality.

One of the National League for Nursing (NLN) objectives is "to promote the preparation of a nursing workforce that contributes to healthcare quality and safety" (NLN, 2015). The NLN supports nursing education and improvement in nursing education to ensure graduates can provide care that meets the healthcare professions core competencies and support the NLN's core values of caring, diversity, integrity, and excellence by providing educator resources and training and nursing education accreditation standards.

Educating Nurses: A Call for Radical Transformation

Educating Nurses is a landmark report of a study that examined the status of nursing education (Benner, Sutphen, Leonard, & Day, 2010). The sample for this qualitative study includes several nursing programs and provides extensive data and analysis with recommendations for nursing education. The results call for change and improvement in nursing education in order to ensure that education is in sync with practice needs and healthcare delivery. As Benner and colleagues (2010) state, "New nurses need to be prepared to practice safely, accurately, and compassionately, in varied settings, where knowledge and innovation increase at an astonishing rate. They must enter practice ready to continue learning" (p. 1). The researchers note that nurses practice in a *dysfunctional* environment (a descriptor also used in the *Quality Chasm* reports). This nursing education report supports the common messages from the *Quality Chasm* reports emphasizing the need for healthcare quality, but to accomplish this we need competent healthcare providers, nurses, and others. To meet this demand means nursing education must also change and improve.

The Future of Nursing: Leading Change, Advancing Health

This report has had a significant impact on the nursing profession and consequently healthcare delivery (IOM, 2010). Its content was influenced by the previous *Quality Chasm* reports on quality care, emphasizing that to maintain safe, patient-centered care across settings, nursing education also needs to improve. Along with the need for improvement in education, nurses need to be full partners in the healthcare delivery system and in CQI—assuming responsibility for identifying problems, participating in measurement and analysis of care problems, and developing interventions/strategies to prevent errors and care quality problems or to resolve them. The competencies discussed in *The Future of Nursing* report relate to the healthcare professions core competencies. Additional discussion of this report is found in several chapters in this text.

American Nurses Association Practice Standards

The ANA includes standards of practice for generalist and advanced practice nurses and also for a number of specialties. Some nursing specialty organizations offer standards that pertain to their specialty focus. All of these standards emphasize the need for CQI and the role and responsibilities of nurses to practice in a manner to ensure quality care, supporting the healthcare professions core competencies. These standards are reviewed and revised as needed. Nurses need to be aware of the standards that pertain to them and apply them in their practice. HCOs need to ensure that their staff follow them. Standards are discussed in more detail in other sections of this text; however, in this chapter it is important to note that standards relate not only to practice but also to education.

National Council of State Boards of Nursing Simulation Study

In 2009, the National Council of State Boards of Nursing (NCSBN) began a national, multisite, longitudinal study to better understand simulation outcomes in pre-licensure nursing programs (NCSBN, 2015). Use of simulation had been increasing and continues to do so today, but we needed to know more about it. In addition, this study began after the publication of significant reports about healthcare professions education and the need for quality improvement.

This study was conducted in three phases. Phase I focused on a survey of pre-licensure programs to provide more information on the use of simulation. Phase II was a randomized controlled trial examining the outcomes of using different levels and amounts of simulation in place of clinical site competencies. Data from 10 schools of nursing (5 associate degree and 5 baccalaureate programs) included student perceptions of meeting their learning needs in clinical and in simulation experiences and compared their licensure (NCLEX) pass rates. This study collected and analyzed data from assessment of nursing knowledge and clinical experience. Phase III followed new graduates through the first 6 months of their first clinical positions as registered nurses, focusing on their competency in practice (clinical competency, critical thinking, readiness for practice). This part of the study included data from the new graduates' nurse managers, adding an important factor, the healthcare delivery perspective of management. Data collection for Phase III concluded in June 2014.

The results provide strong evidence that when up to 50% of traditional clinical experiences in pre-licensure programs were replaced by simulation, there was no significant difference in educational outcomes (Hayden, Smiley, Alexander, Kardong-Edgren, & Jeffries, 2014). The researchers note that best practices for high-quality simulation should be incorporated by nursing programs, including use of consistent terminology; clear participant objectives; inclusion of professional integrity applied to participants/students; and use of active facilitation with a facilitator, debriefing process, and participant assessment and facilitator evaluation

(IACSL, 2013). When changes are made in nursing education, it is important to support the changes with evidence to ensure that students will get the learning experiences they need.

The AHRQ also supports the use of simulation and provides resources about simulation, noting the following:

> When applied properly, simulation-based training allows the opportunity to learn new skills, engage in deliberate practice, and receive focused and real-time feedback. The goal of simulation-based training is to enable the accelerated development of expertise, both in individual and team skills, by bridging the gap between classroom training and real-world clinical experiences in a relatively risk-free environment. (HHS, AHRQ, PSNET, 2015)

Simulation was first used in education programs for healthcare professions students, but now it is also found to be useful in developing teamwork, particularly for interprofessional teams; applying human factors engineering to patient safety in simulated experiences; and testing new equipment and technology in real-world situations. Systematic reviews of simulation provide evidence that it is an effective educational method (HHS, AHRQ, PSNET, 2015). Simulation is also used in part of the medical licensure exams and for specialty anesthesiology exams. At this time, it is not yet used for registered nurse licensure exams.

National League for Nursing Simulation Innovation Resource Center

The NLN's Simulation Innovation Resource Center (SIRC) provides resources for nurse educators (SIRC, 2015). It is described as an interactive global simulation community, launched in 2008. SIRC is also involved in offering courses and conferences and supporting simulation-focused research. Both this initiative and the extensive study done by NCSBN indicate the importance of simulation to nursing education, and it is also expanding for other healthcare professions. Simulation is an education experience that can effectively integrate CQI and also teamwork—both included in the healthcare professions core competencies. To accomplish this goal, schools of nursing need to plan and implement initiatives to actively increase content and simulation experiences related to CQI and teamwork.

American Organization of Nurse Executives Competencies and Guiding Principles

The American Organization of Nurse Executives (AONE) is the major organization for nurse leaders and managers in HCOs. It strongly supports active nursing involvement in CQI and the need to develop nursing competencies that are discussed in this chapter. The AONE identifies the need for nursing leadership, teamwork, improved care, effective use of informatics, and patient-centered care. The organization provides standards and a framework for nursing leadership that focus on effective leadership and management, improving practice and care, resources, training opportunities, and conferences. Additional content about the AONE, CQI, and leadership content can be found in other chapters in this text.

Nursing Education and CQI

As discussed previously, nursing education standards include the need for students to gain competency in CQI. However, more needs to be done to integrate effective learning experiences throughout pre-licensure education and also within graduate programs. CQI is not a topic reserved for one level of nursing education. This text provides information to move toward CQI competency. As nurses practice, they then build on this knowledge and competency to practice with an emphasis on CQI. As noted in this chapter, there have been a number of initiatives to improve nursing education; however, this must be a continuous process as we adjust to a rapidly changing healthcare environment and expansion of knowledge.

Staff Education and CQI

The ANA standards *Nursing Professional Development: Scope and Standards of Practice* (ANA, NNSDO, 2010) are important standards that are used to guide nursing staff education in HCOs. The goal is to orient staff and support ongoing learning so that staff are competent to provide quality care. As is true for all of the ANA standards, the central point of the standards is the protection of the public and provision of quality care. HCOs invest a lot of their budget in staff orientation and education. Some HCOs also include support for staff to attend conferences and in some cases continue academic education, such as to obtain a baccalaureate or a graduate degree, thus supporting the recommendations found in *The Future of Nursing* report (IOM, 2010).

Along with education provided by HCOs for their staff, there is also need for a more effective model of continuing education (CE) for nurses and other healthcare professions. *Redesigning Continuing Education in the Health Professions* (IOM, 2009) is a report that examines CE from an interprofessional perspective. Currently, typical methods used for CE include attending a conference or presentation, completing an evaluation form, and then getting the CE credit. In some states academic credits may also be used for nursing CE credit. A third method is to complete an online course, which is often short and may require completion of a brief quiz and often can be repeated. A question that is often asked is how do we know that the healthcare professional applies what is learned and the impact of the learning experience on care outcomes? The report states the following:

> [CE] is the process by which health professionals keep up to date with the latest knowledge and advances in health care. However, the CE "system" . . . is so deeply flawed that it cannot properly support the development of health professionals. CE has become structured around health professional participation instead of performance improvement. This has left health professionals unprepared to perform at the highest levels consistently, putting into question

whether the public is receiving care of the highest possible quality and safety. (IOM, 2009, p. ix)

Following this 2009 report, the AACN and the American Association of Colleges of Medicine (AACM) held a conference on lifelong learning for medicine and nursing. The vision statement from the two organizations noted the following:

> We envision a continuum of health professional education from admission into a health professional program to retirement that values, exemplifies, and assesses lifelong learning skills; emphasizes interprofessional and team-based education and practice; employs tested, outcomes-based continuing education methods; and links health professional education and delivery of care within the workplace. (AAMC & AACN, 2010, p. 3)

This all sounds familiar, as it is another example of support for the healthcare professions core competencies; however, in this case, the vision statement emphasizes the competencies not only in academic programs but also in lifelong learning for the healthcare professions. This report describes the problems and issues but does not recommend specific strategies to improve lifelong learning. More work is needed to address regulation, accreditation, education, and certification for all healthcare professions and to develop and improve strategies. The content of this report focuses on the following (AAMC & AACN, 2010, pp. 6, 7, 19, 20, 22, 27):

- **Lifelong learning** is voluntary and self-motivated pursuit of knowledge for either personal or professional reasons. The report notes the need to meet the following key competencies: an understanding of evidence-based health care and critical appraisal, familiarity with informatics and literature search and retrieval strategies, practice-based learning and improvement methods, self-reflection and assessment, and other skill sets related to knowledge management,
- **Continuing education** has long acted as a major support to lifelong learning through CE offerings. CE is formal transmission of a predetermined body of knowledge. These activities are frequently provided with designated accreditation and generate "credits" for practitioners, necessary for most state licensure and other credentialing processes.
- **Interprofessional education** is education for individuals from different professions offered together during all or part of the professional training and in practice—in order to promote collaborative teamwork in their professional practice.
- **Workplace learning** is a way in which individuals or groups acquire, interpret, reorganize, change, or assimilate a related cluster of information, skills, and feelings, and a means by which individuals construct meaning in their personal and shared organizational lives. The report notes that workplace learning has an impact on prevention of errors, staff

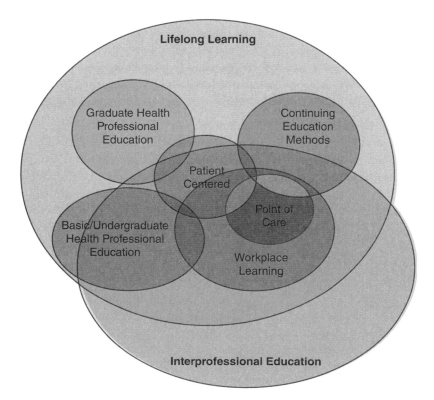

Figure 3-9 Finalized
Key Constructs for
Lifelong Learning.
Reproduced from American
Association of Colleges of Nursing
and Association of American
Medical Colleges. (2010). *Lifelong
learning in medicine and nursing:
Final conference report.* Retrieved
from http://www.aacn.nche
.edu/education-resources
/MacyReport.pdf

self-reflection on performance, and improvement of individual and
organization performance outcomes.

- **Point-of-care learning** is a subset of workplace learning that occurs at the
time and place (whether virtual such as simulation or actual) of a health
professional–patient encounter.

The report ties together the various types of education for healthcare professions
and illustrates the incorporation of patient-centered care, as described in **Figure 3-9**.

Interprofessional Education and CQI

Several years after the *Health Education Professions* report was published, there was
more examination of interprofessional education (IPE). This work flowed from the
identification of healthcare professions core competencies (IOM, 2003a). In 2011, a
report was published about IPE that was developed by a collaborative of healthcare
professions organizations: American Association of Colleges of Nursing, American
Association of Colleges of Osteopathic Medicine, American Association of Colleges
of Pharmacy, American Dental Education, Association of American Medical
Colleges, and Association of Schools and Programs of Public Health (IPECEP, 2011).

This collaboration of many different healthcare professions indicates the importance of this topic to health care and the preparation of different healthcare professions. The report identifies four competency domains (IPECEP, 2011, p. 16):

1. Values/ethics for interprofessional practice (patient-centered, community/ population orientation; shared purpose and commitment)
2. Roles/responsibilities (understanding of different roles and responsibilities and how they complement each other)
3. Interprofessional communication (support collaborative practice and teams)
4. Teams and teamwork (team player, cooperation, coordination, shared decision-making)

We have basic competencies for all, but we also now need to determine how to apply more IPE to develop and improve interprofessional competencies and teamwork within healthcare professions education and staff education. It is easy to view IPE as a course in which different healthcare professions students are enrolled, and they sit next to each other in the classroom. This is not IPE. Students need to engage in the learning process together, participating in learning activities that require them to interact and work together. The World Health Organization has published a number of reports on the need for IPE that describe IPE in the following manner: "[IPE] occurs when two or more professionals learn about, from, and with each other to enable effective collaboration and improve health outcomes" (WHO, 2010, p. 13). This collaborative approach is not simple to accomplish. Schools of nursing that are not near other healthcare professions programs have major problems providing IPE. Simulation is also effective in bringing together different students for teamwork and can also be used in interprofessional staff education. Understanding of roles and responsibilities—differences and similarities—is a critical part of IPE. It is best achieved when students or staff interact with one another and collaborate on their learning. The core competency of working in interprofessional teams is difficult to accomplish if students cannot experience interprofessional interactions before they enter practice.

The report notes that there needs to be greater connection between changes in the redesign of practice and healthcare professions education. A change in one impacts the other. There is also greater need for widespread adoption of IPE. There is need for a framework to measure IPE interventions and their outcomes; collaborative behavior is critical (IOM, 2015, pp. 26, 29). The components of healthcare professions education (pre-licensure and graduate), workplace education, and continuing education need to be linked and improved to include IPE. **Figure 3-10** provides a model for the interprofessional-learning continuum. These components should be directed at learning outcomes that address reaction, attitudes/perceptions, knowledge/skills, collaborative behavior, and performance in practice. The learning outcomes are influenced by and also influence health and system outcomes associated with individual health, population/public health, organizational change, system efficiencies, and cost effectiveness. Enabling or interfering factors that impact the

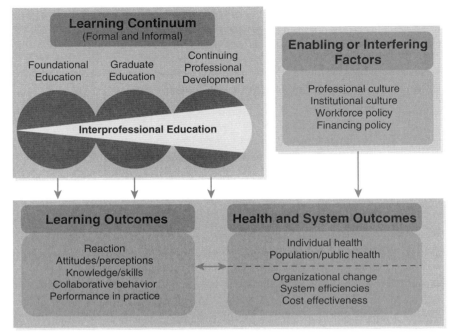

Figure 3-10 The Interprofessional Learning Continuum (IPLC) Model.

Reproduced with permission from Institute of Medicine and Committee on Patient Safety and Health Information Technology Board on Health Care Services. (2012). *Health IT and patient safety: Building safer systems for better care.* Washington, DC: National Academies Press. Courtesy of the National Academies Press, Washington, DC.

health and system outcomes are professional culture, institutional (organizational) culture, workforce policy, and financing policy.

Stop and Consider #3

Interprofessional education is needed, but it is difficult to accomplish.

Conclusions

Since the publication of the *Quality Chasm* landmark report on health professions education recognizing that to reach the goal of improving care we must consider the competency of the staff providing care, there has been more concern about healthcare professions education and staff competency. As discussed in this chapter, the five core competencies have been adapted by nursing in the QSEN initiative (Cronenwett et al., 2007; 2009); however, this does not negate the need to follow the recommended core competencies that focus on interprofessional needs. In meeting the five core competencies, healthcare professionals practice from the same core base of competencies, even though there are differences in practice per profession. With the growing need to improve care and practice, healthcare professions education and continuing education have also been examined and require improvement. This text is about quality improvement, and education is a critical strategy for improving care.

Apply CQI

Chapter Highlights

- The NAS/HMD has been very active in the CQI movement by examining problems and providing recommendations. One of its major recommendations is the need for a consistent base of core competencies for all healthcare professions. In this approach, competencies are not identified for a specific profession; rather they apply to all healthcare professions.
- The Quality and Safety Education for Nurses (QSEN), a nursing initiative, focuses on improvement. It adapted the NAS/HMD core competencies to nursing, emphasizing knowledge, skills, and attitudes (KSAs).
- QSEN provides resources, training, and research for nursing education.
- Nursing education programs must integrate the competencies, CQI content, and new approaches to learning, such as simulation.
- Professional continuing education (CE) is also more important today than ever before. Evaluation of outcomes indicates that CE needs to be improved, although accomplishing this is not easy. Attendance is the major evaluation criterion and in some cases a brief quiz. In addition, more CE should be interprofessional to support effective use of interprofessional teams.
- There is greater emphasis today on interprofessional education within healthcare profession degree programs, although it is a challenge to accomplish.

Critical Thinking and Clinical Reasoning and Judgment: Discussion Questions and Learning Activities

1. What impact do you think having core competencies may have on healthcare delivery?
2. Compare and contrast the five NAS/HMD core healthcare competencies with the QSEN competencies. Provide examples for each competency and how it relates to your practice.
3. Attend a continuing education offering. Critique the experience and what you observe. If the offering was interprofessional, what impact might this approach have had on the content and attendees? If it was not interprofessional, how could it have been changed to an interprofessional focus? Identify how greater emphasis on IPE might impact practice. Review *Core Competencies for Interprofessional Collaborative Practice* (2011) and relate this content to your experience.
4. Access *The Future of Nursing* report and review the sections on education and competence. Summarize the key points in a list of items you want to remember. Identify why the items are important.

Connect to Current Information

- American Association of Colleges of Nursing (AACN)
  http://www.aacn.nche.edu
- National League for Nursing (NLN)
  http://www.nln.org
- Quality and Safety Education for Nurses (QSEN)
  http://qsen.org/
- American Organization of Nurse Executives (AONE)
  http://www.aone.org/
- *Core Competencies for Interprofessional Collaborative Practice* (2011)
  http://www.aacn.nche.edu/education-resources/IPECReport.pdf
- *Redesigning Continuing Education in the Health Professions* (2009)
  http://www.nap.edu/catalog/12704/redesigning-continuing-education-in-the-health-professions
- Accelerating Change and Transformation in Organizations and Networks (ACTION) (2015)
  http://www.ahrq.gov/research/findings/factsheets/translating/action/index.html

EBP, EBM, and Quality Improvement: Exemplar

Hayden, J., Smiley, R., Alexander, M., Kardong-Edgren, S., & Jeffries, P. (2014). The NCSBN national simulation study: A longitudinal, randomized, controlled study replacing clinical hours with simulation in pre-licensure nursing education. *Journal of Nursing Regulation, 5*(2), Supplement. Retrieved from https://www.ncsbn.org/JNR_Simulation_Supplement.pdf

This extensive study focuses on the critical issue of the value of simulation and clinical learning experiences.

Questions to Consider

1. What is the design used for this study, including research question(s), sample, interventions, data collection, and analysis?
2. What are the results of the study?
3. How might these results be applied to nursing education in academic programs and staff education?

Evolving Case Study

You are one of the staff education instructors in a 500-bed acute care hospital. The department staff includes the director and four instructors. Each clinical unit has a designated staff member who assists with staff education and collaborates with the staff education department. With the increased concern about quality of care in the hospital and an error rate that does not meet the desired standard, it has been a stressful time. Sometimes you feel like "the dump department"; if there is a problem, staff education will fix it. However, not all problems can be fixed with education alone, and for some problems this is not even a realistic strategy. During your weekly meeting with the director and other instructors, you are all having a difficult discussion as again the department is asked to fix it.

Case Questions A

The following questions relate to the staff meeting.

1. One of the instructors says, "I don't understand why they think we are the ones to fix the error rate." Why do you think this might be a common response from the hospital administration?
2. How might you engage the staff on the units who offer unit education in this discussion?
3. How does the core competency focused on quality improvement relate to your conversation and interprofessional teams and education?

Case Questions B

You have moved past the venting, and you are trying to understand the problem so that you can move to action.

1. The department decides to prepare a brief summary of issues that the hospital should consider related to staff education and CQI. How would you design this document, and what content would you include?
2. Describe specific strategies the department will use to ensure that CQI is integrated in staff education.
3. Describe how the department will assess outcomes. What measures will it use?
4. When issues and problems are outside its domain, how will the department communicate this to administration?

References

American Association of Colleges of Nursing (AACN). (2006). *The essentials of doctoral education for advanced nursing practice.* Washington, DC: Author.

American Association of Colleges of Nursing (AACN). (2008). *The essentials of baccalaureate education for professional nursing practice.* Washington, DC: Author.

American Association of Colleges of Nursing (AACN). (2011). *The essentials of master's education in nursing.* Washington, DC: Author.

American Nurses Association (ANA). (2015). *Nursing: Scope and standards of practice* (3rd ed.). Silver Spring, MD: Author.

American Nurses Association (ANA) & National Nursing Staff Development Organization (NNSDO). (2010). *Nursing professional development: Scope and standards of practice.* Silver Spring, MD: Author.

Association of American Medical Colleges (AAMC) & American Association of Colleges of Nursing (AACN). (2010). *Lifelong learning in medicine and nursing: Final conference report*. Retrieved from http://www.aacn.nche.edu/education-resources/MacyReport.pdf

Benner, P., Sutphen, M., Leonard, V., & Day, L. (2010). *Educating nurses: A call for radical transformation*. San Francisco, CA: Jossey-Bass.

Cosgrove, D. (2012). A CEO checklist for high-value health care. Washington, DC: The Institute of Medicine. Retrieved from http://www.ncbi.nlm.nih.gov/books/NBK207215/

Cronenwett, L., Sherwood, G., Barnsteiner, J., Disch, J., Johnson, J., Mitchell, P., . . . Warren, J. (2007). Quality and safety education for nurses. *Nursing Outlook, 55*(3), 122–131.

Cronenwett, L., Sherwood, G., Pohl, J., Barnsteiner, J., Moore, S., Taylor Sullivan, D., . . . Warren, J. (2009). Quality and safety education for advanced nursing practice. *Nursing Outlook, 57*(6), 338–348.

Dolansky, M., & Moore, S. (2013). Quality and safety education for nurses (QSEN): The key is systems thinking. *OJIN: The Online Journal of Issues in Nursing, 18*(3). Retrieved from http://www.nursingworld.org/Quality-and-Safety-Education-for-Nurses.html

Finkelman, A., & Kenner, C. (2012). *Teaching IOM. Implications of the Institute of Medicine reports for nursing education* (3rd ed.). Silver Spring, MD: American Nurses Association.

Hayden, J., Smiley, R., Alexander, M., Kardong-Edgren, S., & Jeffries, P. (2014). The NCSBN national simulation study: A longitudinal, randomized, controlled study replacing clinical hours with simulation in pre-licensure nursing education. *Journal of Nursing Regulation, 5*(2), Supplement. Retrieved from https://www.ncsbn.org/JNR_Simulation_Supplement.pdf

Healthy People. (2015). About healthy people. Retrieved from https://www.healthypeople.gov

Institute of Medicine (IOM). (2001). *Crossing the quality chasm*. Washington, DC: The National Academies Press.

Institute of Medicine (IOM). (2003a). *Health professions education: A bridge to quality*. Washington, DC: The National Academies Press.

Institute of Medicine (IOM). (2003b). *Keeping patients safe: Transforming the work environment for nurses*. Washington, DC: The National Academies Press.

Institute of Medicine (IOM). (2007). *The learning healthcare system: Workshop summary*. Washington, DC: The National Academies Press.

Institute of Medicine (IOM). (2008). *Knowing what works in health care: A roadmap for the nation*. Washington, DC: The National Academies Press.

Institute of Medicine (IOM). (2009). *Redesigning continuing education in the health professions*. Washington, DC: The National Academies Press.

Institute of Medicine (IOM). (2010). *The future of nursing: Leading change, advancing health*. Washington, DC: The National Academies Press.

Institute of Medicine (IOM). (2011a). *Learning what works: Infrastructure required for effectiveness research: Workshop summary*. Washington, DC: The National Academies Press.

Institute of Medicine (IOM). (2011b). *Finding what works in health care: Standards for systematic reviews*. Washington, DC: The National Academies Press.

Institute of Medicine (IOM). (2012). *Health IT and patient safety: Building safer systems for better care*. Washington, DC: The National Academies Press.

Institute of Medicine (IOM). (2015). *Measuring the impact of interprofessional education on collaborative practice and patient outcomes*. Washington, DC: The National Academies Press.

International Association for Clinical Simulation & Learning, Board of Directors (IACSL). (2013). Standards of best practice: Simulation. *Clinical Simulation in Nursing, 9*(6), S1–S32.

Interprofessional Professional Education Collaborative Expert Panel (IPECEP). (2011). *Core competencies for interprofessional collaborative practice*. Retrieved from www.aacn.nche.edu/education-resources/IPECReport.pdf

Kovner, A., & Rundall, T. (2009). Evidence-based management reconsidered. In A. Kovner, D. Fine, & R. D'Aquila (Eds.), *Evidence-based management in healthcare* (pp. 53–78). Chicago, IL: Health Administration Press.

Melnyk, B., & Fineout-Overholt, E. (2010). *Evidence-based practice in nursing and healthcare* (2nd ed.). Philadelphia, PA: Lippincott Williams & Wilkins.

National Council State Boards of Nursing (NCSBN). (2015). Simulation study. Retrieved from https://www.ncsbn.org/685.htm

National League for Nursing (NLN). (2015). About NLN. Retrieved from http://www.nln.org/about

Odell, E. (2011). Teaching quality improvement to the next generation of nurses: What nurse managers can do to help. *Journal of Nursing Administration, 41*(12), 553–557.

Pearlman, E. (2006). Robert I. Sutton: Making a case for evidence-based management. Retrieved from http://www.cioinsight.com/c/a/Expert-Voices/Robert-I-Sutton-Making-a-Case-for-EvidenceBased-Management/

Quality and Safety Education for Nurses (QSEN). (2014a). About QSEN. Retrieved from http://qsen.org/about-qsen/

Quality and Safety Education for Nurses (QSEN). (2014b). Press release: Phase I (November 2005). Retrieved from http://qsen.org/about-qsen/project-overview/project-phases/

Quality and Safety Education for Nurses (QSEN). (2014c). Press release: Phase II (April 2007). Retrieved from http://qsen.org/about-qsen/project-overview/press-release-phase-ii/

Quality and Safety Education for Nurses (QSEN). (2014d). Press release: Phase III (February 2009). Retrieved from http://qsen.org/about-qsen/project-overview/press-release-phase-iii/

Quality and Safety Education for Nurses (QSEN). (2014e). Press release: Phase IV, (March 2012). Retrieved from http://qsen.org/about-qsen/project-overview/press-release-phase-iv/

Quality and Safety Education for Nurses (QSEN). (2014f). Pre-licensure KSAs. Retrieved from http://qsen.org/competencies/pre-licensure-ksas/

Rundall, T., Martelli, P. F., McCurdy, R., Graetz, I.. & Arrayo, L. (2009). Using research evidence when making decisions: Views of health service managers and policymakers. In A. Kovner, D. Fine, & R. D'Aquila (Eds.), *Evidence-based management in healthcare* (pp. 3–16). Chicago, IL: Health Administration Press.

Simulation Innovation Resource Center (SIRC). (2015). History of the SIRC. Retrieved from http://sirc.nln.org/mod/page/view.php?id=347

U.S. Department of Health and Human Services (HHS), Agency for Healthcare Research and Quality (AHRQ). (2015). Accelerating change and transformation in organizations and networks III: Fact sheet. Retrieved from http://www.ahrq.gov/research/findings/factsheets/translating/action3/index.html

U.S. Department of Health and Human Services (HHS), Agency for Healthcare Research and Quality (AHRQ) & Patient Safety Network (PSNET). (2015). Simulation training. Retrieved from https://psnet.ahrq.gov/primers/primer/25/simulation-training

U.S. Department of Veterans Affairs (VA), Center for Organization Leadership and Management Research. (2015). National Center for Organization Development. Retrieved from http://www.choir.research.va.gov/

Walshe, K., & Rundall, T. (2001). Evidence-based management: From theory to practice in healthcare. *The Milbank Quarterly, 79*(3), 429–457.

World Health Organization (WHO). (2010). Framework for action on interprofessional education and collaborative practice. Retrieved from http://whqlibdoc.who.int/hq/2010/WHO_HRH_HPN_10.3_eng.pdf

Change and Healthcare Delivery

CHAPTER OBJECTIVES

At the conclusion of this chapter, the learner will be able to:

- Examine change as a process and understand its relationship to continuous quality improvement.
- Discuss the role of stakeholders in the change process.
- Examine the change process.
- Analyze the barriers to change and strategies to overcome the barriers.
- Apply methods to assess and describe the need for change and develop solutions.

OUTLINE

KEY TERMS

Brainstorming

Change

Change agent

Decision tree

Delphi technique

GANTT chart

Groupthink

Nominal group

Pass the problem

Plan-do-study-act

PERT chart

Proactive change

Reactive change

Six hat method

Solution analysis

Stakeholder

Introduction

Change is discussed in the first section of this text because it is a critical element of healthcare delivery and continuous quality improvement (CQI). The healthcare system is not a static system and undergoes changes daily as care is provided. As we have discussed, the system is in need of improvement in all sectors and among all healthcare practitioners. Achieving this improvement requires change, and change is not something most people like to experience. This truth applies to healthcare organizations (HCOs), where effective change is often resisted. *Effective* is a key term here, as not all change effects positive outcomes. Put another way, even though improvement requires change, not all changes represent improvement. Negative responses to change are often due to past negative experiences with the change process and/or results. However, when healthcare practitioners come to understand the vital role of change in the CQI process, they will be more apt to buy in. All managers and staff should be engaged in change—looking for opportunities to change, participating actively to integrate changes, and evaluating changes that are made and then using these insights to effect further change. The overall goal should be to adapt the common perspective of change from a dreaded experience to an opportunity. Change agents, or those who work to bring about change, are important to success.

Change: An Ongoing Experience in Healthcare Delivery and Quality Improvement

Maureen Bisognano, president and CEO of the Institute for Healthcare Improvement, identified the first factor in influencing improvement as that of "building will" (HHS, AHRQ, June 2015): She explains this idea as follows:

> When someone is tired, when they implemented change and they haven't seen dramatic results, or when they find resistance in their peers or they find problems in the supply chain—when they come up against those walls, I believe it's our obligation to help them to see the end result. And that is to tell the story of the patient. Often I think when we have a team that's demoralized or tired or overloaded by too many projects, the sense making that can come from telling a story and combining that with data is very powerful. (HHS, AHRQ, June 2015)

Patient-centered care is emphasized throughout the CQI decision process and changes within the healthcare system. To **change** is to do something to cause something to be different—for the patient, system, healthcare services, and so on. This concept seems simple enough to accomplish, but it is not. Bringing about change is a complex process. Every human being experiences changes. HCOs also change daily. There is change that just happens, and then there is change that is planned, implemented, and evaluated, which may or may not be connected to quality improvement. As staff work, they have to make decisions, and the outcome of these decisions may lead to small or major changes. This chapter primarily focuses on the process of change as a basis for further understanding and application in CQI and CQI planning.

There is no doubt that whether change just occurs or it is planned, equilibrium (individual and organizational) is disturbed. Change may involve eliminating something (e.g., process, procedure, program service) or improving or enhancing current activities, which may include adding new approaches, or it may involve a combination of these approaches. Change can be negative or positive, and while HCOs and healthcare providers can learn from both types, CQI supports positive change. The vision of the healthcare system and the aims for improvement, as identified by major quality initiatives, all involve changes. With the rapidly changing healthcare delivery system and health knowledge, along with the expansion of health informatics and technology (HIT), *change* is an everyday experience for those who work in health care.

Factors Influencing Change

So, with change being such a natural occurrence in health care, one might wonder, where does it come from? Change occurs daily in the healthcare delivery system, both on the macrolevel (national, state, local) and on the microlevel (HCOs of all types). Some of the influences that have a major impact on healthcare delivery include the following:

- Patient needs
- Demographic changes
- Expansion and change in medical knowledge including influence of research
- Changes in treatment (e.g., pharmaceuticals, procedures)
- Healthcare reform (e.g., Affordable Care Act)
- Healthcare reimbursement
- Health policy and legislation
- Government programs such as Medicare and Medicaid
- Use of multiple CQI methods leading to identification of change needs based on gaps
- Greater emphasis on primary care
- Population health
- Local, state, and national economics (e.g., fluctuating economy that impacts HCO reimbursement and budgets)
- Increase in aging population
- Health promotion and prevention
- Changing healthcare roles and new degrees, such as in nursing

- Greater use of interprofessional collaborative teams
- Increase in chronic disease across the life span
- Increased emphasis on patient-centered care
- Increase in errors and decreased quality of care
- Expansion of HIT
- Expansion of medical technology
- Greater emphasis on performance outcomes requiring better monitoring of care
- Staffing concerns (e.g., level, mix, shortage, expertise and competence, retention of staff, burnout and stress)
- The uninsured and underinsured
- Patient confidentiality and rights
- Healthcare legal and ethical issues
- Access to care
- Government initiatives to improve care
- Changing vulnerable populations
- Healthcare profession changes
- Healthcare industry changes (e.g., merges, hospital closures, development of national healthcare corporations, shortage of services, financial issues)
- Need for improvement in healthcare professions education
- Global health concerns (e.g., Ebola virus and other infectious diseases)

This list is not exhaustive, but it provides a view of how many influences may impact the healthcare delivery system and healthcare professionals. For each of the examples, there are multiple possible changes that might occur.

Sometimes it can be very tiring trying to cope and adjust, but there is no avoiding it. Change can lead to positive experiences and outcomes, and it can lead to difficult and even negative experiences and outcomes. A key factor to supporting successful experiences with change is to understand change and how it works. In addition, it is important to use self-reflection and understand how you respond to change and how you might improve your coping with change. Within an HCO, each staff member impacts the organization change process; thus, how each staff member responds to the change process can have an impact. For example, if the staff member is in a leadership position and is hesitant to engage in change, this has a major impact. If some staff members do not engage in the process and try to block change, the power of the group can have an impact. Later in this chapter, stakeholders are described. Stakeholders have power to move change forward positively or negatively.

Why is change important? Consider what people, organizations, and situations would be like if there were no change. There would be no way to improve: limiting recognition of new ideas, adding new people and positions, and providing different services and meeting new needs. History is all about change. Individuals and families experience change across the life span. Communities experience change in demographics, economic status, safety, health services, and so on. Government changes to meet new needs and discard old approaches. People often question how or when the government should make these changes, but if there were no changes, government would no longer meet the many needs of the citizens. As changes are made in an organization, the organization's vision, mission, and objectives need to be considered. Changes should align with the current view of the organization, unless one of the changes is actually to alter the organization's vision, mission, or objectives.

Understanding the potential landmines of change is important to success, but there are also many benefits to change. It can invigorate us. We do not know all of the answers, and we often confront new issues and problems, but this should not stop us from valuing change. Complacency and isolationism lead us to becoming stale and reduce ability to respond to situations in an effective and timely manner. Isolationism, doing our work and trying to just maintain it with no interferences, can become comfortable for us. When we avoid isolationism, however, we are provided with more opportunities to develop innovative responses. Isolationism often brings rigidity, which only diminishes creativity. Then when a critical need for change occurs, as it will, we will not be ready to deal with it.

The idea of change may elicit an emotional reaction, such as the following:

- A person may laugh and say, "Not again, another change!"
- A person may express frustration and not know where to begin.
- A person may fear the change will blow up in his or her face.
- A person may complain about more paperwork, confusion, and poor communication.
- A person may become depressed and less productive.
- A person may become angry with management personnel who "don't know what they're doing."

None of these responses are helpful, but within the organization's culture, they may become more common than is embracing change. It is important to recognize that change is personal; everyone has an experience with it and a personal view of it. Leaders of change need to understand these personal reactions to better prevent barriers to change. Even leaders of change have their own personal experiences and reactions to change that need to be recognized.

Change Theories and Models

A successful change begins as an idea that is shaped and molded through the change process and, ideally, should be preplanned. Leadership needs to consider the process carefully. The outcome(s) should be clearly identified so that outcomes can guide the evaluation of the change. There are many theories and models that address change and the change process. Many were developed several decades ago but are still applied today. The following represent some of these theories and models.

Lewin's Force Field Theory

The force field model of change focuses on the change team identifying, analyzing, and then adjusting as needed based on the driving and restraining forces (Lewin, 1947). This model applies one of three strategies to determine feasibility. The team can increase the number or strength of the driving forces, decrease the number or strength of the restraining forces, or combine these two strategies. The model includes three stages. In the *unfreezing stage*, the major issue is increasing knowledge and awareness of the problem and then identifying and decreasing any forces that do not allow change, or if required, maintenance of the current situation. The *moving stage* ensures that the problem is clearly described and that the team identifies change outcomes based on the problem. As the name of the stage implies, this is an active stage of implementing interventions/strategies to reach the identified outcomes. The final stage is *refreezing* when the change is "hardwired" or becomes part of the HCO and the culture. For many changes, refreezing is not easy to accomplish, as there is risk of a return to the way things were or some back and forth for a time until the change is truly integrated into the system. A criticism of this model is that it does not emphasize feelings and attitudes enough, but it is still commonly used and can be combined with other models of change that would consider more of these elements. Lewin's model emphasizes the impact of the group over individuals. With today's increasing emphasis on interprofessional collaborative teams, this focus on the group is critical. **Figure 4-1** describes this model.

This model also assumes a more episodic approach. Episodic changes are mostly infrequent, discontinuous, and intentional. In this situation, the HCO is not adapting to its needs, and the result is ineffectiveness and pressure to change. This type of change takes more time, and often staff do not feel the change process is really

Figure 4-1 Force Field Analysis.

completed because another change usually begins. The organization experiences disequilibrium and then the change moves on to a new equilibrium. Avoiding disequilibrium requires planned change. Lewin's model is one of the most commonly applied models used to make deliberate changes.

Weick and Quinn (1999) also identify the importance of continuous change or a series of fast mini-episodes of change. Change is brought about by the need to adapt, but in reality change never starts or stops. This view is helpful in appreciating how change is a part of everything and is ongoing; however, as will be discussed here, one can still look at specific change efforts, the process, and results that lead to decisions. As Weick and Quinn (1999) explain, "When change is continuous, the problem is not one of unfreezing [as is described by Lewin] The problem is one of redirecting what is already under way" (p. 379). Quinn has also described "slow death" and "deep change." These terms are quite visual. If your HCO does not make needed changes, then the organization accepts "what is" as the best it can be. In these organizations, staff often experience this as a status quo approach, and this can limit staff enthusiasm and drive, impacting performance and productivity. Deep change often leads to significant readjustment within the HCO.

Human factors cannot be ignored in the process, whether it is episodic change or continuous change. Although presented here, the process of change may seem to be a single process or episodic, but in reality HCOs have multiple, organized, ongoing change processes occurring all the time. Waiting for one change process to complete before beginning another change is a luxury few have today in thriving HCOs. In the background, there always is continuous change.

Havelock's Theory

Many theories and models build on one another. Havelock's theory expands Lewin's theory by focusing more on the management of change—planning and monitoring change. This theory includes the following steps (Havelock, 1973):

1. Building relationships
2. Diagnosing the need for change
3. Getting the resources needed for change
4. Selecting the best option to respond to the change and implementing it
5. Establishing and accepting change
6. Maintaining and stabilizing

The steps need to be clear and include typical steps attributed to planning. When comparing this theory/model with other theories/models, the steps or stages are different. For example, the stages in Lewin's model focus on increasing and decreasing forces that influence the problem and change.

Kotter's Change Model

Kotter's model focuses on a culture of change, with emphasis on vision and leadership and greater emphasis on the implementation stage rather than the entire process (Kotter, 1996). A change needs to become part of the HCO culture. The stages in this model begin with an important consideration: It is easy to become complacent—we like the way it is; we have time to make adjustments—but this response is not helpful. Kotter's model involves eight stages:

1. Establish a sense of urgency.
2. Create a guiding coalition.
3. Develop a vision and strategy.
4. Communicate the change vision.
5. Empower broad-based action.
6. Generate short-term wins.
7. Consolidate gains and produce more change.
8. Anchor new approaches in the culture.

This model is similar to Havelock's theory, but it describes more than just planning steps, as it includes process, leadership elements, attitudes, and responses.

Juran's Trilogy Model

Juran's model focuses on the customer; that is, the product must meet the customer's needs. In the case of health care, the most important customer is the patient. There are, however, other customers. For example, the HCO also views insurers as customers, or when a laboratory provides services for a nurse or physician, the laboratory views the the nurse or physician as a customer in addition to the patient (Juran & Defeo, 2010). The laboratory would be concerned with satisfaction in their services for both the patient and providers. The Juran trilogy includes the following elements:

1. *Quality planning.* Identify the customers, determine customer needs, and develop a product/service that addresses the needs.
2. *Quality improvement.* Develop a process to produce the product/service and optimize the process.
3. *Quality control.* Prove that the process will result in the product/service with minimal oversight, and transfer the change process to HCO operations.

This model emphasizes first identifying major concerns about change and then deciding what should be done to address the concerns.

Appreciative Inquiry

Appreciative inquiry provides a perspective of change that is important to consider and can alter staff perception of dread when change is mentioned. This approach focuses on what is working well, considers why this is the case, and then applies this information to continue with what is going well (Whatis.com, 2015). Typically, the change approach taken is to first identify problems rather strengths, but it is then easy to lose sight of what works. In comparison, appreciative inquiry applies to long-term rather than short-term strategy and does not focus on dysfunction, but rather on building strengths (Swearingen, 2008). It is important to view the positive as well as what needs improvement. Appreciative inquiry involves the following four stages (Fallon, Begun, & Riley, 2013):

1. *Discovery stage.* This stage focuses on appreciating the current status from a positive point of view.
2. *Dream stage.* In this stage, participants ask the question, "What might be?" This is positive visualization. As with the first stage, the goal is to get participants to be positive.
3. *Designs for change stage.* In this stage, participants ask questions such as, "What do we need to do to make needed change?" and "How can we best get to where we want to be?" This stage is the work stage—making the changes.
4. *Destiny stage.* This stage focuses on sustaining the change.

The order in which these stages occur may vary from that described here, and some stages may not formally occur. As described by Fallon and colleagues (2013), appreciative inquiry

> draws upon people's desire for positivity and optimism. It emphasizes collaboration and participation by all members of the organization and its stakeholders. It values continuity with the past while moving the organization forward. [Appreciative inquiry] has a system thinking orientation because it approaches change as a journey that unfolds, rather than as a planned event. (pp. 326–327)

This is an important perspective to use when the change process is then applied to CQI.

Proactive Versus Reactive Change

The discussions in this chapter and in other chapters support the use of **proactive change**, change that is planned based on assessment of need. This approach to change is much more effective than is **reactive change**. When we wait for something to happen that might require change, we often miss the opportunity to be effective. Looking ahead—projecting needs and then planning—is better than trying to handle a problem that was not foreseen, which often leads to a response that is insufficiently planned and lacks clear objectives to evaluate outcomes. The change theories and models discussed in this chapter are based on proactive change.

Stop and Consider #1

CQI cannot occur without change.

Stakeholders

A **stakeholder** is any party that has a strong enough interest in an issue to want to give input and engage in actions relating to the issue. Such parties can be an individual (e.g., patient, staff member), a patient's family or significant others, groups/teams, staff, management, communities, government agencies, professional organizations, nonprofit organizations, insurers, or businesses.

Identification of Stakeholders

There are many possible stakeholders that might be involved in the change process. Stakeholders may be internal and external to the HCO. The identification of specific stakeholders depends on the change issue and the healthcare setting. If stakeholders are not identified, then they may act as barriers to success, as they feel left out of the process.

Engaging Stakeholders

The change process requires that stakeholders be convinced the change is needed, and when a solution is selected, stakeholders need to be committed to it. Often, approaches used to convince stakeholders to participate are political, requiring use of influence, but it is critical to have all key players on board with the change. When talking to others and getting their support, the information collected in earlier steps may help later in the process. For some, the support may be just that they are not going to block the change. Others may provide support by doing something specific to help implement the change. Stakeholders may provide different views of a problem, assessments of solutions, evaluation of actions taken, and new information and may identify potential barriers that need to be considered during the change process. It can also be useful to include staff who are negative about a planned change on the planning team. If the team hears only positive comments, then they may be missing important factors necessary to understand the "real-world" view of the problem. In addition, listening is very important as change proponents engage stakeholders, even if they disagree with the stakeholder's view.

Stop and Consider #2

Nurses are stakeholders in the CQI change process.

The Change Process

The process of change is a living process in that it is not exactly the same every time a change is planned. It requires careful balancing with the many factors that are involved, even with a simple change. It is important to remember that not all change is planned, and in fact most change is not planned. It happens. Unplanned change can get organizations into trouble because the change process may not be controlled and staff usually then feel more frustration and stress.

The change process includes multiple steps that influence each other. Steps may merge into future steps, particularly if all the tasks related to a step in the process are not completed. It is easy to underestimate the amount of training and time it will take. In addition, it is important to know when more help is needed, either to guide the planning or to implement the change. Data may change what might be needed to understand a problem, requiring flexibility rather than rigidity to a change approach. Rigidity is a barrier to effective CQI projects.

The focus in this chapter is understanding change as an important process within healthcare delivery and making response to change as effective as possible. As discussed in other chapters, systems and processes are very important in improving care and in developing CQI plans. System-level factors that need to be kept in mind during the change process are identified in **Figure 4-2**.

Identification of the Need for Change

It is key that the issue, problem, or need for change is understood in order to develop the best response. If not, then there may be energy and resources wasted in an effort

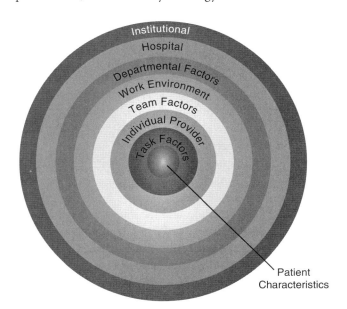

Patient
Characteristics

Figure 4-2

System-Level Factors that Impact Safety.
Reproduced from Agency for Healthcare Research and Quality (AHRQ). (June 2015). Collaborative Unit-Based Safety Program (CUSP) toolkit: Learn about CUSP. Retrieved from http://www.ahrq .gov/professionals/education /curriculum-tools/cusptoolkit /modules/learn/index.html

that will not progress long term. The first step is to identify the issue or problem, but often more information is needed to fully describe it, which leads to step 2. It is during the first step that change leaders decide if the effort should continue, and in steps 2 and 3 the final decision is made to complete the entire process or to stop the process if it is not needed. This type of approach may also be called proactive planning, particularly if the goal is to avert a problem. The objectives are clarified, which should be in line with the overall goal or outcome. Other chapters expand on CQI approaches and planning used in the improvement process, which apply the change process.

The Team: Leadership and Followership

Today, teams, both intraprofessional and interprofessional, are important in health care. Nurses have long worked on nursing teams, but they now must become more involved in interprofessional teams, too. Other chapters in this text discuss teamwork in greater detail; however, teamwork needs to be recognized as a part of an effective change process. Change within an HCO does not happen with one leader or manager or with one staff member. Using a team with an effective leader and team members (followers) is the best approach for an effective change process. TeamSTEPPS is discussed in other chapters as an effective approach to improving teamwork. **Figure 4-3** provides a description of the steps in the process to ensure effective team functioning, leadership, and followership.

Analysis and Description of the Problem

The amount of information or data needed to fully describe a problem or issue can vary a great deal depending on the problem or issue. For example, if a hospital is instituting use of an electronic medical record (EMR) or electronic health record (EHR), the amount of information needed is greater, such as information about software choices, customization of possible software, advantages and disadvantages of the software options, and type of information required for the EMR/EHR to ensure that all documentation needs are met. In addition, consideration must be given to the HCO's typical CQI problems and how the EMR/EHR might help to improve care, software cost, maintenance requirements, staff education to implement the change, and so on. A smaller project that might require less information to fully describe the problem or issue might be to extend clinic hours by one hour. In this case, the HCO would need to understand what could be done in the extra hour that is different from the current schedule, and the impact the change might have on staffing, budget, space, parking needs, and issues such as better lighting for night hours, security, response of stakeholders (healthcare providers, nonclinical staff, and patients), and so on. Other decisions might have greater impact on the HCO, such as a decision to develop a home care service. This type of service requires extensive marketing information, budget analysis, consideration of the impact on other HCO

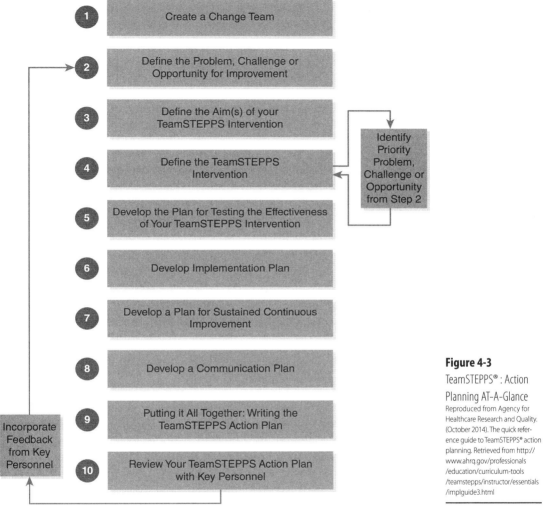

Figure 4-3

TeamSTEPPS® : Action
Planning AT-A-Glance
Reproduced from Agency for
Healthcare Research and Quality.
(October 2014). The quick reference guide to TeamSTEPPS® action
planning. Retrieved from http://
www.ahrq.gov/professionals
/education/curriculum-tools
/teamstepps/instructor/essentials
/implguide3.html

services, input from community stakeholders, and so on. All of these examples are changes. Some may be directly related to CQI in that CQI data indicate a problem in quality exists; others may be responding to changing trends and community needs. All represent change.

The description of data should allow decision makers to review the information and better understand the problem or issue. The result should include a clear description of the issue or problem and should connect to the predicted expected outcomes. Failure to present this information clearly can be one of the biggest barriers to effective change. Decisions must be based on the description of the issue or problem. Jumping to conclusions or selecting the most obvious description, which may seem like the easier route, may lead to problems later. Often we tend to consider the initial information or data we hear as the most important, when it may not be. More in-depth discussion of measurement and data is provided in other chapters.

Readiness Assessment

Readiness for change is also an important factor to describe. It is critical that management and the change team understand the current status of the HCO and its staff and how this impacts their ability to handle change. This readiness is not necessarily focused on a specific change but rather on the ability to engage in the change process. Some staff are more ready to handle change than are others. How is the HCO functioning? Effective planning to respond to change is more difficult for dysfunctional organizations. Does the organization have the resources available such as financial resources, physical space, equipment, supplies, informatics technology, and staffing levels and expertise? Have there been other recent changes, and what are their status and staff response? Is there effective leadership within the HCO to guide the change process? What is the history of changes in the HCO?

Past experiences with change have a direct impact on current change; for example, if the HCO has had a difficult experience with a change, then staff may be reluctant to get involved in another change. The U.S. Department of Health and Human Services, Health Resources and Services Administration (2015), offers advice for getting staff on board with the change process:

> Change is always challenging, but since redesigned systems typically are improvements, these changes are easier than most. It is important to reinforce why the change is essential and to support staff that may have difficulty. It is also important to communicate to staff the data that illustrates the benefit of the change—improved outcomes for patients as an example. Emphasizing that all team members' contributions are important to making the redesigned system work is also helpful.

It could be that it is just not the right time to make a particular change. One can never be sure that change will be successful; it is risky (Finkelman & Kenner, 2016). Knowing how much the organizational culture can handle at one time can make a difference in how difficult it will be to even get the change process moving. How critical the problem or issue becomes is a major factor in determining if this change must be made now. For example, 10 years ago, instituting use of EMR/EHRs was not so important, although many hospitals did begin to use EMR/EHRs. Today, this is different. There is more evidence supporting the need for EMR/EHRs and their impact on reducing errors. The federal government is pushing for use across the country in all types of healthcare settings. In the case of this issue, an HCO would not spend a lot of time debating the readiness for this change.

Budget is also an important factor in readiness for change. If an organization does not have the money to cover the expenses, then change should not happen. Budget issues are not just organization focused. State and national economic issues impact HCO budgets, as does reimbursement for healthcare services. All of these considerations must be figured into a discussion about readiness.

Another readiness factor is leadership. If an organization has undergone major changes in critical leadership positions, these changes will impact the types of changes the organization is able to handle. Changes in leadership positions are major concerns in any HCO and need to settle some before other major changes are started. New leadership, however, often means that the leaders themselves will be moving to make changes, often to demonstrate their own leadership to staff and to higher-level leadership within the HCO. Many staff have experience working with new leaders who are eager to make changes, often with limited understanding of the new organization and staff or use of effective planning. Staff may then feel like every time they turn around there is a new change. This scenario is not effective planning for change or effective leadership. Leaders who use evidence-based management (EBM) tend to make more effective decisions about change, as they review and apply best evidence to problems and use this to determine possible solutions.

Assessment of readiness for change should lead to a change process plan. The plan describes how a change will occur and is critical for success of the change process. This plan of action should be written and clear to all who may be involved. Guidelines to creating a change process plan include the following:

- Clearly describe the issue or problem (the focus of the change process).
- Identify specific goals and objectives, and describe the major intervention(s) or solution(s) (the change), with rationale to support the change.
- Identify the policies and procedures needed to apply the recommendations.
- Describe the implementation phases.
- Specify the timeline in sufficient detail so that all concerned understand the due dates.
- Designate responsibilities, including specific names.
- Develop the budget.
- Describe the evaluation methods; create a timeline that includes both short-term and long-term evaluation markers.

The goals and outcomes should be measurable and achievable. The timeline is important, and it should be reasonable. Can the goals and outcomes be met in the time frame described? Moving too fast or even too slowly can interfere with meeting outcomes. The timeline may need adjustment as the change process occurs; however, frequent adjustments indicate a weak timeline and plan.

Selection and Development of the Solution(s): Using Best Evidence

When plans are developed, EBM—and when necessary evidence-based practice (EBP)—should be used to select and develop solution options. The following are typical steps used to identify solution options and apply the best solutions:

1. *Prepare staff for the change.* Education about the need for change and the process of change is important for all staff that will be affected by the change. It is best that this effort is planned so that all information is covered and all those concerned are included. Leaving people out leads to resistance and impacts effective implementation and outcomes.

2. *Test the solution(s).* Ideally, the change process includes pilot tests to implement a change before it is used in a broader way in the HCO. Some changes are not implemented throughout the HCO, as the change is too specific; for example, the HCO may change the procedure for admitting newborns to the neonatal unit to improve the assessment process, although there may still be a testing time designated to identify potential problems, get staff and parent feedback, and so on. For other changes, a rollout plan is more effective (e.g., the institution of the EMR/EHR in a hospital). The hospital may choose to begin use of the EMR/EHR in certain departments, divisions, or units first and then expand to other areas. This approach allows for corrections before the entire hospital is moved to the new system. The difficulty with this approach is initially the hospital would be using two documentation systems. For some changes, this approach may not be useful (e.g., the development of home care services). The hospital needs to weigh the pros and cons of the best method to use. Testing can be very important to work out the kinks and create more effective change. Pilot tests need to be time limited and carefully evaluated by those who best understand the change and its need and by stakeholders.

3. *Implement the change (solution).* Implementing the change means all the steps necessary to start the change solution are begun as planned. Timing is important; it is particularly important to determine the best start time and the timeline for major steps in the process. During the implementation of the solution(s), change leaders should pay attention to feedback, which may be important in preventing problems. Perceiving staff feedback as resistance or mere complaining may lead to serious mistakes. In fact, building in feedback as part of the implementation step is important. This engages staff in the process and increases commitment. Staff, however, also have the responsibility of communicating concerns in a clear and timely manner.

4. *Spread improvement.* Supporting the integration of change within the organization is a critical part of the process. The goal is to make the change a part of the system. Many factors can impact the success of a change,

such as staff attitude and preparation, staffing levels, staff issues such as morale and frequent turnover, changes in leadership/management, work environment and the culture of safety, communication, diversity issues, collaborative approach, empowerment, commitment, budget, standards and regulations, equipment and supplies, and other changes that are ongoing. Timing is critical, and making several major changes at one time should be avoided when possible. Staff get tired of constantly coping with changes. It is stressful, and strain impacts work productivity and quality. Even as changes are implemented, work continues, and it is important to avoid decreasing productivity and quality whenever possible. Evaluation needs to be integrated through the implementation phase and at the conclusion. The evaluation data should be used to make needed adjustments and to learn about the change process for the next time change is needed.

Best practices to improve the change process, especially during major change projects, include the following (Robinson-Walker, 2011, p. 11):

- Encourage self-care by helping staff be reasonable about what needs to be done and not get overwhelmed.
- Recognize that change can lead to staff unhappiness when staff experience lack of understanding, lack of information, and/or fear about the future.
- Communicate. Even when one thinks something has been communicated, repeat if needed. Use emails, newsletters, meetings, and so on to share. Provide opportunities for dialogue (two-way discussion); promote trust and respect of others.
- Avoid asking specific staff or managers to keep secrets. This leads to distrust and rumors. Rumors are very destructive to the process.
- Be visible; leaders should be engaged.
- Consider how changes in titles and positions cause stress.
- Accept that change is inevitable.
- Understand how you respond to change, how you might block change, and how to improve your response to change.
- Planned change is best, but you have to learn to cope with unplanned change.
- Lead change when needed, but also be an effective follower in the change process.
- Recognize that some change efforts are not effective; learn how to effectively work to make it a positive experience rather than just blocking change negatively.
- Communicate and collaborate with your team and organization.
- Use critical thinking effectively.
- Be willing to recognize a poor decision, admit it, and learn from it.
- Work collaboratively with others.

McCannon, Schall, and Perla (2008) pose some useful questions to consider when developing and implementing change projects: "How will your system for spreading change foster learning and create value for participants every single day? How will you collect and quickly redistribute insight from the front lines?" (p. 11). Here are some other useful questions to consider: Will you need to collect new data for the project? How can you generate information that is useful to front-line teams?

Roles and Responsibilities

The **change agent**, who may be an individual or a team, focuses on the problem or change issue and possible approaches to take. Change agents may be in formal leadership positions, such as a nurse manager, the chair of a task force leading a CQI project, or the administrator responsible for development of a new service, or may have no formal position. Even if the change agent is not in a formal leadership position, the change agent needs to use leadership to accomplish tasks. The change agent is the driver of change; however, do not assume that this person or team is the only relevant party in the change process. All staff and managers are involved in change, ideally working together and not against one another. Consider the following questions when you think about the organization in which you work and the role of the change agent.

- What happens when staff make suggestions?
- Are staff suggestions used, and if so, are their contributions acknowledged?
- When new staff are oriented, is the value of staff involvement and creativity in the organization discussed and, if so, in what manner?
- During orientation, are new staff given examples of how staff participate in organization changes? Are potential staff members asked about their typical responses to change?
- How are critical thinking and clinical reasoning and judgment used in your organization? When and by whom?
- How is the change process applied in your organization?

Evaluation and Follow-up

Evaluation is often the weakest part of the change process. It may be because change leaders and staff are tired, or it could be that no one wants to listen to outcomes. However, evaluation is critical. First, it is important to know if the change solution is working. Are the outcomes met? If not, what went wrong? Feedback from staff who are involved in the solution is an important element of the evaluation plan. It is common to think that if evaluation is performed at the end of implementation, then the requirement for evaluation has been satisfied. The best approach, however, is to use continuous evaluation throughout implementation and then at the end.

For example, evaluation points might be at month 1, month 3, and so on, and then at the conclusion of implementation with a clearly identified date.

It is important to determine any adjustments needed and implement them as needed during implementation and evaluation. With the example of implementation of changes to EMR/EHR, more than likely there will be many adjustments required, and the need for adjustments will span a long period. Due to the critical nature of documentation for patient care, quality care, reimbursement, and in general communication, waiting to make some adjustments might be highly risky.

Stop and Consider #3

Given that change is inevitable in the work environment and a critical part of CQI, Consider how you respond to change, your experience with it, and how you can improve your response.

Barriers to Change and Strategies to Prevent or Overcome Barriers

As planning is begun, it is important to identify barriers to and support for change. As barriers and support may change, adjustments should continue throughout the planning and implementation of a change.

Barriers

As noted earlier, restraining forces are important (Figure 4-1). Sometimes staff who are involved in a change process are reluctant to explore the barriers that may be blocking the change process, but understanding them can prevent problems later when change is planned and implemented.

Resistance

Using empathy or putting yourself in the shoes of others will help to better understand staff. As noted by Senge, "Resistance to change is natural, expected, and difficult. . . . It is a balancing force designed to maintain the status quo within a system. Resistance arises from threats to traditional norms and ways of doing things" (HHS, HRSA, 2015; Senge, 1990). Staff (clinical and nonclinical) resistance to change is common. Change disturbs people and the environment in which they work. For many changes, the disturbance may be minor or last only a short time, but for other changes, it can last years. Feeling comfortable with the way things are does not typically move an organization forward.

Why might staff resist a specific change? This is what needs to be understood. It could be just general resistance to all change, but it may also be something about the specific change. Staff may not understand why the change is necessary, may feel concerned about its effect on work processes, may fear that it will result in a loss (e.g., job, responsibility and authority, ranking or status, pay, working with a specific team, work schedule, friends within the work setting, job enjoyment and satisfaction), or may consider the change to be a personal criticism of job performance.

How change has been experienced in the past, either in the same organization or in another, can lead staff to be highly resistant, particularly if the change process was poorly planned and implemented and no one listened to the staff. Another issue related to resistance is the amount and level of change. An HCO can handle only a certain amount and level of change at one time before the change begins to negatively impact operations. Change leaders need to recognize this risk and consider it carefully. This can be a major barrier to effectively implementing a change. Typically, barriers can be classified as (1) emotional reactions, (2) perceptual issues or view of the situation, (3) economic threat or loss, and (4) social threat or loss. Better understanding of the barriers can lead to a plan to address them up front rather than waiting for additional problems to occur.

Not only may staff be resistant to change, but also HCOs as organizations can be resistant to change. HCOs that are bureaucratic, highly structured, and heavily dependent on following policies and procedures may be less likely to change easily. Khator (2014) identified four attitudes that often get in the way of coping with and effectively managing the change (pp. 4.2–4.3):

- *Ignorance.* "When did that happen?" This reaction may indicate that staff feel as though things are moving too fast and are too complicated to manage.
- *Arrogance.* "We have been doing this our way a long time and we know best." Staff often do not know what is best for the HCO as a whole and may not have the insights needed to anticipate disruption until faced directly with it. Everything seems fine to them, so why rock the boat?
- *Victimization.* "Why are they doing this to us?" Disruptions are a real part of business; they are not personal.
- *Panic.* "We have to do something! Anything! And quickly!" Panic creates a fragmented, inefficient work environment; effecting positive change requires a supportive, unified work environment.

Support for change is also important to understand. Change leaders need to identify stakeholders who will support the change process because they believe in it. Stakeholders can help to identify barriers and ways to resolve barriers through effective strategies. For example, a staff member who fears suffering a professional setback due to a proposed change might actually get a promotion, more pay, a better work team, a better work environment, or a better work schedule. Change leaders may help the stakeholder recognize, and consequently rectify, this misunderstanding where the stakeholder lacks such insight.

The work environment should facilitate productivity and ensure patient and staff safety. Many changes can improve the work environment, though some can make it more difficult. Change leaders need to consider the impact of the planned change on the work environment. They must identify solutions in order to solve or improve the problem. In this step, the planning moves from collecting data and information to putting the information together so that solutions can be identified. For most problems or issues, there are multiple options. The more that is known about them, the more likely that the best approach to the change will be selected.

Inadequate Leadership

Leaders need to think ahead and engage in planning. This includes developing effective infrastructure, staff training, effective information systems, policies and procedures, and performance appraisal that includes rewards. Quinn's work on change and leaders emphasizes that often the major issue with organizational change is the leaders' fears about what might happen to them due to the change (Quinn, 1996, 2000). Effective change requires leaders who are challenged by change and do not pull away from it, as noted by Quinn, recognizing the need to engage in the heroic journey.

Groupthink

Groupthink occurs when group members go along with a proposed idea as a group. There is, however, at least one member who may disagree with the idea, but when this member sees that no one is sharing negative views, this member then keeps quiet and goes along with the group. This type of response is not that unusual and acts as a major barrier to creativity and shared ideas. It blocks an open communication environment. If members speak up and present minority views, they may fear retaliation or be concerned they will not be viewed as a member of the group. This dynamic is not part of a functional organizational culture, nor is it effective teamwork. Teamwork does not mean everyone must agree, but rather that everyone works together to arrive at best solutions, considering multiple viewpoints. Team members need to understand that compromise may be required.

Inadequate Planning

Not all change is successful. We know change is disruptive and causes stress for staff, but why does change sometimes fail? The following are possible reasons failure is associated with planning for change. Understanding why change fails also makes a difference in successfully managing change in the future (Ponti, 2011, p. 43).

- *Lack of urgency.* Urgency is a critical change driver. Leadership and staff need to feel it is really important that a change is made. If this is not felt, moving change forward is difficult. Another problem is when the leader thinks there is urgency, but there is not. A third problem is when the leader does not take the time to work through the need for change and lead others to understand the need for change (the urgency).
- *Lack of coalition.* Who are the key people who need to be driving the change and forming a coalition? Sometimes the wrong people are chosen, or someone critical is left out.
- *Lack of vision.* A plan for change requires a clear vision. It provides the goal(s) and the meaning of the change.
- *Ineffective communication.* Limited information and understanding about urgency, vision, and the plan will lead to problems. Communication needs to be clear, timely, and consistent and needs to support the sharing of information.
- *Vision obstacles.* Obstacles to change are inevitable. When possible, they need to be prevented. If they cannot be prevented, then they need to be dealt with or adjusted to ensure that change occurs as planned.
- *Lack of short-term wins.* Often the focus is on the end point; however, most change takes time. It is important to also celebrate and recognize the accomplishment of interim short-term goals.
- *Declaring victory too soon.* Leaders have to be careful about prematurely pronouncing the change a success. Determining the status requires careful analysis.
- *Not anchoring changes.* Making sure the change is part of the culture and "the way things are done" is critical. It is easy to assume this has occurred when it has not, and this can then result in losing momentum in ensuring that the change is part of the organization.

Strategies to Prevent or Overcome Barriers

Empowering staff to make decisions is a sign of an effective, healthy organization. If all decision-making power is in the top or middle level of management, this impacts how the organization functions. Staff need some power to make decisions where decisions count and when needed, at the direct site of work. For healthcare providers, this may mean at the bedside or on the unit. Teams are critical, and teams make decisions. If they cannot make decisions, then there is not much reason to have teams.

Trust is also an issue. During change, predictability and capability have an impact on trust. Staff feel most comfortable, as do many managers, when work expectations, schedules, processes, and so on are clear and predictable. Often during change, this predictability is lost. Capability relates to whether or not the HCO can do what needs to be done, and this also then impacts roles and responsibilities. During the change process, the HCO's capability may not be clear all the time. As a consequence, if predictability and/or capability are in flux, staff and managers may have reduced trust. This atmosphere of distrust impacts empowerment, both in managers "trusting" staff with power to make decisions or follow-through and with staff "trusting" managers. The following is a checklist of some strategies to consider when responding to resistance.

- *View resistance as a friend.* This makes you pay attention in case you are headed in the wrong direction.
- *Allow others to tell their stories.* Listen, as you may learn something important.
- *Look at resistance as a "cue."* It is difficult to listen to negative feedback, but these comments may reveal issues that may be important to further understand an issue or problem.
- *Use "no" as a connecting point.* Stop and find out why someone disagrees.
- *Stop doing what is not working.* It could be that this approach needs revision.
- *Include staff in the change process.* Particularly include some staff that are not 100% for the change to provide different views.
- *Identify the driving and restraining forces in language that can easily be understood.* Use the method suggested in Lewin's theory to decrease restraining forces and/or increase driving forces. First, however, you need to identify the restraining and driving forces.
- *Establish a safe environment where staff feel comfortable expressing their concerns.* Avoid letting negativity become the main theme.

The Nursing Organizations Alliance (The Alliance) believes that a healthful practice/work environment, an environment that is able to cope with change, is supported by the presence of the following elements (The Alliance, 2004):

1. *Collaborative practice culture.* The culture is marked by respectful collegial communication and behavior, team orientation, presence of trust, and respect for diversity.
2. *Communication-rich culture.* Communication is clear and respectful, open and trusting.
3. *A culture of accountability.* Role expectations are clearly defined; everyone is accountable.
4. *The presence of adequate numbers of qualified nurses.* Nurses are able to provide quality care to meet patients' needs; work–home life is balanced.
5. *The presence of expert, competent, credible, visible leadership.* Leaders serve as an advocate for nursing practice, support shared decision-making, and allocate resources to support nursing.

6. *Shared decision-making at all levels.* Nurses participate in system, organizational, and process decisions; formal structure exists to support shared decision-making; nurses have control over their practice.

7. *The encouragement of professional practice and continued growth/ development.* Continuing education/certification is supported/ encouraged; participation in a professional association is encouraged; an information-rich environment is supported.

8. *Recognition of the value of nursing's contribution.* Nurses are rewarded and paid for performance; they are afforded career mobility and expansion.

9. *Recognition by nurses for their meaningful contribution to practice.* Nurses need to understand how they can make a difference and to use their position and competencies effectively.

The American Organization of Nurse Executives also endorses these elements. They represent an important part of change within nursing. Much work needs to be done to ensure nursing staff and leadership are able to respond to delivery and organizational issues, supporting the type of environment described in this list. Inevitably, this involves change.

Stop and Consider #4
Barriers to change can be turned into positive factors.

Examples of Methods to Assess and Describe the Need for Change and Develop Solutions

Data have become very important in health care, having a direct impact on healthcare delivery, change, and CQI. Medical education has begun to address this issue, noting the need for physicians to use "health data to not only improve community-wide health but also to make a difference for their individual patients" (Frieden, 2015). Frieden (2015) interviewed **Marc Triola,** director of the Institute for Innovations in Medical Education, who had the following to say:

> We're at this amazing time where federal and local governments are releasing health data through initiatives like data.gov, and medical schools have access to data about the health care delivered by doctors in the community. . . . With the changes happening in health care and the changing role of technology and data, teaching these [data analysis] skills seems more important than ever.

Nurses also need this same improvement. HCOs use a variety of methods to better understand problems and changes that organizations need to make, such as questionnaires or surveys, observation, and interviews, which are discussed in content about measurement. Examples of other methods that are often used are described below. The Connect to Current Information section at the end of the chapter provides links to sites that describe figures for some of these methods.

Solution Analysis

Deciding on the best solution requires a structured approach. The **solution analysis** method considers each of the possible solutions and then ranks them according to how effective the solution might be in meeting the objective, cost, time, and feasibility. It is often referred to as SWOT analysis, with SWOT representing the four key elements of solution analysis—the **s**trengths, **w**eaknesses, **o**pportunities, and **t**hreats of a situation. This approach may be used to analyze each possible solution. During this process, all involved need to check their assumptions carefully, think through the process, and continue to increase knowledge about the issue or problem. Sometimes it is important to use intuition when appropriate and step away from rigidity. Do not overemphasize that decisions are final, as most are not; and consider timing and its impact.

Plan-Do-Study-Act

Plan-do-study-act (PDSA) is an example of a rapid-cycle change method. The PDSA—also referred to as the Deming cycle, after its inventor—is a common method used by HCOs today to assist in responding to change and in planning. The PDSA cycle can be used to help with the following (Value Based Management.net, 2011):

- Daily routine management, for the individual and/or the team
- Problem-solving process
- Project management
- Continuous development
- Human resources development
- New product or service development
- Process trials

A few key questions are first asked when applying this cycle: (1) What are we trying to accomplish? (2) How will we know that a change is an improvement? (3) What changes can we make that will result in improvement? After this consideration, the cycle is applied (IHI, 2012; Langley et al., 2009):

1. *Plan.* In step 1, the team describes a plan for the change. Objectives are clarified, and predictions of what will happen are identified. The team plans for the test of change. Planning should consider the five *W*s: (1) who, (2) what, (3) when, (4) where, and (5) why data.
2. *Do.* In step 2, the change is pilot tested using a smaller perspective—for example, on one unit.

3. *Study.* In step 3, the focus is on collecting and analyzing data in order to better understand outcomes. Compare the data with the predictions made in step 1. If the prediction was there would be a certain percentage of staff complaints or errors, was this met? Was it lower or higher, and why? The data are summarized so that the data can be understood and communicated. Note that some who use PDSA have changed the "S" to a "C," or check impact of the change (Sollecito & Johnson, 2013, p. 37).

4. *Act.* In step 4, the change may be adjusted based on what has been learned in the pilot test or trial. Then the next pilot test is planned, or the decision is made to apply the change to the larger system based on the specific purpose of the change initiative.

Brainstorming

Brainstorming is a method used to identify as many ideas as possible so that the ideas can then be assessed to determine if they can be used or should be eliminated. In the beginning of the process, all ideas are considered relevant; they are "put on the table" for consideration and there is no "right" or "wrong" answer, but rather an open forum to explore ideas options. This approach requires input from a variety of people. It is a quick way to identify new ideas. Brainstorming might focus on identifying what the change is that needs to be considered; factors impacting the change; and solutions. Brainstorming may be unstructured or structured. Unstructured brainstorming methods use open discussion and anyone can add ideas at any time, as there is no specific order or process. Brainstorming does not really require any preparation and may be used at any point during meetings to get ideas from the team.

Typically, the risk with asking the team for ideas is that some members may participate more than others do. Structured brainstorming methods use a specific process to elicit the ideas and increase participation, reducing the chance of staff not participating. This type of process uses a leader or facilitator who guides the process. The following are some methods used in structured brainstorming.

Delphi Technique

The **Delphi technique** is easy to use when it is difficult for staff to meet or when anonymity may be needed, such as if staff are concerned that speaking out might have a negative impact on them. Staff are provided with a questionnaire that focuses on a particular problem, and they are asked to identify possible solutions. After the results are compiled, staff who participated in the first round are given a copy of the results. This can be done on the computer; however, if anonymity is a concern and respondents can be identified, another method may need to be used. The respondents are then asked to comment on results from round 1, and these new comments are added to the round 1 results. This activity can continue for many rounds, and the information changes based on discussion results and the deletion or addition of new ideas. This method is time consuming, and participants do not get immediate feedback. Since this is a structured method, it allows time for thought and further examination of the issue or problem.

Nominal Group

The **nominal group** is another method used in brainstorming. It requires participation from all group or team members, avoiding the problem of several members controlling the brainstorming (Fallon et al., 2013). The process works as follows: All members are informed of the process, and the facilitator shares information about the issue to be discussed. Then each member thinks about his or her own ideas related to the issue with no sharing of this information. After this phase, members write down their ideas and submit them to the facilitator. All of the ideas are then documented, numbered, and shared with the entire group or team, leading to a discussion about the proposed ideas and a vote on them. Items with the largest number of votes are considered to be the most important ideas. In some cases, there may be additional rounds and voting. The goal is to ensure that all relevant staff contribute to the change process to reach the most effective decision possible.

Pass the Problem

Pass the problem is a method used after a problem has been described and possible causes identified. The steps are as follows:

1. Staff are divided into groups or could be identified by work teams.
2. The leader creates a folder for each identified problem and potential root causes and gives one folder to each group.
3. Each group generates as many strategies as possible to address the problem in 10 minutes (time frame may vary but should not be long). The strategies are written and added to the folder.
4. Then each group passes its folder to the group on its right. This means each group has a new problem with some potential strategies with some potential strategies to examine.
5. The new group then adds to and refines the existing list of strategies. (Steps 4 and 5 are done several times based on the number of small groups.)
6. After all groups have responded, the last round concludes by having the groups input the list on a PowerPoint slide(s).
7. The PowerPoint slides per problem are then shared.
8. As each problem and its lists of strategies are presented to the entire group, the group discusses each problem and its associated possible strategies one at a time.

Six Hat Method

The **six hat method** is a brainstorming method used by teams to better understand proposals for change (Fallon et al., 2013). During the process, team members assume one of the roles (hats) and discuss the proposal from that perspective. One role/ hat is the facilitator. Using this method helps team members step away from their usual perspectives and better understand all aspects of the proposal as they assume different hats representing different roles.

Stop and Consider #5

Consider how you were involved in change today, in the past week, and in the past month, and reflect on methods that were used to assess and describe the change.

Examples of Methods Used to Describe Planning for Change

The following are a few examples of methods used in planning to describe actions needed, decision processes, and timelines. Additional information is found in other chapters. The Connect to Current Information section at the end of the chapter provides links to sites with examples of some of these methods.

GANTT and PERT Charts

Effective change requires a clear implementation plan with a timeline. A **Gantt chart** may be used to display progress in a project over time. This type of chart is an important part of the plan for change.

Sometimes this type of chart is referred to as a **PERT chart**, where PERT is an acronym for **p**rogram **e**valuation **r**eview **t**echnique. The PERT chart is a visual or graphic representation describing a project or a process using boxes and arrows to illustrate sequence of tasks. It is particularly useful for viewing sequential relationships of project tasks (Langley et al., 2009).

Decision Tree

The **decision tree** is a method that helps to identify alternatives. After a problem is identified, solutions and their potential positive and negative outcomes are identified. The goal is to identify the best solution that will yield the most positive outcomes and the least negative outcomes. The process should include staff involved in the issue or problem.

Conclusions

Now, you may still be thinking, why bother with the topic of change? The truth is you have no choice. Change is a fact of life, and certainly it is a fact of life for an

HCO and its staff. Consider these quotes and note their wide range of dates and the variety of people who have been intrigued by this subject:

- *Nothing is permanent but change.*
  (Heraclitus 535–475 BCE, pre-Socratic Ionian philosopher)
- *Chaos often breeds life, when order breeds habit.*
  (Henry Brooks Adams 1838–1919, American writer and historian)
- *It's been a long time coming. But I know a change is gonna come.*
  (Sam Cooke 1931–1964, American musician)
- *People don't resist change. They resist being changed!*
  (Peter Senge, 1947–, writer focused on management and famous for identifying the concept of the learning organization)
- *I am personally convinced that one person can be a change catalyst, a "transformer" in any situation, any organization. Such an individual is yeast that can leaven an entire loaf. It requires vision, initiative, patience, respect, persistence, courage, and faith to be a transforming leader.*
  (Stephen R. Covey, 1932–, business consultant focusing on leadership; his book *Seven Habits of Highly Effective People* was listed in 2011 as one of the 25 most influential management books)

Apply CQI

Chapter Highlights

- Effective CQI requires use of the change process.
- Not all changes are improvement.
- Change is an ongoing experience in HCOs.
- Critical change theories and models include Lewin's force field theory, Havelock's theory, Kotter's change model, Juran's trilogy model, and appreciative inquiry.
- Many factors—both internal and external to an HCO—influence the need for change.
- Stakeholders need to be identified and engaged in the change process.
- The change process includes the following steps: identification of need, development and engagement of the team requiring leadership and followership, analysis and description of the problem, readiness assessment, selection and development of the solution(s) based on best evidence, testing and implementation of the solution(s), spreading improvement, identification of roles and responsibilities, and evaluation and follow-up.
- Barriers to change need to be identified and addressed.

- Typical barriers to change are lack or readiness, inadequate leadership, groupthink, and inadequate planning.
- The planning for change needs to include interventions/strategies to address current and potential barriers.
- Examples of methods to assess and describe the need for change are solution (SWOT) analysis, the plan-do-study-act (PDSA) approach, and brainstorming, such as the Delphi, nominal group, and pass the problem techniques.
- Examples of methods used to describe planning are GANTT and PERT charts and decision trees.

Critical Thinking and Clinical Reasoning and Judgment: Discussion Questions and Learning Activities

1. Develop a visual that includes a minimum of three of the change theories and models discussed in the chapter. The visual (poster, PowerPoint slides, or other methods) should include the key points in each of the theories/models.
2. After reviewing the change process, apply the information to a change you think should be made in a clinical situation. This can be for a problem you have identified in your clinical experience or based on a new idea you have read about that you think should be applied. Describe what would need to be done for each step of the change process.
3. Based on your response to the preceding exercise, identify the key stakeholders and why they would be considered stakeholders.
4. Assess how you respond to change. Provide several examples in your assessment. What might you do to improve your response to change?
5. Review each of the elements that the Nursing Organizations Alliance believes support a healthful practice/work environment. Provide examples that illustrate the elements from the practice environment that you have observed.

Connect to Current Information

- Examples of SWOT
  http://images.search.yahoo.com/search/images?_adv_prop=image&fr=moz35&va=SWOT
- Examples of decision trees
  http://images.search.yahoo.com/search/images?_adv_prop=image&fr=moz35&va=decision+tree

- Examples of GANTT charts
  http://images.search.yahoo.com/search/images?_adv_prop=image&fr=
     moz35&va=GANTT
- Examples of PERT charts
  https://images.search.yahoo.com/yhs/search?p=Pert+Chart

EBP, EBM and Quality Improvement: Exemplar

Varkey, P., & Antonio, K. (2010). Change management for effective quality improvement:
A primer. *American Journal of Medical Quality, 25*(4), 268–273.
   This article examines change, change management, and quality improvement.

Questions to Consider

1. According to this article, what is the relationship between change
   management and quality improvement?
2. What does the article recommend to better manage change and quality
   improvement?
3. How does the information in the article apply to nursing?

Evolving Case Study

As a staff member who serves on the Quality Improvement Planning Committee,
you are at a meeting to discuss the best way to share information about recent
CQI data so that staff in the hospital can appreciate the value of the data. You
need to identify pros and cons of methods the committee might use to assess
and describe data for planning purposes.

   The committee is mostly new, so some members have limited experience. You
and two other members have the most experience, so you three volunteer to help
the others get up to speed as quickly as possible so that decisions can be made
about steps to take with the data and you can get to decisions about strategies.
You make clear to the other committee members that (1) this is a team effort
and (2) the team must engage hospital staff at all levels. You comment, "We have
tried to keep this to ourselves, thinking only we knew the best approaches, and
we failed." Staff do not feel engaged in CQI and complain about the extra work
for which they see no value.

Case Questions A

The following questions relate to the committee's discussion.

1. What are some of the barriers that could be influencing limited staff
   engagement?
2. What strategies might be used to overcome these barriers?

Case Questions B

Now the committee must move to the work they must do.

1. What are pros and cons to the methods used to assess and describe the need for change (discussed in this chapter)?
2. What are the common reasons staff resist change?
3. How might the committee use GANTT and PERT charts and/or decision trees?

References

Fallon, L., Begun, J., & Riley, W. (2013). *Managing health organizations for quality performance.* Burlington, MA: Jones & Bartlett Learning.

Finkelman, A., & Kenner, C. (2016). *Professional nursing concepts: Competencies for quality leadership* (3rd ed.). Burlington, MA: Jones & Bartlett Learning.

Frieden, J. (2015, August 13). The changing face of medical education: Big data, self-paced learning. Retrieved from http://healthleadersmedia.com/content/HR-319604/The-Changing-Face-of-Medical-Education-Big-Data-SelfPaced-Learning

Havelock, E. (1973). *The change agent's guide to innovation in education.* Englewood Cliffs, NJ: Technology Publication.

Institute for Healthcare Improvement (IHI). (2012). How to improve. Retrieved from http://www.ihi.org/knowledge/Pages/HowtoImprove/default.aspx

Juran, J., & Defeo, J. (Eds.). (2010). *Juran's quality handbook* (6th ed.). Columbus, OH: McGraw-Hill Companies.

Khator, R. (2014). Innovate or perish: The future is here. In M. Fennell & S. Miller (Eds.), *Presidential perspectives, 2014–2015 series: Inspirational innovation* (pp. 4.1–4.4). Philadelphia, PA: Aramark.

Kotter, J. (1996). *Leading change.* Boston, MA: Harvard Business School Press.

Langley, G., Moen, R., Nolan, K., Nolan, T., Norman, C., & Provost, L. (2009). *The improvement guide: A practical approach to enhancing organizational performance* (2nd ed.). San Francisco, CA: Jossey-Bass Publishers.

Lewin, K. (1947). Group and social change. In T. Newcomb & E. Hartely (Eds.), *Readings in social psychology.* New York, NY: Holt, Rinehart, and Winston.

McCannon, C., Schall, M., & Perla, R. (2008). *Planning for scale: A guide for designing large-scale improvement initiatives.* IHI Innovation Series white paper. Cambridge, MA. Retrieved from http://www.ihi.org/resources/pages/ihiwhitepapers/planningforscalewhitepaper.aspx

Nursing Organizations Alliance (The Alliance). (2004). *Principles and elements of a healthful practice/work environment.* Retrieved from http://www.aone.org/resources/healthful-practice-work

Ponti, M. (2011). Why change fails. *Nurse Leader, 9*(8), 41–43.

Quinn, R. (1996). *Deep change: Discovering the leader within.* San Francisco, CA: Jossey-Bass.

Quinn, R. (2000). *Change the world: How ordinary people can accomplish extraordinary results.* San Francisco, CA: Jossey-Bass.

Robinson-Walker, C. (2011). Managing an onslaught of change. *Nurse Leader, 9*(7), 10–11.

Senge, P. (1990). *The fifth discipline: The art and practice of the learning organization.* New York, NY: Doubleday.

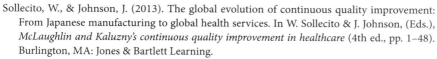

Sollecito, W., & Johnson, J. (2013). The global evolution of continuous quality improvement: From Japanese manufacturing to global health services. In W. Sollecito & J. Johnson, (Eds.), *McLaughlin and Kaluzny's continuous quality improvement in healthcare* (4th ed., pp. 1–48). Burlington, MA: Jones & Bartlett Learning.

Swearingen, J. (2008, August 18). What is appreciative inquiry? CBS money watch. Retrieved from http://www.cbsnews.com/news/what-is-appreciative-inquiry/

U.S. Department of Health and Human Services (HHS), Agency for Healthcare Research and Quality (AHRQ). (2015, June). In conversation with... Maureen Bisognano. Retrieved from http://webmm.ahrq.gov/perspective.aspx?perspectiveId=178

U.S. Department of Health and Human Services (HHS), Health Resources and Services Administration (HRSA). (2015). Quality improvement. Retrieved from http://www.hrsa.gov/quality/toolbox/methodology/qualityimprovement/part3.html

Weick, K., &. Quinn, R. (1999). Organization change and development. *Annual Review of Psychology, 50*, 361–386.

Whatis.com. (2015). Appreciative inquiry. Retrieved from http://whatis.techtarget.com/definition/Appreciative-inquiry-AI

Value Based Management.net. (2011) The Deming cycle. Retrieved from http://www.valuebasedmanagement.net/methods_demingcycle.html

Section II

Understanding the Healthcare Environment to Improve Care

"No, no! The adventures first, explanations take such a dreadful time."

Lewis Carroll, *Alice's Adventures in Wonderland* (1865)

© Mopic/Shutterstock

The goal of the maze is to reach a state of quality care. The maze may not be clear enough for you to fully appreciate quality improvement. To do this you must engage in continuous quality improvement planning and the measurement process within the healthcare environment. Neither is easy to understand and takes time. It is at this time that the patient enters and is the center of all activities. How do you find the information you need to understand all of this, and where does the information take you? To an effective CQI plan and measurement that meets CQI outcomes.

CHAPTER 5

Entering the Quality Improvement World

CHAPTER OBJECTIVES

At the conclusion of this chapter, the learner will be able to:

- Compare and contrast examples of quality care theories, models, and approaches.
- Analyze the impact of the blame culture.
- Examine the impact of a culture of safety on continuous quality improvement.
- Appraise the process for assessing and planning to implement a culture of safety.

OUTLINE

KEY TERMS

Accountability	Healthcare disparity	Rapid cycle model
Blame culture	Healthcare equity	Reliability
Code of silence	Healthcare inequality	Science of improvement
Consonant culture	High-reliability organization	Six Sigma
Cultural competence	Just culture	Social determinants of health
Culture	Lean approach	STEEEP®
Culture of safety	Linguistic competence	Triple aim
Dissonant culture	Organizational culture	

Introduction

In 2015, Dr. Gandhi, Chief Executive of the National Patient Safety Foundation (NPSF), looked back over the development of patient safety and quality since *To Err Is Human* (IOM, 1999) was published (IHI, 2015b). This review has relevance to this chapter as we begin to examine the continuous quality improvement (CQI) world—what it is and approaches that might be taken to provide a framework for the CQI work that is done by individual healthcare providers and healthcare organizations (HCOs). Dr. Gandhi notes that the first focus was to convince us we had a problem—we lacked the level of quality care we should have. This effort is ongoing, but the focus now is more on answering the questions, how do we improve and what type of **culture** and leadership are needed to accomplish improvement? Since 1999, the culture has changed, engaging the staff, including frontline workers, and incorporating health informatics technology (HIT). Change has been discussed and will continue to be a theme throughout this text. Engaging staff begins with knowledge; a major goal of this text is to provide more information and resources for nurses, and as noted earlier, healthcare professions education must include more content about CQI and its relationship to HIT. This is an expanding area, providing us with more data, better analysis methods, and more timely communication. This chapter discusses issues related to the current focus.

Creating a Vision of Quality Care: Theories, Models, and Approaches

There are many references that could be used to introduce this section about the vision of quality care. Since this text focuses on nurses and their engagement in CQI, we will turn to the *Quality Chasm* report *Keeping Patients Safe: Transforming the Work Environment of Nurses* (IOM, 2004a). Looking at the title of the report, there are two critical messages: (1) The patient is mentioned first, and (2) the term *transforming* is used. These choices communicate a message of positive change focused on patients. The nurse's work environment is also included in the title, and this consideration is critical if we are to meet required patient outcomes. The 2004 report makes five recommendations that nursing must consider (IOM, 2004a):

- Implementing evidence-based management
- Balancing tension between efficiency and reliability
- Creating and sustaining trust
- Actively managing the change process through communication, training, feedback, sustained effort and attention, and worker involvement
- Creating a learning organization

As noted in the discussion about the healthcare professions core competencies in other sections of this text, these competencies do not separate out safety from quality. Safety is a "central aim of quality" (The Joint Commission, 2015), a part of quality care. Typically, HCOs do have a structural component such as an organizational unit (e.g., department, service) focused on quality improvement, and that work includes safety for staff and patients. In the end, quality must become a systemwide attribute—so much a part of the system that it is never thought of as a separate aspect of an organization.

Current quality improvement frameworks/models tend to emphasis the six dimensions of quality care noted in the earlier *Quality Chasm* reports (IOM, 1999, 2001). The dimensions are safety, timeliness, effectiveness, efficiency, equity, and patient-centeredness (STEEEP). Even with these dimensions, quality is not a static concept (Powell, Rushmer, & Davies, 2009). The dynamic (changing) nature of health care is demonstrated in the various current models of quality improvement. There are key similarities but also some differences in these models. Some of the models were developed specifically for health care, and others are borrowed from other industries and then adapted as needed and applied to health care. Quality improvement is also viewed as a journey, implying movement and change; data are collected, and when needed, changes are initiated (Storme, 2013). According to the Health Resources and Services Administration of the U.S. Department of Health and Human Services (HHS), "An organization that implements a quality improvement program experiences a range of benefits," including the following (HHS, HRSA, 2011b, p. 6):

- *Improved patient health (clinical) outcomes that involve both process outcomes (e.g., provide recommended screenings) and health outcomes (e.g., decreased morbidity and mortality).*
- *Improved efficiency of managerial and clinical processes.* By improving processes and outcomes relevant to high-priority health needs, an organization reduces waste and costs associated with system failures and redundancy. Often quality improvement processes are budget-neutral, where the costs to make the changes are offset by the cost savings incurred.
- *Avoided costs associated with process failures, errors, and poor outcomes.* Costs are incurred when nonstandard and inefficient systems increase errors and cause rework. Streamlined and reliable processes are less expensive to maintain.
- *Proactive processes that recognize and solve problems before they occur ensure that systems of care are reliable and predictable.* A culture of improvement frequently develops in an organization that is committed to quality because errors are reported and addressed.
- *Improved communication with resources that are internal and external to an organization, such as, funders and civic and community organizations.*

A commitment to quality shines a positive light on an organization, which may result in an increase of partnership and funding opportunities. When successfully implemented, a quality improvement infrastructure often enhances communication and resolves critical issues.

Dailey (2013) offers a useful description of quality, saying, "Quality is a concept. It expresses people's perceptions of what makes something seem better or worse in some way that can only be measured by proxy, comparison, or using some abstract metric." The following are principles on which quality is based (Galt, Paschal, & Gleason, 2011, p. 8):

1. Healthcare professionals are intrinsically motivated to improve patient safety because of the ethical foundation, professional norms, and expectations of our respective disciplines.
2. Organizational leaders are responsible for setting the standards for achieving safety at the highest level and in response to societal expectations.
3. Consumers are becoming increasingly aware of healthcare safety problems and are not accepting of it.
4. There is substantial room for improvement of healthcare systems and practices that will result in a reduction in both error potential and harm.

There are a variety of models and theories that apply to quality improvement. HCOs typically use one of them, a combination, or adapt one or two to serve as a guide for their quality improvement program. The following discussion describes some of the common models and theories.

Science of Improvement

According to the Institute for Healthcare Improvement (IHI) (2015c):

The **science of improvement** is an applied science that emphasizes innovation, rapid-cycle testing in the field, and spread in order to generate learning about what changes, in which contexts, produce improvements. It is characterized by the combination of expert subject knowledge with improvement methods and tools. It is multidisciplinary—drawing on clinical science, systems theory, psychology, statistics, and other fields.

It requires clear goals, which implies a plan and measurement. The science of improvement focuses on three questions that the HCO should ask (IHI, 2015c).

1. *What are we trying to accomplish?* This question focuses on assessment, description of issues, and development of goals and a plan.
2. *How will we know that a change is an improvement?* This question is based on using the plan as a guide to identify outcomes and measurements required.

3. *What changes can we make that will result in improvement?* This question considers changes/interventions/strategies that will lead to improvement.

The **rapid cycle model** is associated with the science of improvement and related to these three key questions. The approach is used to pilot test small changes recommended by frontline staff and actively engage staff in the CQI process, recognizing that small changes can impact the HCO with positive outcomes. The plan-do-study-act (PDSA) model is used to respond to needs and move toward improvement. PDSA is discussed in other sections of the text. Using this approach emphasizes frontline staff identification of needs for change and actively engages staff; there is then less need to "force" changes on staff (Powell et al., 2009).

Improvement capability needs to be considered to ensure that the science of improvement focuses on CQI to reach improvement outcomes. Efforts include the following (IHI, 2015a):

- Building science-based improvement capability at individual, organizational, and system levels
- Arming future doctors and nurses and others preparing for careers in health care with quality improvement knowledge and skills before they enter the workforce
- Expanding the capability of middle managers and other operational leaders to use advanced improvement methods to guide and support frontline improvement
- Developing learning networks to accelerate implementation, spread, and scale-up of innovative approaches to improve health outcomes
- Providing a clear road map for how organizations applying the lean approach and Six Sigma (discussed later) can use the science of improvement to accelerate results
- Providing individuals, professional groups, organizations, and whole systems with the right "dose" of improvement capability to drive results

The Triple Aim

In 2008, the IHI proposed a framework for CQI, which is called the **triple aim** (Stiefel & Nolan, 2012). Since its development, it is now used globally, and it had an impact on the Affordable Care Act of 2010 (ACA). It is also a critical part of the National Quality Strategy (NQS), which is discussed in multiple chapters of this text (Whittington, Nolan, Lewis, & Torres, 2015). The triple aim is to (1) improve the patient experience of care (including quality and satisfaction), (2) improve the health of populations, and (3) reduce the per capita cost of health care (IHI, 2015d). **Figure 5-1** describes the triple aim framework as it relates to STEEEP.

Figure 5-1. Triple Aim:
Experience of Care

The triple aim framework acknowledges that all three aims must be pursued together, as they are interdependent, and HCOs should clarify responsibilities for these aims. Meeting these aims requires a systems approach to change.

The triple aim considers constraints that require a balance in the CQI process; for example, when considering costs and who gets care, there should be equity of care. As Berwick, Nolan, and Whittington (2008) state, "The gain in health in one subpopulation ought not to be achieved at the expense of another subpopulation. But that decision lies in the realms of ethics and policy" (p. 760). Diversity and disparities in health care remain a critical concern, and when one gets into this area, ethics becomes even more important. Berwick and colleagues comment that the United States has the technical methods for data collection, measurement, and analysis to monitor and improve care to meet the triple aim, but the biggest barrier is whether or not there is drive to make changes in HCOs and maintain them.

Structure, Process, Outcomes Model

The *Quality Chasm* reports' definition of quality care incorporates the model of healthcare quality described many years ago by Donabedian (1980). This model, described in **Figure 5-2**, focuses on three aspects of the healthcare delivery system: structure, process, and outcomes. Most types of healthcare settings have used this model to understand and evaluate quality. Structure focuses on how the organization is organized—the system and its parts, including its facilities, finances, supplies

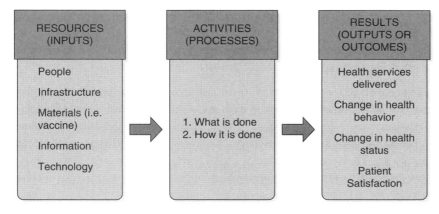

Figure 5-2. Inputs/Structure, Processes, and Outputs/Outcomes
Reproduced with permission from Donabedian, A. (1980). *Explorations in quality assessment and monitoring, Volume 1: The definitions of quality and approaches to its assessment.* Ann Arbor, MI: Health Administration Press. Reproduced with permission from Health Administration Press.

and equipment, informatics (hardware and software), staff and staffing, clinical expertise, and so on. Process considers how the parts interact and function and also the interaction with patients and healthcare providers, including assessment and diagnosis, coordination, patient education, delivery of care, and use of HIT. Outcomes should indicate that care meets the STEEEP criteria and should include long-term outcomes to improve functioning and quality of life (Lawless & Proujansky, 2006). As stated by Donabedian, (1988), "Good structure increases the likelihood of good process, and good process increases the likelihood of good outcomes" (p. 1147).

CQI: A Systematic Approach

CQI is the approach that is now recommended for all HCOs and providers. Sollecito and Johnson (2013) define CQI as "a structured organizational process for involving personnel in planning and executing a continuous flow of improvements to provide quality healthcare that meets or exceeds expectations" (p. 4). They go on to define the following characteristics of CQI (Sollecito & Johnson, 2013, pp. 4–5):

- A link to key elements of the organization's strategic plan
- A quality committee made up of the institution's top leadership
- Training programs for personnel
- Mechanisms for selecting improvement opportunities
- Formation of process improvement teams
- Staff support for process analysis and redesign; staff engagement and commitment

- Personnel policies that motivate and support staff participation in process improvement
- Application of the most current and rigorous techniques of the scientific method and statistical process control

The goal of CQI is to improve or streamline activities, which should be a continuous process. This model focuses on data, leadership, and active participation from all relevant staff levels. Applying CQI means the HCO manages its performance, motivates improvement among staff, and learns from its experiences. As the Health Resources and Services Administration (2011) explains, "It is an ongoing effort to improve the efficiency, effectiveness, quality, or performance of services, processes, capacities, and outcomes." The following key strategies are often used in CQI (Draper, Felland, Liebhaber, & Melichar, 2008, p. 3):

- Having supportive hospital leadership and keeping them actively engaged in the work
- Setting expectations for all staff—not just nurses—that quality is a shared responsibility
- Holding staff accountable for individual roles and responsbilities
- Inspiring and using physicians and nurses to champion efforts
- Providing ongoing, visible, and useful feedback to engage staff effectively

The main elements of this model are to first know the customer (patient) well and connect this understanding with the daily functions of the HCO. Secondly, there is need to develop the HCO culture through leadership emphasizing commitment, pride in the HCO, and use of scientific thinking. The third element is to use organized methods to collect and analyze data and make decisions based on this measurement (Berwick, 1999). Empowerment of staff is critical, as is controlling variation. Healthcare professionals usually like to be in control, which sometimes makes coping with patient variations difficult, impacting reliability and quality. In a systematic review focused on quality improvement models, the authors note the following strengths of CQI:

> It emphasizes determining and meeting the needs and wishes of patients or customers; it aims at a holistic approach to quality improvement based on identifying the underlying causes of poor performance; it emphasizes fact-based management and scientific methodology and may therefore be culturally compatible with the values of health professionals; and it emphasizes the need to improve quality on a daily basis. (Powell et al., 2009, p. 27; Shortell, Bennett, & Byck, 1998)

Culture of Accountability

HCOs want to effectively use evidence-based practice (EBP) and evidence-based management (EBM) to support individual staff in learning and engaging in CQI.

To do this, HCOs must adopt a culture of accountability (O'Hagan & Persaud, 2009). **Accountability**, or being responsible for what you do and the outcomes, should be integrated into the HCO and supported in performance requirements, orientation and staff education, and ongoing performance measurement. Increasing staff accountability means staff are more tuned into value and costs such as working toward reducing overuse, misuse, and underuse of resources. Change is present and should be dealt with routinely by staff.

STEEEP®: Pursuit of Excellence

STEEEP® is a framework that is based on the six aims identified in the *Quality Chasm* series (safety, timeliness, effectiveness, efficiency, equity, patient-centeredness) (IOM, 2001). This framework was developed and trademarked by Baylor Scott & White Health (Texas). It integrates Kotter's change model, discussed in this text, and applies PDSA (Baylor Scott & White, 2014; Mayberry, Nicewander, Qin, & Ballard, 2006). It is based on four principles: Develop a strong customer focus, apply CQI, engage staff, and use data to improve decision-making. A performance improvement team is used to ensure accountability and improvement. Resources on the website for this framework provide support to implement the framework (Baylor Scott & White, 2014). The implementation plan includes the plan itself, organization or structure to meet the plan, communication, required education, motivation strategies, and measurement and review of performance.

The Lean Approach to Quality Improvement

The **lean approach** in healthcare quality improvement focuses on value to the customer, the patient, with efforts made to reduce waste in time, effort, and cost—doing more with less (Litvak & Bisganon, 2011; Powell et al., 2009). This approach was adopted from Toyota and later applied to healthcare delivery. As the Health Resources and Services Administration (2011a) explains, "This model defines value by what a customer (patient) wants. It maps how value flows to the customer, and ensures the competency of the process by making it cost effective and time efficient" (p. 8). The ACA and other government requirements now focus more on value and cost. This leads to a more lean perspective and strategies (Johnson, Smith, & Mastro, 2012).

A concern that staff may have with this model is its emphasis on reducing costs, and this might have major implications for staffing and the work environment (Powell et al., 2009). It might also develop healthcare systems that are more structured and less flexible. To avoid this response, HCOs need to assess themselves periodically to ensure that they are not overemphasizing reducing cost and failing to view the larger perspective and needs. A published review of 34 studies on the use of the lean approach with Transforming Care at the Bedside (TCAB), examined the impact of eliminating non-value-added activities on direct care or time at the bedside (Brackett, Comer, & Whichello, 2013). The review concludes the following:

> Although Lean and TCAB processes may be effective in the improvement of specific outcomes, there is no direct relationship with the implementation of these processes and time spent at the bedside. Furthermore, it is evident that organizations must be in a position to commit valuable time and resources to the implementation of these strategies. (Brackett et al., 2013, p. 13)

If the lean model is used, leaders need to be open about its purpose and allow staff time to discuss their fears, which may not be based on reality. The typical wastes within HCOs that need to be assessed are unnecessary motion, unnecessary transportation (movement of supplies, equipment, people, information throughout the HCO), defects and errors, waiting, inadequate inventory, processing waste, overproduction, and unused human potential (Six Sigma, 2015). Within every process, there are opportunities to eliminate lean waste. The acronym DOWNTIME illustrates these wastes; for example, waste during the hospital discharge process may exist in these eight forms (HHS, AHRQ, 2011):

- *Defects, or failure modes.* Examples: omission of discharge order, omission of follow-up appointment, incorrect selection of medication, failure to provide discharge prescriptions, incomplete discharge instructions, failure to assess patient comprehension, and omission of home medical equipment order
- *Overproduction.* Example: overproduction of printed discharge teaching sheets that are not individualized or that become outdated
- *Waiting.* Examples: wait times for patient information prior to discharge; staff waiting for medications for discharge patients
- *Non-value-added processing.* Examples: rework and redundancies
- *Transportation.* Example: too few wheelchairs creating discharge delays
- *Inventory.* Example: over- or undersupply of medical treatment supplies needed to prepare patients for discharge
- *Motion.* Examples: having to go to another location to retrieve discharge materials instead of having them nearby or at the point of service;stooping, stretching, pulling, or pushing inappropriately
- *Employee (i.e., underutilizing or not using staff-based knowledge).* Example: not including staff members who perform the actual work as part of the problem-solving process

The lean approach does not support use of workarounds, a subject discussed in other chapters, and looks to resolve problems at their root (Brackett et al., 2013). In doing this, it is believed that inefficient processes can be improved.

Six Sigma

Six Sigma is a measurement-based strategy, and it is another approach that began outside of health care. It includes three key elements (Fallon, Begun, & Riley, 2013, p. 265): (1) Measure work output, (2) apply the process throughout all departments in an organization, until it eventually becomes part of the organization's culture, and (3) maintain a goal of no more than 3.4 errors per 1,000,000 operations. This framework focuses more on statistical methods that are used to identify and remove errors (Kelly, Johnson, & Sollecito, 2013). A defect is "an outcome that does not meet the requirements of its customers" (Ramaswamy & Barker, 2013, p. 548). Reducing process variability increases opportunity to reduce defects. Examples of defects might be long wait times for an appointment, long wait time in the emergency department for inpatient admission, medications not arriving on time from the pharmacy, and communication barriers. CQI projects are conducted using DMAIC (define, measure, analyze, improve, control) and DMADV (define, measure, analyze, design, verify) to guide development of new processes (HHS, HRSA, 2011a, p. 8). These methods are discussed in other chapters. Some HCOs combine the lean model with Six Sigma, calling it Lean Six Sigma, with both models using small changes tested over time, focusing on analyzing processes and use of mapping to achieve improvement.

High-Reliability Organization

High-reliability organizations (HROs) have become more common in health care. HROs are HCOs that use a three-step approach to high reliability (Nolan, Resar, Haraden, & Griffin, 2004). The six dimensions of quality health care are integrated into HROs. What is **reliability?** It is the state of being failure-free that develops in an environment over time. "Over time," as mentioned here, is a critical aspect, as it is not a one-time viewpoint of quality, but rather consistent, effective performance, which ties in with CQI. The concept of "over time" also applies to the HCO and individual patient trajectories.

Reliability is measured by the following formula:

$$\text{Reliability} = \text{Number of actions that achieve the intended result} \div \text{Total number of actions taken}$$

HROs are *mindful* organizations in that they are concerned about processes, how they work, and their results" (Nolan et al., 2004, p. 3). Average or low-performing organizations are typically described as bureaucratic and reactive (with managers and leaders focused on self), risk averse, and oriented around control and lack of information at the managerial level (Ettinger, 2006, p. 125). To implement and retain reliability requires concentrated effort. Leaders in HROs commit to actively developing and maintaining CQI (Fallon et al., 2013). **Table 5-1** provides information about critical characteristics of HROs.

TABLE 5-1 Characteristics of High-Reliability Organizations	
Characteristic	**Description**
Preoccupation with failure	Everyone is aware of and thinking about the potential for failure. People understand that new threats emerge regularly from situations that no one imagined could occur, so all personnel actively think about what could go wrong and are alert to small signs of potential problems. The absence of errors or accidents leads not to complacency but to a heightened sense of vigilance for the next possible failure. Near misses are viewed as opportunities to learn about systems issues and potential improvements, rather than as evidence of safety.
Reluctance to simplify	People resist simplifying their understanding of work processes and how and why things succeed or fail in their environment. People in high-reliability organizations (HROs) understand that the work is complex and dynamic. They seek underlying rather than surface explanations. While HROs recognize the value of standardization of workflows to reduce variation, they also appreciate the complexity inherent in the number of teams, processes, and relationships involved in conducting daily operations.
Sensitivity to operations	Based on their understanding of operational complexity, people in HROs strive to maintain a high awareness of operational conditions. This sensitivity is often referred to as "big picture understanding" or "situation awareness." It means that people cultivate an understanding of the context of the current state of their work in relation to the unit or organizational state—i.e., what is going on around them—and how the current state might support or threaten safety.
Deference to expertise	People in HROs appreciate that the people closest to the work are the most knowledgeable about the work. Thus, people in HROs know that in a crisis or emergency the person with greatest knowledge of the situation might not be the person with the highest status and seniority. Deference to local and situation expertise results in a spirit of inquiry and de-emphasis on hierarchy in favor of learning as much as possible about potential safety threats. In an HRO, everyone is expected to share concerns with others, and the organizational climate is such that all staff members are comfortable speaking up about potential safety problems.
Commitment to resilience	Commitment to resilience is rooted in the fundamental understanding of the frequently unpredictable nature of system failures. People in HROs assume the system is at risk for failure, and they practice performing rapid assessments of and responses to challenging situations. Teams cultivate situation assessment and cross monitoring so they may identify potential safety threats quickly and either respond before safety problems cause harm or mitigate the seriousness of the safety event.

Reproduced with permission from AHRQ Patient Safety Network, Lyndon, A., Wachter, R.M., & Hartman, E.E. (September 2015). Patient safety primer: High reliability. Retrieved from https://psnet.ahrq.gov/primers/primer/31.

Other chapters discuss CQI measurement and improvement interventions/ strategies in more detail; however, to provide a better description of HROs, one might ask what would this organization do to meet the three-step approach? The Agency for Healthcare Research and Quality's Patient Safety Network (2015) explains, "HROs cultivate resilience by relentlessly prioritizing safety over other performance pressures." These HCOs use systems thinking throughout the organization, with recognition that the HCO is not static and change is ongoing. The goal is to create and maintain an environment "in which potential problems are anticipated, detected early, and virtually always responded to early enough to prevent catastrophic consequences" (HHS, AHRQ, PSNet, 2016).

The following are recommended levels of interventions/strategies to develop and maintain an HRO (Nolan et al., 2004).

1. Prevent failure (a breakdown in operations or functions).
2. Identify and mitigate failure (identify failure when it occurs and intercede before harm is caused, or mitigate the harm caused by failures that are not detected and intercepted).
3. Redesign the process based on the critical failures identified.

Accomplishing these strategies requires HCO leadership, an active safety culture, and an effective process of improvement initiative that supports reliability. Since reliability was first used in non-healthcare industries, this is another example of applying methods and approaches used by other industries.

In an HRO, management and staff might use standardization, for example, by using checklists and actively providing staff feedback. The HCO also uses structured communication methods with patients and staff such as calling patients to remind them of appointments or making sure communication is clear when using abbreviations and numbers to avoid errors. The organization might apply failure modes and effects analysis (FMEA) as a method to improve structure and processes. FMEA is discussed in other chapters.

Chassin and Loeb (2011) discuss the complex nature of care delivery and its impact on reliability: "As new devices, equipment, procedures, and drugs are added to our therapeutic arsenal, the complexity of delivering effective care increases. Complexity greatly increases the likelihood of error, especially in systems that perform at low levels of reliability" (p. 563). HROs are driven to ensure that the organization functions at its best level despite this complexity. Many new approaches to improve care have been developed and applied. In this text, many of these approaches are discussed. The field requires more collective mindfulness, with every individual, the HCO as whole, and all its parts working to identify potential failures that can lead to adverse events. One approach supported by the IHI emphasizes that "applying reliability principles to health care has the potential to help reduce 'defects' in care or care processes, increase the consistency with which appropriate care is delivered, and improve patient outcomes" (Nolan et al., 2004, p. 3). Connecting reliability to several of the *Quality Chasm* reports' healthcare system aims, the following are important to consider: "effectiveness (where failure can result from not applying evidence), timeliness (where failure results from not taking action in the required time), and patient-centeredness (where failure results from not complying with patients' values and preferences)" (Nolan et al., 2004, p. 3).

The Agency for Healthcare Research and Quality: Quality Improvement Process

The Agency for Healthcare Research and Quality (AHRQ) is the major agency in the HHS that guides national efforts toward improving quality. The NQS, discussed in other chapters, is the current major initiative that it is expected to guide efforts to meet this goal. The AHRQ not only sets a model or framework, but also works with stakeholders in implementation efforts to improve care (Dixon & Shofar, 2006). The agency is also concerned with ensuring that evidence from research is implemented into practice when appropriate—to fill the gap in knowledge (EBP and EBM). With the expansion of research and the concern for use of best practice evidence falling through the cracks, this in itself is a major effort. The AHRQ supports the development of HROs and the CQI process based on STEEEP.

The AHRQ focuses its CQI process on various healthcare settings, such as the hospital. The process uses administrative and clinical data to assess quality, identify problems or concerns that require more examination, and determine what needs to be monitored over time (HHS, AHRQ, 2014). When implementing the CQI process, the AHRQ recommends applying the following, which are not only supported by the government but also healthcare professional groups (HHS, AHRQ, 2015a):

- *Place a priority on encouraging communication, engagement, and participation.* Include the stakeholders involved with or affected by the changes required by your CQI work. Look for ways to help them embrace the changes and begin to take ownership of them.
- *Start your implementation of improvements with small-scale demonstrations.* Small-scale demonstrations are easier to manage than are large-scale changes. They also allow you to refine the new processes, demonstrate their impact on practices and outcomes, and build increased support by stakeholders. Some HCOs refer to this as pilot testing.
- *Keep in mind and remind others that CQI is an iterative process.* You will be making frequent corrections along the way as you learn from experience with each step and identify other actions to add to your strategy.

Stop and Consider #1

There are multiple theories and models about quality improvement that an HCO can choose to apply.

The Blame Culture and Its Impact

The *Quality Chasm* reports noted that were there problems not only with the quality of care, but also with responses to errors. The reports indicated that HCOs emphasized a work culture that focused on blame.

Organizational Culture

Organizations have their own cultures, and the culture impacts how the organization is structured and functions. **Organizational culture** is the values, beliefs, traditions, and communication processes that bring a group of people together and characterize the organization. The culture also impacts teams and teamwork within the HCO. As explained by Heathfield (2012), "Culture is a powerful element that shapes your work enjoyment, your work relationships, and your work processes. But, culture is something that you cannot actually see, except through its physical manifestations in your workplace."

An organization's culture is complex. There is the overall organizational culture, such as the culture of a hospital. Then within an organization, there are differences in culture within its units, divisions, or departments and with staff groups, such as nurses, physicians, nonclinical staff, management, and so on. Ideally, all should reflect the overall organizational culture, but this is typically not the case. Lack of an overall organizational culture may actually lead to conflict if there are major differences in values, attitudes, and behaviors. Sometimes these differences are due to differences in leadership style, and sometimes it comes more from the staff. Organizational culture does change over time and is influenced by changes in high-level leadership and the organization's vision, mission, and goals. Communication is a critical element in an organization's culture, and it is complex, with many levels and a great number of staff and services. Organizational culture includes language, decision-making, symbols, stories and legends, and daily work practices (Heathfield, 2012).

Organizational culture may be described as consonant and dissonant. A **consonant culture** implies that the organization's culture is effective. A **dissonant culture** acts as a block to effectiveness and thus has a negative impact on the development of a collaborative team environment. How does one identify a dissonant organization? The following characteristics of a dissonant culture were identified in Sovie (1993) and were described again in Jones & Redman (2000, p. 605). Added to these characteristics are comments about the current relevance of the characteristics:

- *Focus on serving the providers and not the patients.* This focus would be in conflict with the movement today to increase patient-centered care.
- *Lack of clarity about individual and department expectations.* Staff who do not know what is expected may become frustrated, and this lack of clarity may also impact staff burnout, productivity, and outcomes.

- *Failure to regularly measure quality of services.* There is more measurement of quality today with the increased emphasis and concern about problems in quality of care; however, the effectiveness of the measurement and response varies. We have need for much improvement and development of more effective measurement.
- *Lack of patient involvement in decision-making.* Patient-centered care requires patient involvement in decision-making; however, we have much to do to improve. Some providers are not as committed as they should be to ensuring patient participation, or there may be other barriers to patient involvement.
- *Limited concern about employee satisfaction.* This can be a major problem and lead to problems of staff frustration and burnout, recruitment and retention issues, lower productivity, and a culture that is not seen as caring of staff.
- *Limited education/training programs for employees.* This can lead to the same problems noted for employee satisfaction but may also have a major impact on quality of care and increasing errors.
- *Frequent turf battles.* This is clearly a sign of an organization that is not functioning well, demonstrating lack of cohesiveness (i.e., no clear vision, mission, and goals), poor communication, and lack of collaboration.
- *Failure to recognize staff accomplishment.* This leads to poor relationships between upper and middle management and staff, decreasing trust and commitment to the organization.

Improving the culture so that the organization is a place where people want to work makes a major difference in how the organization functions and its outcomes. However, this is not something that is solely in the hands of upper or even middle management. All staff must work to improve the organization's culture. This requires taking risks, being clear about perspectives, and communicating needs and goals effectively. Effective teams exist in effective organizational cultures.

Description of a Blame Culture

The publication of *To Err Is Human* led to significant consideration of the approach HCOs had been taking toward errors (IOM, 1999). The report suggested a tendency of HCOs to examine errors with a focus on assigning blame to individuals. This approach results in what is often referred to as a **blame culture**. It is clear that this approach has not worked; errors continue to rise and quality care continues to decrease. The blame culture has led to a work environment in which staff fear blame when "things go wrong." Being assigned blame may lead to punishment, such as forcing staff to attend a medication administration course or identifying staff "at fault" in some way. There are situations where individuals are the reason for an error, but many errors are system errors, and individual staff are merely involved in the system. Effective CQI requires that both system and individual factors be considered.

Stop and Consider #2

The blame culture impacts nursing practice and continuous quality improvement.

Culture of Safety

Following the identification of a healthcare system that uses a blame culture to respond to errors in HCOs, the *Quality Chasm* reports and other experts recommended a change to a culture of safety, also known as a no blame culture or a just culture.

Description

Bashaw, Rosenstein, and Launsbury (2012) describe a **culture of safety** as

> a system of shared accountability that supports the safest hospital environments for patients, staff, and visitors. Organizations that adopt the just culture model accept that errors will occur, with or without negative outcomes. Each type of error is equally important to disclose because error identification and reporting promote trust, transparency, high-quality care, and patient safety across disciplines . . . . [A culture of safety] embraces system failures, errors, and weaknesses for the purpose of turning them into opportunities for improvement and learning" (2012, p. 38)

A related term is **just culture**. According to the AHRQ's Patient Safety Network, this culture recognizes that

> many individual or active errors represent predictable interactions between human operators and the systems in which they work. However, in contrast to a culture that touts "no blame" as its governing principle, a just culture does not tolerate conscious disregard of clear risks to patients or gross misconduct (e.g., falsifying a record, performing professional duties while intoxicated). (HHS, AHRQ, PSNet, 2015)

This culture supports staff behaviors throughout the HCO that result in "safe, reliable, and productive performance," meeting four critical dimensions of a culture of safety (Drenkard, 2011, pp. 28–29):

- A strategic focus at the top levels in the organization on cultural improvements and error reduction
- A comprehensive assessment of past, present, and future human performance leading to a prioritized improvement plan

- Systematic implementation of improvement initiatives using proven prevention, detection, and correction methods
- An appreciation that maintaining a strong safety culture is a lifelong endeavor for the organization

Some refer to the culture of safety as a no blame culture because the focus moves away from individual blame; however, this reluctance to assign blame can go too far. This type of work culture should not imply that there is no individual accountability (Wachter & Pronovost, 2009). Healthcare providers are still responsible for following their professional standards and regulatory requirements, such as their states' Nurse Practice Acts and HCO standards, policies, and procedures, and need to acknowledge when they lack knowledge or expertise. The goal is to develop leadership and staff commitment to quality care. Within this culture, strategies are used to increase staff self-awareness; improve staff education about quality, errors, and error reporting to improve performance; and meet standards set by healthcare professions, government, accreditors, and insurers. Meeting these objectives requires effective communication and interprofessional teamwork.

The American Nurses Association (ANA) entered the discussion about just culture in 2010 when it published a position statement on this topic (ANA, 2010). The goal was to understand the concept and implications for nurses. The ANA supports the use of just culture in HCOs and initiatives to support its use. There is recognition that a threatening and punitive approach to errors results in limited staff reporting of errors. The ANA position statement emphasizes system errors but does not negate the importance of individual accountability. A culture of safety or just culture views errors from three perspectives (ANA, 2010):

1. Human error, which refers to inadvertently making an error or doing something that should not have been done
2. At-risk behavior that may lead to errors
3. Behavior that does not consider standards and expectations

The focus should be on reducing errors in an environment that is open and allows staff to discuss issues. Nurses should be actively involved in the culture of safety and serve as leaders. Nurses should have input into the HCO structure, processes, and outcomes—for example, ensuring staffing levels for more effective care, participating in policy and procedure development that is based on EBP, engaging in CQI responsibilities as an individual provider, and participating in HCO-organized CQI activities. Individual staff need to feel comfortable reporting concerns, which relates to the staff's sense of accountability for system improvement. The overall result for the HCO should be "an organization-wide mindset that positively impacts the work environment and work outcomes" (ANA, 2010, p. 6). **Figure 5-3** describes data published in 2015 that the AHRQ collected to better understand hospital patient safety culture.

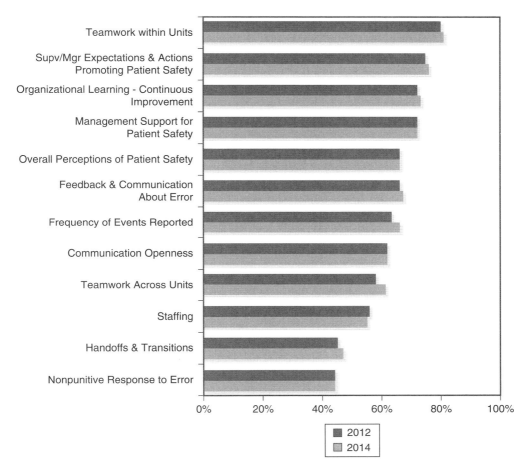

Figure 5-3. Hospital Patient Safety Culture Survey Results
Reproduced from Agency for Healthcare Research and Quality. (April 2015). 2014 national healthcare quality and disparities report: Chartbook on patient safety. AHRQ Publication No. 15-0007-2. Retrieved from http://www.ahrq.gov/sites/default/files/wysiwyg/research/findings/nhqrdr/2014chartbooks/patientsafety/2014nhqdr-ptsafety.pdf

System and Individual Concerns

An example of system concern can be found in a 2015 AHRQ decision to update its Hospital Survey of Patient Safety Culture, which was developed in 2004. After feedback and further development, a pilot test of the revised survey was conducted in 2016. There are also surveys for nursing homes, ambulatory outpatient medical offices, community pharmacies, and ambulatory surgery centers. The AHRQ provides a database so that HCOs can compare their data with data from similar HCOs. Using this comparative approach provides information about the HCO's strengths and helps to identify opportunities for improvement of the patient safety culture. The following describes the objectives for the 2015 changes and provides examples of how this initiative considered multiple factors that might lessen the blame focus in the survey questions (HHS, AHRQ, 2015b):

1. Shift to a just culture framework for understanding responses to errors.
2. Reduce the number of negatively worded items.
3. Add a "Does not apply/Don't know" response option.
4. Reword complex and/or difficult-to-translate items.
5. Reword items to be more applicable to physicians and nonclinical staff.
6. Align the Hospital Survey on Patient Safety Culture with the other AHRQ patient safety culture surveys.
7. Reduce survey length.
8. Develop a supplemental item set.

The development, implementation, and revision of this survey offered through the AHRQ illustrate the importance of having a culture of safety in HCOs and assessing the culture routinely.

The North Carolina Board of Nursinga culture of safety assessment instrument, the Complaint Evaluation Tool (CET), is an example of the impact of individual nursing concerns and recognition of the importance of a culture of safety (Burhans, Chastain, & George, 2012). Why did a board of nursing develop this type of tool or even have interest in a culture of safety? Regulation and performance are associated with one another. Traditionally, when errors and performance concerns have been reported to a board of nursing, the response has been similar to the blame culture found in some HCOs, with individual nurses identified at fault for the error followed by some type of punitive measure. The purpose of the CET is different. As explained by Burhans and colleagues (2012), its purpose is to

> provide a standard by which the employer and the [board of nursing] can work collaboratively and communicate openly in reviewing practice errors or deficiencies. It also provides a framework to apply expectations for accountability and behavioral choices consistently, while treating nurses respectfully and fairly. (p. 44)

The CET identifies several views of human error. A human error may result in situations when a staff member has no prior supervisory issues related to practice. It may also occur when the staff member demonstrates required knowledge, skills, and ability, and in these cases the event could be described as accidental or an oversight. The third descriptor for human error is there was no policy, standard, or requirement that staff should have followed, and the error is considered to be unintentional. A rating scale is used to rate at-risk behavior and reckless behavior.

A culture of safety requires that HCOs be transparent systems that report errors and openly discuss and consider types of errors, analysis of errors, and steps taken to prevent errors (IOM, 2001). This transparency not only communicates that it is acceptable to be open about errors so that they can be understood and care improved, but it also leads to individual staff learning more about safety and how to prevent errors—how to identify and analyze errors in a manner that leads to a more effective healthcare system. Each nurse is tuned in to practice actions as they occur and is focused on assessing quality outcomes.

Dangers of a Code of Silence

As noted earlier, ANA and other organizations joined in on the need to examine the HCO culture and its connection to patient and staff safety. In 2005, the American Association of Critical Care Nurses and the Association of periOperative Registered Nurses joined with VitalSmarts® to conduct a study. The conclusions from the study note that tools and warnings about safety are helpful, but if staff do not feel safe in speaking up even when staff know something is wrong and do not get others to act to improve, then the culture will not really be changed. This **code of silence** exists in our HCOs and acts as a major barrier for improvement, setting up a work environment that is not positive or healthy for the staff. Recognizing that nurses need to assume greater responsibility and leadership in CQI includes standing up and speaking out when an organizational culture requires improvement.

Diversity Within a Culture of Safety

As noted in other parts of this text, the *National Healthcare Quality Report* and the *National Healthcare Disparities Reports* are now combined into one report (*NQD*). The *NQD* is an important data resource used to track quality care and disparities. A culture of safety needs to consider the impact of diversity on its functioning and the outcomes. The World Health Organization (2015a) defines the **social determinants of health** as the

> conditions in which people are born, grow, live, work, and age, including the health system. These circumstances are shaped by the distribution of money, power, and resources at global, national, and local levels, which are in and of themselves influenced by policy choices. The social determinants of health are mostly responsible for health inequities.

This definition recognizes the importance of culture and diversity. Other key definitions that help to understand culture and disparities include the following:

- **Health inequality** is the difference in health status or in the distribution of health determinants between different population groups (WHO, 2015b).
- **Healthcare disparity** relates to "differences in the quality of health care that are not due to access-related factors or clinical needs, preferences, and appropriateness of interventions. These differences would include the role

of bias, discrimination, and stereotyping at the individual (provider and patient), institutional, and health-system levels" (IOM, 2003, p. 32).

- **Health equity** is attainment of the highest level of health for all people. Achieving health equity requires valuing everyone equally, with focused and ongoing societal efforts to address avoidable inequalities, right historical and contemporary injustices, and eliminate health and healthcare disparities (Healthy People, 2015).
- **Cultural competence** is a set of congruent behaviors, attitudes, and policies that come together in a system or agency or among professionals, enabling effective work in cross-cultural situations (HHS, OMH, 2015).
- **Linguistic competence** is the capacity of an organization and its personnel to communicate effectively and convey information in a manner easily understood by diverse audiences, including persons of limited English proficiency, those who have low literacy skills or are not literate, and those with disabilities (HHS, OMH, 2015).

What can we do to improve? We need to develop partnerships with stakeholders to arrive at best strategies to improve and decrease health inequities. HCOs and healthcare professional education programs need to integrate cultural and linguistic competencies in health professions education and in practice, including adding this information to position descriptions and performance evaluation.

Health literacy has become a critical component of quality improvement frameworks due to the need to respond to healthcare disparities problems. The *Health Literacy* report discusses three intervention points in its framework describing the impact of health literacy on health outcomes and costs (IOM, 2004b). The first intervention point is multifactorial: Culture and the society in which a person lives and works impact ability to understand, think, and respond. Factors such as age, ethnicity, gender, race, socioeconomic status, education, native language, and so on are important to consider. The second intervention point is the health system, and the third is the education system. Health literacy impacts the health system: patient–provider interactions and communication, individual patient and HCO outcomes, access to care, and so on. The education system and its outcomes are crucial to individual literacy and numeracy skills, which impact health literacy. The following are examples of interventions or strategies that may be used to improve health literacy; healthcare diversity within communities, HCOs, and the healthcare delivery system in general; and health outcomes (HHS, OMH, 2011, pp. 1–2).

1. Develop and disseminate health and safety information that is accurate, accessible, and actionable.
2. Promote changes in the healthcare system that improve health information, communication, informed decision-making, and access to health services.

3. Incorporate accurate, standards-based, and developmentally appropriate health and science information and curricula in child care and education through the university level.

4. Support and expand local efforts to provide adult education, English language instruction, and culturally and linguistically appropriate health information services in the community.

5. Build partnerships, develop guidance, and change policies.

6. Increase basic research and the development, implementation, and evaluation of practices and interventions to improve health literacy.

7. Increase the dissemination and use of evidence-based health literacy practices and interventions.

Barriers to a Culture of Safety

Developing and maintaining a culture of safety or a just culture is not easy. Barriers exist in all HCOs. A lack of understanding of the meaning of a culture of safety or just culture is a significant barrier. Key leaders within the HCO need to understand it to ensure that it is communicated effectively to all staff, and all need to be committed to the culture of safety. It is easy to emphasize sharing this concept with clinical staff; however, all staff within the organization (e.g., staff from housekeeping, office support, dietary, maintenance, informatics technology) need to be engaged or efforts will fail.

It is also easy for some staff to view a just culture as an opportunity for the individual staff member to relinquish accountability for his or her actions, and this is not the case. This misperception can represent a major barrier. We still must be able to ask staff to explain what they did and why. There are times when a staff member's performance, not the system, may be the reason for an error, even though most events are system-based.

Many staff members may feel that the HCO's culture is fine and does not need to be changed, or that things have been done one way for so long that there is no chance the HCO will actually change. In some situations, surface changes are made, but underneath, the HCO still has a blame culture. HCO factors such as major budgetary problems, lack of effective leadership or too many management positions in flux, inadequate staffing levels and/or inadequate expertise, major organizational changes such as merging with other organizations, the addition or elimination of services, the need for major facility improvements such as renovation, and so on impact changing organizational culture.

The central feature of a culture of safety is the recognition that events or incidents are opportunities for improvement. We know there will be events that are not acceptable, but this does not mean we treat all who might be involved negatively. Dekker (2007) recommends the following strategies to better ensure a just culture or culture of safety and other strategies that have been recognized as important:

- Focus the culture on concern for system factors that impact CQI; however, recognize there is need for accountability and times when cause may relate primarily to individual performance.
- Remove all penalties that have been associated with events or incidents.
- Monitor stigmatization of staff who are involved in these events; prevent stigmatization when possible.
- Provide support to staff involved in an event.
- Institute debriefing; if already using it, then evaluate it and make changes as needed to support a culture of safety or just culture.
- Develop an effective quality improvement program with staff committed to a culture of safety or just culture and ensure that it is demonstrated in actions throughout the HCO.
- Include the culture of safety or just culture as an important part of staff orientation, orientation for healthcare professions students who are at the HCO for clinical experiences, and routine staff education.
- Ensure that staff know their rights and responsibilities related to events or incidents.
- Include implementation and engagement in the culture in all position descriptions and performance appraisal.
- Build trust at all levels of the organization.
- Identify clear descriptions of roles and responsibilities, including who makes decisions when events or incidents occur.
- Integrate local, state, federal, and healthcare professional requirements and standards into the culture of safety or just culture. Clearly demonstrate how this integration is accomplished.
- Determine the HCO policy and procedure for patient disclosure, and consult with HCO legal experts as needed.

Leadership to Support a Culture of Safety

Leadership is required for effective CQI. This includes developing and maintaining a culture of safety. Leadership in an HCO includes the board of directors, senior management, and all other levels of managers. Assessing the effectiveness of a culture of safety is not easy to accomplish; for example, in a systematic review of 4,239 references, only 16 studies could be selected for review. More research is required to better assess effectiveness (Parmelli et al., 2011).

Clear communication has a positive impact on the culture of safety. Leadership within an HCO must ensure that communication at all levels is clear and should ensure improvement when necessary. This includes formal procedures such as incident reporting, sharing of feedback (from management to staff and vice versa), and a transparent HCO. The culture of an HCO cannot be changed without effective communication and leadership. Part of this effort must be a discussion with all staff about the need for a culture of safety, their views of what this culture might entail, management and staff roles and responsibilities, and methods that will be used to ensure that a culture of safety is maintained over time. Leaders in the HCO need to drive this effort and maintain it.

Stop and Consider #3
A culture of safety requires much effort to implement and maintain.

Conclusions

Weston and Roberts (2013) offer a summary of the current trends in healthcare CQI:

> Quality and performance improvement initiatives are driving significant changes in the U.S. healthcare system. In anticipation of the full implementation of national health reform over the next several years, the pace of these changes has been increasing. The goals of these quality initiatives mirror the National Quality Strategy's three aims, which include better care, Healthy People/Healthy Communities, and ACA.

There are many theories and models used to describe quality improvement, several of which are discussed in this chapter. Along with greater development of approaches to CQI, the culture of safety or just culture is now a critical aspect of CQI and the CQI process. This is a change from the view of the blame culture, moving away from individual blame to greater consideration of system factors.

Apply CQI

Chapter Highlights

- There are many visions of quality improvement; some integrate multiple views of quality.
- The science of improvement focuses on innovation, rapid-cycle testing of change, and lessons learned from changes.
- The triple aim (to improve the patient experience; improve the health of populations; and reduce the per capita cost of health care) is now used in many of the quality improvement models/theories.
- Models built around structure (how organizations are organized as a system), process (how organization functions), and outcomes (results) were

introduced in the 1980s and continue to influence quality improvement models/theories.

- CQI emphasizes a systematic approach that is ongoing.
- STEEEP® is based on the triple aim and the *Quality Chasm* reports. The focus is on customers/patients and CQI; data are important in making decisions.
- The lean approach emphasizes value and cost.
- Six Sigma is a measurement-based strategy.
- High-reliability organizations emphasize reducing operation failure and errors to reduce harm. Redesign of processes is used when necessary.
- The blame culture led to a healthcare work environment in which individual staff members were blamed for errors and system issues were not effectively addressed in improving care and reducing errors.
- A culture of safety or just culture is now recommended to replace the blame culture. Though it still recognizes individual accountability, it turns the focus to systems.
- Diversity (patients and staff) is an important factor in a culture of safety.
- Leadership is required to guide the development and maintenance of a culture of safety.

Critical Thinking and Clinical Reasoning and Judgment: Discussion Questions and Learning Activities

1. Compare and contrast the examples of theories and models described in this chapter. Summarize your comparison in a visual format such as a figure, table, poster, and so on. Discuss your visual with a group of your classmates.
2. What is your opinion of the change from a blame culture to a culture of safety or just culture?
3. Assess a clinical organization in which you are working, or previously worked, for clinical experiences. How would you describe its culture of safety? If it is not a culture of safety, why does it not meet the criteria for this type of culture? Is it a culture in which you would like to work? Why or why not?

Connect to Current Information

- Graphics of models of improvement
  http://www.bing.com/images/search?q=graphics+of+models+of+improvement&qpvt=graphics+of+models+of+improvement&qpvt=graphics+of+models+of+improvement &FORM=IGRE

- AHRQ improvement resources
  http://www.ahrq.gov/professionals/quality-patient-safety/quality-resources
     /index.html
  http://www.hrsa.gov/quality/toolbox/methodology/qualityimprovement/
- Surveys on Patient Safety Culture (AHRQ)
  http://www.ahrq.gov/professionals/quality-patient-safety/patientsafetyculture
     /index.html

EBP, EBM, and Quality Improvement: Exemplar

Collier, S., Fitzpatrick, J., Siedlecki, S., Dolansky, L., & Less, M. (2016). Employee engagement and a culture of safety in the intensive care unit. *Journal of Nursing Administration, 46*(1), 49–54.

   This article describes a study that focuses on the relationship between employee engagement and the culture of safety in an intensive care unit.

Questions to Consider

1. What is the design used for this study, including research question(s), sample, interventions, data collection, and analysis?
2. What are the results of the study?
3. How might you apply these results to a clinical setting to engage staff and improve care?

Evolving Case Study

After conducting a survey about the hospital culture and CQI, your hospital has moved to developing a culture of safety. There are broad guidelines for this change, but ultimately each unit must make the adjustment. As nurse manager of the obstetrical service, you are confronted with where to begin. Your services cover predelivery admissions, labor and delivery, nursery care, postpartum care, and clinics. It is a very busy specialty with overworked staff, and there is a problem with registered nurse retention and turnover. You have been manager for 2 years. Errors have increased by 10% in the 2 years, and staff have become more reluctant to report incidents through the required system. They complain that when staff make errors they are penalized. This complaint is also common within other areas of the hospital. You go to the following website to get information and resources: http://www.ahrq.gov/professionals/quality-patient-safety/patient-safety-resources/resources/esrd/cultureofsafety.html.

Case Questions A

You first need to understand more about the change.

1. What is a culture of safety, and how does it compare to the current culture?
2. How will you demonstrate and convince your staff that this change is real and will make a positive difference?

Case Questions B

After you understand the problem better, you move to planning.

1. Develop a plan to foster a culture of safety. Specify tools you will use and the reason for their use. Develop your process. (See online resources and the chapter content for help.)
2. How will you engage staff in the development of the plan and its implementation? Be specific.
3. How will you assess your outcomes? Be specific.

References

American Nurses Association (ANA). (2010). *Position statement: Just culture.* Retrieved from http://nursingworld.org/psjustculture

Bashaw, E., Rosenstein, A., & Launsbury, K. (2012). Culture trifecta: Building the infrastructure for Magnet® and just culture. *American Nurse Today, 7*(9), 35, 38, 41.

Baylor Scott & White. (2014). STEEEP® improvement toolkit. Retrieved from http://www.baylorhealth. edu/Documents/SGI/Baylor%20Improvement%20Toolkit%20Booklet%202014%20print.pdf

Berwick, D. (1999). Controlling variation in health care: A consultation with Walter Shewhart. *Medical Care, 29*(12), 1212–1225.

Berwick, D., Nolan, T., & Whittington, J. (2008). The triple aim: Care, health, and cost. *Health Affairs, 27*(3), 759–769.

Brackett, T., Comer, L., & Whichello, R. (2013). Do lean practices lead to more time at the bedside. *Journal for Healthcare Quality, 35*(2), 7–14.

Burhans, L., Chastain, K., & George, J. (2012). Just culture and nursing regulation: Learning to improve patient safety. *Journal of Nursing Regulation, 2*(4), 43–49.

Chassin, M., & Loeb, J. (2011). Ongoing quality improvement journey: Next stop, high reliability. *Health Affairs, 30*(4), 559–568.

Dailey, M. (2013). Overview and summary: Health care and quality: Perspectives from nursing. *OJIN: The Online Journal of Issues in Nursing, 18*(3). Retrieved from http://www.nursingworld. org/MainMenuCategories/ANAMarketplace/ANAPeriodicals/OJIN/TableofContents/Vol-18-2013/No3-Sept-2013/OS-Healthcare-and-Quality.html

Dekker, S. (2007). *Just culture. Balancing safety and accountability.* Burlington, VT: Ashgate Publishing Company.

Dixon, N., & Shofar, M. (2006). Patterns, culture, and reliability. *Health Services Research, 41*(4), Part II, 1618–1632.

Donabedian, A. (1980). *Explorations in quality assessment and monitoring, Volume 1: The definitions of quality and approaches to its assessment.* Ann Arbor, MI: Health Administration Press.

Donabedian, A. (1988). The quality of care. How can it be assessed? *JAMA, 260*(12), 1743–1748.

Draper, D., Felland, L., Liebhaber, A., & Melichar, L. (2008). The role of nurses in hospital quality improvement. Center for Studying Health System Change. *Research Brief,* (3), 1–8.

Drenkard, K. (2011). Magnet momentum: Creating a culture of safety. *Nurse Leader, 9*(4), 28–31, 46.

Ettinger, W. (2006). Basic tools for quality improvement. In D. Nash & N. Goldfarb (Eds.), *The Quality Solution* (pp. 115–132). Sudbury, MA: Jones & Bartlett Publishers.

Fallon, L., Begun, J., & Riley, W. (2013). *Managing health organizations for quality and performance.* Burlington, MA: Jones & Bartlett Learning.

Galt, K., Paschal, K., & Gleason, J. (2011). Key concepts in patient safety. In K. Galt & K. Paschal (Eds.), *Foundations in patient safety for health professionals,*(pp. 1–14). Burlington, MA: Jones & Bartlett Learning.

Heathfield, S. (2012). Culture: Your environment for people at work. Retrieved from http://humanresources.about.com/od/organizationalculture/a/culture.htm

Healthy People. (2015). Healthy people 2020. Retrieved from http://www.healthypeople.gov

Institute for Healthcare Improvement (IHI). (2015a). Improvement capability: Overview. Retrieved from http://www.ihi.org/Topics/ImprovementCapability/Pages/Overview.aspx

Institute for Healthcare Improvement (IHI). (2015b, June 12). Interview with Tejal Gandhi: New directions in patient safety. Retrieved from http://www.ihi.org/communities/blogs/_layouts/ihi/community/blog/ItemView.aspx?List=0f316db6-7f8a-430f-a63a-ed7602d1366a&ID=51&Web=1e880535-d855-4727-a8c1-27ee672f115d

Institute for Healthcare Improvement (IHI). (2015c). Science of improvement. Retrieved from http://www.ihi.org/about/Pages/ScienceofImprovement.aspx

Institute for Healthcare Improvement (IHI). (2015d). The IHI triple aim. Retrieved from http://www.ihi.org/Engage/Initiatives/TripleAim/Pages/default.aspx

Institute of Medicine (IOM). (1999). *To err is human.* Washington, DC: The National Academies Press.

Institute of Medicine (IOM). (2001). *Crossing the quality chasm.* Washington, DC: The National Academies Press.

Institute of Medicine (IOM). (2003). *Unequal treatment.* Washington, DC: The National Academies Press.

Institute of Medicine (IOM). (2004a). *Keeping patients safe: Transforming the work environment of nurses.* Washington, DC: The National Academies Press.

Institute of Medicine (IOM). (2004b). *Health literacy: A prescription to end confusion.* Washington, DC: The National Academies Press.

Johnson, J., Smith, A., & Mastro, K. (2012). From Toyota to the bedside. Nurses can lead the lean way in healthcare reform. *Nursing Administration Quarterly, 36*(3), 234–242.

Jones, K., & Redman, R. (2000). Organizational culture and work redesign: Experiences in three organizations. *Journal of Nursing Administration, 30*(12), 604–610.

Kelly, D., Johnson, S., & Sollecito, W. (2013). Measurement, variation, and CQI tools. In W. Sollecito & J. Johnson (Eds.), *McLaughlin and Kaluzny's continuous quality improvement in healthcare* (4th ed., pp. 75–116). Burlington, MA: Jones & Bartlett Learning.

Lawless, S., & Proujansky, R. (2006). The provider's role in quality improvement. In D. Nash & N. Goldbarb (Eds.), *The quality solution* (pp. 135–154). Sudbury, MA: Jones & Bartlett Publishers.

Litvak, E., & Bisganon, M. (2011). More patients, less payment: Increasing hospital efficiency in the aftermath of health reform. *Health Affairs, 30*(1), 76–80.

Mayberry, R., Nicewander, D., Qin, H., & Ballard, D. (2006). Improving quality and reducing inequities: A challenge in achieving best care. *Baylor University Medical Center Proceedings, 19*(2), 103–118.

Nolan, T., Resar, R., Haraden, C., & Griffin, F. (2004). Improving the reliability of health care. Retrieved from http://www.ihi.org/resources/Pages/IHIWhitePapers/ImprovingtheReliabilityofHealthCare.aspx

O'Hagan, J., & Persaud, D. (2009). Creating a culture of accountability in health care. *The Health Care Manager, 28*(2), 124–133.

Parmelli, E., Flodgren, G., Schaafsma, M., Baillie, N., Beyer, F., & Eccles, M. (2011). The effectiveness of strategies to change organizational culture to improve healthcare performance. The Cochrane Collaborative, Wiley Publishers. Retrieved from http://onlinelibrary.wiley.com/doi/10.1002/14651858.CD008315.pub2/abstract

Powell, A., Rushmer, R., & Davies, H. (2009). A systematic narrative review of quality improvement models in health care. NHS Quality Improvement Scotland. Retrieved from http://www.healthcareimprovementscotland.org/previous_resources/hta_report/a_systematic_narrative_review.aspx

Ramaswamy, R., & Barker, P. (2013). Quality improvement in resource-poor countries. In W. Sollecito & J. Johnson (Eds.), *McLaughlin and Kaluzny's continuous quality improvement in healthcare* (4th ed., pp. 537–570). Burlington, MA: Jones & Bartlett Learning.

Shortell, S., Bennett, C., & Byck, G. (1998). Assessing the impact of continuous quality improvement on clinical practice: What will it take to accelerate progress. *The Milbank Quality, 76*(4), 593–624.

Six Sigma. (2015). 8 wastes of lean. Retrieved from http://www.isixsigma.com/dictionary/8-wastes-of-lean/

Sollecito, W., & Johnson, J. (2013). The global evolution of continuous quality improvement: From Japanese manufacturing to global health services. In W. Sollecito & J. Johnson (Eds.), *McLaughlin and Kaluzny's continuous quality improvement in healthcare* (4th ed., pp. 1–48). Burlington, MA: Jones & Bartlett Learning.

Sovie, M. (1993). Hospital culture: Why create one? *Nursing Economics, 11*(2), 69–75.

Stiefel, M., & Nolan, K. (2012). A guide to measuring the triple aim: Population health, experience of care, and per capita cost. Institute for Healthcare Improvement (IHI). Retrieved from http://www.ihi.org/resources/Pages/IHIWhitePapers/AGuidetoMeasuringTripleAim.aspx

Storme, T. (2013). Healthcare analytics for quality and performance improvement. Hoboken, NJ: John Wiley & Sons, Inc.

The Joint Commission. (2015, July). Comprehensive accreditation manual for hospitals. Oakbrook IL: Author.

U.S. Department of Health and Human Services (HHS), Agency for Healthcare Research and Quality (AHRQ). (2011). Defining lean waste and potential failure modes. AHRQ Project RED (Re-Engineered Discharge) Training Program. Retrieved from http://archive.ahrq.gov/professionals/systems/hospital/red/leanwaste.html

U.S. Department of Health and Human Services (HHS), Agency for Healthcare Research and Quality (AHRQ). (2014, October). Chapter 8. What's next? Action planning for improvement. Retrieved from http://www.ahrq.gov/professionals/quality-patient-safety/patientsafetyculture/hospital/2011/hosp11ch8.html

U.S. Department of Health and Human Services (HHS), Agency for Healthcare Research and Quality (AHRQ). (2015a). Three tips for facilitating the quality improvement process. Retrieved from http://www.ahrq.gov/cahps/quality-improvement/improvement-guide/4-approach-qi-process/index.html

U.S. Department of Health and Human Services (HHS), Agency for Healthcare Research and Quality (AHRQ). (2015b). Update on the hospital survey on patient safety culture. Retrieved from http://www.ahrq.gov/professionals/quality-patient-safety/patientsafetyculture/hospital/update/index.html

U.S. Department of Health and Human Services (HHS), Agency for Healthcare Research and Quality (AHRQ), Patient Safety Network (PSNet). (2016). High reliability. Retrieved from https://psnet.ahrq.gov/primers/primer/31/high-reliability

U.S. Department of Health and Human Services (HHS), Health Resources and Services Administration (HRSA). (2011a). Quality improvement. Retrieved from http://www.hrsa.gov/quality/

U.S. Department of Health and Human Services (HHS), Health Resources and Services Administration (HRSA). (2011b). *Quality improvement.* Retrieved from http://www.hrsa.gov/quality/toolbox/508pdfs/qualityimprovement.pdf

U.S. Department of Health & Human Services (HHS), Office of Minority Health (OMH). (2015). Cultural and linguistic competency. Retrieved from http://www.minorityhealth.hhs.gov/omh/browse.aspx?lvl=1&lvlid=6

U.S. Department of Health & Human Services (HHS), Office of Minority Health (OMH), National Partnership for Action to End Health Disparities. (2011). National stakeholder strategy for achieving health equity. Retrieved from http://minorityhealth.hhs.gov/npa/templates/content.aspx?lvl=1&lvlid=33&ID=286

Wachter, R., & Pronovost, P. (2009). Balancing "no blame" with accountability in patient safety. *New England Journal of Medicine, 361*(14), 1401–1406.

Weston, M., & Roberts, D. (2013). The influence of quality improvement efforts on patient outcomes and nursing work: A perspective from chief nursing officers at three large health systems. *OJIN: The Online Journal of Issues in Nursing, 18*(3). Retrieved from http://www.nursingworld.org/Quality-Improvement-on-Patient-Outcomes.html

Whittington, J., Nolan, K., Lewis, N., & Torres, T. (2015). Pursuing the triple aim: The first seven years. *Milbank Quarterly, 93*(2), 263–300.

World Health Organization (WHO). (2015a). Glossary of terms used. Retrieved from http://www.who.int/hia/about/glos/en/index1.html

World Health Organization. (WHO). (2015b). Social determinants of health. Retrieved from http://www.who.int/social_determinants/en/

Patient and Family Engagement in Quality Improvement

CHAPTER OBJECTIVES

At the conclusion of this chapter, the learner will be able to:

- Examine the relationship of patient-centered care and patient/family engagement in continuous quality improvement (CQI).
- Explain the need to consider reimbursement when reviewing patient-centered care and CQI.
- Summarize the role of the patient in CQI.
- Apply methods to increase patient/family engagement in CQI.
- Explain the importance of technology to patient-centered care.
- Examine efforts to monitor and measure patient satisfaction and engagement in CQI.
- Critique examples of patient-centered initiatives.

OUTLINE

KEY TERMS

Advocacy

Collaboration

Collaborative care model

Coordination

Disclosure

Patient-centered care

Self-management

Introduction

Patient-centered care became more important when the *Quality Chasm* reports brought it to the forefront. The reports identified 10 rules to describe an improved health system, and 4 of these rules are directly related to patient-centered care. These rules are as follows: "Care is based on continuous health relationships; care is customized according to patient needs and values; the patient is the source of control; and knowledge is shared and information flows freely" (IOM, 2001, p. 8). These rules also apply directly to continuous quality improvement (CQI). This chapter discusses the need for patient-centered care and its relationship to CQI.

Patient-Centered Care Supports Patient/Family Engagement in CQI

Patient-centered care is a critical element of effective quality care and is described as a dimension of quality in which care is individualized and customized to patients and families. This perspective recognizes that patients, not healthcare providers, have control over their healthcare decisions (Berwick, 2009). As discussed in other sections of this text, the Institute of Medicine (IOM) emphasized patient-centered care in 2001 in the second of the *Quality Series* reports (IOM, 2001). The *Quality Chasm* report defines the healthcare profession competency for **patient-centered care** as follows:

> Identify, respect, and care about patients' differences, values, preferences, and expressed needs; relieve pain and suffering; coordinate continuous care; listen to, clearly inform, communicate with, and educate patients; share decision making and management, and continuously advocate disease prevention, wellness, and promotion of healthy lifestyles, including a focus on population health. (IOM, 2003, p. 4)

It is important for healthcare organizations (HCOs) to incorporate patient-centered care in their views and application of CQI. This issue was introduced because patients expressed concern about their role and inability to participate in decision-making. Health care has long advocated for patient rights; however, this approach had not been implemented very effectively. In 1993, critical dimensions describing quality care were identified, and the following dimensions were then applied in the *Quality Chasm* reports (Gerteise, Edgman-Levitan, Daley & Delbanco, 1993, pp. 5–10):

- *Respect for patients' values, preferences, and expressed needs.* What does the patient think is important? To make effective decisions and participate in planning, the patient needs to be informed. Terms used to describe this effort include *customized* and *individualized care*. Cultural factors are also part of patient-centered care, as they impact who the patient is, what the patient needs and prefers, how capable the patient is of understanding information for informed consent, and how much a patient may or may not want to participate and make decisions. A patient's preferences may change over time, and healthcare providers need to adapt to changes.

- *Coordination and integration of care.* Coordination is also not a new concept in health care, but implementing it has not always been effective. In addition, the patient should be involved, but in many circumstances, he or she is not. Coordinating services to make sure they happen as they should and when they should is critical for positive outcomes. The patient and family need to be able to depend on effective coordination. Transitions from one healthcare provider and setting to another (handoffs) should occur with limited problems, clear communication to reduce errors, and involvement of the patient.

- *Information, communication, and education.* Patients need accurate information and are particularly interested in their diagnoses, instructions on how to stay well, and their prognosis, including details about what can be done to change or manage the prognosis. Patient diversity requires that this information be shared so that care meets individual patient needs. Patients want information they can trust from healthcare providers who are focused on helping them. Confidentiality and privacy are critical components.

- *Physical comfort.* Patients do not always receive the care they need to help with major symptoms such as pain. This care may be given, but it may not be timely, and thus patients suffer unnecessarily.

- *Emotional support—relieving fear and anxiety.* In addition to physical needs, patients have emotional needs. Often these needs are not met. When patients feel disconnected from their care and decisions, this may have a negative impact on patient responses.

- *Involvement of family and friends.* In many situations, the patient's family and significant others are involved with the care and care decisions, but this is not always the case. Including patients in care planning and seeking their approval of decisions have a positive impact on patient outcomes.

These dimensions are recurrent themes in health care and are integrated throughout this text. Nurses and nursing care are critical in ensuring that these dimensions are part of each patient's care.

Quality Improvement: Relationship to Patient-Centered Care

Patient-centered care is important to CQI for a number of reasons. An involved patient has a greater chance of having positive care outcomes. This patient will be more willing to share information with care providers and discuss concerns openly and be engaged in treatment. The patient and provider relationship will be based more on trust. Patients vary a great deal, as do their needs and preferences. The degree to which they want to be involved is highly variable and changes. However, healthcare providers should not assume anything about what the patient wants and proceed in the care process without including the patient.

Because patients are more involved today, they will most likely be more aware of quality care issues; however, one should not assume the involved patient is a demanding or difficult patient, but rather a patient who wants to express his or her needs, preferences, and concerns. To call this patient demanding would deny the relevance of patient-centered care. As Johnson and colleagues (2008) explain, "Patients and families have experience, expertise, insights, and perspectives that can be invaluable to bringing about transformational change in health care and enhancing quality and safety" (p. 1). The physician is responsible for diagnosis and recommending treatment options, and the patient is responsible for identifying goals and concerns, followed by communicating the decision regarding treatment choice to the physician. The physician then implements the plan (Fowler, Levin, & Sepucha, 2011).

For patients to actively participate in their health decisions and make their own decisions, they need to have clear information that they can understand; time to consider the information and concerns, such as risks and benefits of treatment; and interaction with healthcare providers so that they can discuss the information, their questions and concerns, and their own goals or outcomes. These elements are not always important for all patients; however, all healthcare providers need to recognize that patients need the opportunity to consider their health and care carefully and fully within the existing time parameters (Fowler et al., 2011).

The Nursing Alliance for Quality Care (NAQC) considers patient engagement to be critical to effective patient care quality, particularly to nursing care. The NAQC bases this belief on the following assumptions (Sofaer & Schumann, 2013, p. 6):

1. There must be a dynamic partnership among patients, their families, and the providers of their health care, which at the same time respects the boundaries of privacy, competent decision-making, and ethical behavior.
2. This relationship is grounded in confidentiality, where the patient defines the scope of the confidentiality. Patients are the best and ultimate source of

information about their health status and retain the right to make their own decisions about care.

3. In this relationship, there are mutual responsibilities and accountabilities among the patient, the family, and the provider that make it effective.

4. Providers must recognize that the extent to which patients and family members are able to engage or choose to engage may vary greatly based on individual circumstances. Advocacy for patients who are unable to participate fully is a fundamental nursing role.

5. All encounters and transactions with the patient and family occur while respecting the boundaries that protect recipients of care as well as providers of that care.

6. Patient advocacy is the demonstration of how all of the components of the relationship fit together.

7. This relationship is grounded in an appreciation of patient rights and expands on the rights to include mutuality.

8. Mutuality includes sharing of information, creation of consensus, and shared decision-making.

9. Healthcare literacy is essential for the patient, family, and providers to understand the components of patient engagement. Providers must maintain awareness of the healthcare literacy level of the patient and family and respond accordingly. Acknowledgment and appreciation of diverse backgrounds are essential to the engagement process.

Consider how each of these assumptions might impact your nursing practice on a daily basis. Each assumption relates to important aspects of care, and they are interrelated to provide a positive care trajectory for the patient. The assumptions also focus on similar issues such as those found in the rules and description of dimensions of patient-centered care mentioned earlier in this chapter.

Informed Decision-Making: Impact on Quality Care

According to Fowler and colleagues (2011), the healthcare industry has a long way to go in including patients in the decision-making process:

> Consumer rights are also more important today in health care, and the Institute of Medicine's identification of patient-centered care supports consumer or patient rights. Good-quality care requires that procedures, treatments, and tests be not only medically appropriate, but also desired by informed patients. Current evidence shows that most medical decisions are made by physicians with little input from patients. (p. 699)

This type of practice is directly opposite of the view of patient-centered care and patient rights, but it is gradually changing. Patients themselves are demanding more. Patients have rights to informed consent and unbiased information. Withholding information is not the choice of the healthcare provider and is appropriate only if the patient requests to not receive the information. If staff cannot answer patient questions, either because the staff member does not know the answer or because the staff member is not in a position to inform the patient, then the staff member needs to tell the patient that someone will get back to him or her. The staff member needs to inform the appropriate staff member of the patient's questions and follow up to make sure the patient has received the requested information.

Privacy and Confidentiality: Relationship to Quality Improvement

The Health Insurance Portability and Accountability Act (HIPAA) of 1996 focuses on patient privacy and confidentiality. HIPAA identifies protected health information or any information about a patient that connects to an individual patient (e.g., demographic information). Only minimum necessary information may be shared without patient permission. Disclosure of information to others must be monitored. This law and patient rights have an impact throughout the care process, sometimes in ways that staff may think do not relate.

Other patient rights are also identified in HIPAA (Institute for Patient- and Family-Centered Care, 2010). The patient has the right to access medical records, and the healthcare provider must respond within 30 days. If the patient does not think the information is correct or complete, then the patient has the right to amend the medical record. This does not mean the medical record information must be changed, but the patient's comments must be added to the record.

Patient Makes the Decision About Family Engagement

In some cases, HIPAA has become a barrier to the exchange of information with the patient's family (Institute for Patient- and Family-Centered Care, 2010). In the past it was common for healthcare providers to share information with family members without asking the patient for permission, sometimes not even sharing the same information with the patient. HIPAA, which applies to any patient-related information, now makes such practices illegal. If, however, the patient does not state restrictions to healthcare providers, the HCO or healthcare provider may reveal the information. Many patients do not realize they can request restrictions. Patients may request that steps be taken to ensure privacy; for example, they may request that information not be shared by phone messaging, email, or postal mail to the patient's home. These requests must be reasonable. If the patient thinks his or her privacy has been violated, then he or she has the right to report the incident to the healthcare provider (individual or organization), the state licensure board, and the Office of Civil Rights of the U.S. Department of Health and Human Services (HHS) through its website. Providers may be charged a fine for not following HIPAA.

Staff need to clarify sharing of information with each patient. An exception applies if a family member is the legal guardian for the patient. Staff may find it difficult to obey patients requests to not share information with family, as they may view not including family as being in conflict with patient-centered care, but in reality, it strongly supports patient-centered care: The patient decides who gets information and who is involved in healthcare decisions.

Disclosure of Errors and Patient-Centered Care

In the past, HCOs were hesitant to disclose errors to patients, mostly due to legal advice that did not support disclosure. This, however, is changing, and many HCOs now encourage or may require disclosure of errors to patients and, when the patient agrees, to the patient's family (Banja, 2005). Why is disclosure of errors now recommended? As discussed in this text, errors are inevitable even when great effort is made to reduce them. Prevention is important, but it is not enough, as we need to also understand errors and address methods to respond to errors when they occur. Being involved in an error is an emotional experience for the healthcare provider. We do not go into health care to harm the patient, but we are not perfect and systems are not perfect. These incidents leave us with a critical decision as to whether we should inform a patient that an error occurred, assuming the patient does not already know. Doing so is referred to as **disclosure**.

Disclosure of errors has always been a problematic issue. HCOs have worried that informing patients and families that an error almost occurred or did occur will increase the risk of malpractice lawsuits, and as a result, they have often erred toward withholding the information. However, there has been a change in how healthcare providers approach errors with patients. Patient-centered care implies that there is a contract between the patient and the provider, with the patient making decisions about his or her care. If this is the case, then disclosure of errors is a factor that impacts this decision process and errors need to be openly discussed. If we want patients to trust us, then we must reveal the negative events along with the positive. There are increased efforts to describe (1) methods for disclosing errors, (2) by whom, and (3) when. The Agency for Healthcare Research and Quality (AHRQ) provides information on disclosure and notes that the following should be considered by healthcare providers and HCOs (HHS, AHRQ, PSNet, 2014):

- Disclosure of all harmful errors
- An explanation as to why the error occurred
- Minimization of errors
- Physician steps to prevent recurrences

Disclosure is connected to both legal and ethical concerns; both are discussed in other chapters. These principles are relevant to disclosure of errors.

The content of an error disclosure is important. *Full disclosure* of an error incorporates the components found in **Exhibit 6-1**, as well as "acknowledgement of responsibility and an apology by the physician" (Gallagher et al., 2006, p. 1587). Gallagher and colleagues (2006) explain, however, that full disclosure is not always so straightforward:

> There may be a disconnect between physicians' views of ideal practice and what actually happens. For example, most physicians agree that errors should be fully disclosed to patients, but in practice many "choose their words carefully" by failing to clearly explain the error and its effects on the patient's health. (p. 1587)

Full disclosure is an explicit statement, and a *partial disclosure* mentions an adverse event but not an error. *No disclosure* indicates the patient is not told anything about an adverse event or error. In a study on disclosure, it was noted that 56% of the physicians used partial disclosure, 42% full disclosure, and 3% no disclosure (Gallagher et al., 2006).

In addition to what should be shared, it is critical to consider how this communication should occur. The decision to share information about an error with a patient would not be the nurse's responsibility. This responsibility belongs to the physician but should include team input. If the HCO has a policy and procedure on disclosure, and ideally it should, then the policy and procedure must be followed, including any documentation that might be required. The

---

Exhibit 6-1 Content to Include in a Disclosure

- A description of the nature of the error and the harm it caused
- A description of when and where the error occurred
- Consequence of the harm
- Clinical and institutional actions taken to diminish the gravity of the harm
- Identification of who will manage the patient's continuing care
- Identification of systematic elements that contributed to the error
- Identification of who will manage ongoing communication
- Associated costs of the error to be removed from the patient's bill (assuming these costs are known to be related to the error and risk management has been consulted)
- Offer of counseling and support

following is a summary of guidelines for implementing disclosure of errors (Banja & Amori, 2005):

- Plan what will be said (including content, who will inform the patient, best location with privacy, time and patient status, whether the family will be included, and so on).
- Be clear and concise; answer questions truthfully.
- Stop and listen; give the patient time to respond.
- Evaluate response as it develops.
- Respond empathetically.
- Avoid being defensive or identifying blame.
- A meaningful apology may be made.

One should not assume that disclosure of errors prevents lawsuits. Disclosure is not used to prevent a lawsuit, although it may make some patients reconsider whether they will sue the healthcare provider, as they may feel more trust in the healthcare provider who is honest with them. Disclosure is about professional responsibility, accountability, and patient-centered care. Why is patient-centered care important here? Patient-centered care emphasizes the right of patients to know about the care process and outcomes in order to participate in decisions about their health and care, and this patient involvement has an impact on care improvement.

Patient Advocacy

Patient **advocacy** is "the act of pleading for or supporting a course of action on behalf of individuals, families, communities, and population" (Finkelman & Kenner, 2016, p. 43). The American Nurses Association (ANA) *Code of Ethics for Nurses* supports the professional responsibility of each nurse to the patient (ANA, 2015a). The *Scope and Standards of Practice* is also critical in supporting the patient and patient-centered care (ANA, 2015b). The standards of professional practice include the nursing process, and the patient is the center of this process. Another standard on coordination of care emphasizes that effective coordination requires patient involvement. Standards of professional performance focus on a number of factors that influence advocacy and patient-centered care such as culture, communication, collaboration, quality, evidence-based practice, and leadership.

Staff need to feel empowered to advocate for patients, and in the process, empower the patient. Providing clear information should be part of the process. The goal is not to make the patient dependent on the healthcare provider, but rather to work collaboratively with the patient. Effective advocacy requires understanding of patient needs and preferences and recognizing the importance of putting the focus on the patient. The nurse acts as the patient's advocate when the nurse speaks for the patient (individual patient, family, communities/populations). This does not mean the nurse tells the patient what to do, but rather represents the patient. For example, in the CQI process, the nurse acts as the patient's advocate in ensuring that procedures are followed or procedures are improved to reflect best practice. A nurse who stops a surgical procedure due to concern that something is not right is serving as the patient's advocate, or a nurse serving on the quality improvement (QI) committee in an HCO is serving as patient advocate for all HCO patients to ensure quality care. There are many ways a nurse acts as a patient advocate every day. How might this role be demonstrated in your practice?

Stop and Consider #1
Patient-centered care must be part of an effective QI program.

Reimbursement, the Patient, and CQI

For the consumer of health care, reimbursement and the cost of health care have long been concerns of the patient. The Affordable Care Act (ACA) has had an impact on reimbursement and extended access to healthcare insurance. It is still not clear if long-term this legislation will increase or decrease costs to the consumer; for example, there is concern it will increase premiums, deductibles, and co-pays, and thus increase the cost of insurance. The law has eliminated the common third-party payer limitation on preexisting conditions, but consumers are also concerned about their out-of-pocket costs. As noted in other chapters in this text, cost and quality are interrelated; however, spending more money on care does not necessarily mean the care is better. There are countries that spend less than does the United States and yet are ranked higher in health, access, and healthcare services. Another aspect is the cost of QI programs and methods used by the programs—funding, staffing, technology, and so on. CQI does increase costs per HCO and on the macrolevel (local, state, federal). We have also seen an increase in pay-for-performance (P4P) initiatives. This type of approach may improve care, but it is noted that some providers may view P4P as an incentive to use workarounds and limit reporting of problems to give the appearance that outcomes are met. It is important to recognize that most of what would be considered patient-centered care is not reimbursable; healthcare providers and HCOs do not receive payment for many strategies used to ensure patient-centered care. This may have an impact on HCO commitment to make significant changes unless the HCO can see real value in doing so. The consumer (i.e., the patient) no longer is holding back on complaints about healthcare quality and cost, and in the future this outspokenness will most likely increase, particularly if costs continue to rise and quality is still a problem.

Stop and Consider #2

Patients continue to be concerned about reimbursement and cost of care.

Patient, Family, and Staff Responses to a Patient/Family Quality Improvement Role

HCO, government, and nongovernment initiatives to (1) improve care and (2) increase emphasis on patient-centered care developed during the same period. This led to greater recognition that the two goals were connected. A critical question was, and continues to be, what is the patient's role in CQI? One perspective is the patient simply "gets the rewards" from a system that provides quality care, and this is certainly important to the patient and patient's family. There is, however, another important question: Is there a more active role that patients should assume?

Roles and Responsibilities

Many now agree there is an active role in CQI if the patient wants to assume it. Several factors influence this role. First, the healthcare provider and HCO must commit to accepting active participation from the patient and the family in the CQI process. This must be more than verbal acceptance; it must be demonstrated in actions taken to include and listen to the patient. Involving the patient in this manner is not that easy for healthcare providers and HCOs given that historically there has been a more "paternalistic" attitude toward patients, although this has changed over the years.

HCOs must include the patient in their QI programs and plans. How might this be done? Sometimes patient representatives are included on various committees and tasks forces focused on improving care. Patients are asked to complete satisfaction surveys (discussed later in this chapter). The newest method is the most direct. Ask patients to speak up when they have questions or concerns and when they notice problems. This active role puts the patient, and in many cases the family, right in the middle of the care process and the CQI process—stopping care to identify or question something. This patient empowerment can be threatening to staff, so staff education is needed to improve understanding of the need for this approach and how best to respond. Ignoring patient comments or saying broadly "we will look into it" is not enough. Patients must be told that they need to participate, although they cannot be forced to do so. Assisting patients in understanding why their involvement is important is critical, requiring that staff follow the HCO approach of active patient engagement in CQI. Communicating to patients that the HCO is committed to CQI, describing CQI, and noting the value of input from all parties, including the patient, are vital steps toward engaging patients.

Patients also need examples of their role in CQI. Although staff cannot cover all possible scenarios, examples include the following:

- When staff do not wash their hands, the patient should refuse care until hands are washed.
- The patient should ask questions about medications or procedures that may not be in sync with the patient's understanding of his or her treatment.
- The patient should tell staff when there is clutter in his or her room that makes it difficult for the patient to walk safely and ask if it can be removed or moved.
- The patient should identify potential flaws in the discharge plan that will make it difficult to implement the plan in the patient's home.
- The patient should note that informed consent has not been given.

Why might it be difficult for patients to speak up about quality care? Some patients are afraid they will offend staff and that then they may not get the best care or response from staff. Whether or not this concern is justified, this fear is present for many patients. Coordination and **collaboration** are important aspects of care delivery, and patient feedback ensures better outcomes. The IOM (2015) defines collaboration as follows:

> Collaboration is an active and ongoing partnership, often involving people from diverse backgrounds who work together to solve problems, provide services, and enhance outcomes. Collaborative patient-centered practice is a type of arrangement designed to promote the participation of patients and their families within a context of collaborative practice. (p. xi)

In this chapter, we focus on how errors impact patients, how patients might respond to errors, and how patients might help to reduce errors; however, patients also have a role in precipitating errors. This may seem like an unusual statement, but consider the following insight from the AHRQ:

> [Patient] errors may arise from the same underlying causes that contribute to clinicians' errors—while patients may engage in intentionally unsafe behavior, more commonly, patient errors are attributable to the difficulties inherent in an individual's interaction with a complex system. One study classified patient errors into *action errors*, which are errors of patient behavior such as failure to attend a scheduled appointment, and *mental errors*, which include thought process errors such as failing to take a medication as prescribed. (HHS, AHRQ, PSNet, 2015)

Examples of factors that might impact this type of error are health literacy problems and ineffective patient–provider communication. As errors are analyzed, it is important to consider the patient's role, not to blame the patient, but to understand the error, respond to it, and if possible, prevent future errors for the patient and even for other patients. Later in this chapter, strategies are discussed to increase patient engagement in care and CQI. These strategies are also important in reducing the type of error discussed here when the patient is more involved in what led to the error and possible harm.

Effective Communication: Increasing Patient Engagement in CQI

Communication is an element in all that is done during the healthcare process. Staff who listen to the patient, respect the patient, and clearly communicate information the patient needs are much more successful in engaging the patient in CQI with the patient at the center. The patient also needs time to ask questions and feel that staff are listening and willing to answer questions. As is true in all communication, verbal and nonverbal communication are important. Staff need to make sure their nonverbal communication is in sync with their verbal messages. Active listening is critical in the communication process.

Sometimes it may seem that the simple issues are unimportant, but they can be very important. For example, admission staff members often have the first encounter with the patient, and if they begin by addressing the patient with the patient's first name without asking permission to do so, it may have a negative impact. Staff tend to think that calling patients by their first name is more patient-centered, but it is not. What is more patient-centered is asking the patient what he or she wants to be called and using the correct title—for example, "Mr.", "Dr.", and "Mrs." Assumptions get in the way of asking the patient and listening to the patient. Staff need to know details about the patient such as religion and ethnic factors. This information can impact communication with the patient and care.

The following is an example of multiple non-patient-centered communication problems with patients: A patient is recovering from anesthesia after open-heart surgery. The patient's wife is in the room and hears the staff calling her husband "honey" and "baby" as they provide care. The two nurses, including an advanced practice nurse, then try to get the patient to respond by calling him Mr. —. He does not respond, and they appear concerned. The patient is a physician. The patient's wife gets very irritated by the manner of communication and tells the staff not to refer to her husband as "honey" and "baby," as this is insulting, and secondly, it would help if they called her husband Dr. —, as they would get more of a response from him. The nurses followed her instructions, and her husband responded immediately. They had no idea the patient was a physician, although this was in the medical record.

The Patient and Diagnosis

In other chapters, diagnostic errors are discussed; however, in this chapter, the focus is on the patient. Developing strategies to reduce these errors should also involve the patient and communication with the patient, including during the diagnosis process. The patient might help to reduce diagnostic errors, and therein greatly improve their own care, by doing the following (Gruber, 2014, p. 26):

1. Be a good historian. Patients should keep records of their symptoms, when they started, and how they have responded (or not) to treatment.
2. Take advantage of cancer screening.
3. Know test results and keep accurate records of these results. Patients should not assume that no news is good news. They should follow up if they don't receive copies of the results of tests and consults.
4. Speak up! Patients should ask the following questions: (1) What else could it be? (2) What should I expect? (3) When and how should I follow up if symptoms persist or worsen? (4) What resources can I use to learn more? (5) Is this test worthwhile? Can we wait? (More testing does not always mean better care!)
5. Don't assume the healthcare system will adequately coordinate care. Patients should keep their own records and should help coordinate their own care.
6. Provide feedback about diagnostic errors to providers and organizations.
7. Understand that diagnosis always involves some element of uncertainty.
8. Get a second opinion regarding serious diagnoses or unresolved symptoms.
9. Take advantage of help and support: support groups, patient safety staff, patient advocates.

It may seem obvious that the patient is the center of the diagnosis process, but in reality, during this stage, healthcare providers tend to focus more on laboratory tests, exams, history, procedures, and so on. Patients need to be empowered to ask for second opinions and question diagnoses. If errors are made, patients need to report them so that this type of error can be tracked and steps can be taken to improve diagnosing and reduce these errors.

Typical Patient and Family Responses to Engagement in CQI

Patients may respond emotionally as they participate more in their care. They may respond with anger or frustration if they are concerned about care quality. They may also praise staff for their work and feel that they are getting the best of care. The range can vary. The patient's condition and past healthcare experiences are factors that may influence patient responses as well as the relationship they have with healthcare providers and responses they get from healthcare providers. Families, too, may vary in their response. Patients and families need to feel that they can say what they think or feel and ask questions without staff responding defensively and negatively.

Staff Responses to Patient Engagement in CQI

Every staff member, clinical and nonclinical, needs to commit to patient-centered care and take steps in their work to focus on the patient. We tend to focus on clinical staff, but nonclinical staff can make a difference, too. Consider the following nonclinical staff interactions with the patient:

- Dietary staff consider dietary patient needs including religious and ethnic factors and make special arrangements to meet the needs.
- All staff may listen and respond to feedback in all areas of the HCO; for example, staff who clean the patient's room and have a lot of contact with the patient and family have many opportunities to interact and personalize care for the patient.
- Staff transporting patients for procedures or during admission or discharge interact with patients during potentially stressful moments.

These are just a few of the many potential nonclinical staff interactions that may contribute to the patient's experience.

All staff should speak to the patient with respect and recognize when the patient does not want to converse. Acting defensively or with anger is not helpful. It is also easy to "put the patient off"—saying you will get back to the patient or family member later. If staff members do need to delay a response, then they need to go back to the patient or family member to follow up. Not doing so decreases trust and does not support an effective patient–provider relationship.

Stop and Consider #3

Patients should be encouraged to participate in CQI, but they cannot be forced to participate.

Methods to Increase Patient/Family Engagement in CQI

Patients, and their families when patients approve, have roles in the HCO's culture of safety. Many of the elements associated with patient-centered care are described at the beginning of this chapter; however, there are other elements to consider. Implementing patient-centered care in the healthcare delivery system is not easy to accomplish and takes time. It needs to impact the entire culture of the HCO regardless of the type of setting, such as acute care, ambulatory care, urgent care, physician practices, long-term care, home care, and hospice. A critical factor that impacts implementation, as noted earlier, is that much of what is considered to be patient-centered care is not reimbursable; it is considered to be just a part of expected care. Strategies and interventions to support patient-centered care take time and expertise. There are also program costs to integrate patient-centered care effectively and to create partnerships with patients and families to redesign health care and QI. Examples of costs are interpreters, staff training, signage to ensure patients can find their way around, personal attention, which may require more staff, and effective use of an HCO website and other technology to share information with patients and families and improve communication.

Barriers to Patient Engagement

Barriers to engaging the patient and focusing on patient-centered care are typically related to lack of HCO and/or staff commitment to patient-centered care. It may take more time and initiative to accomplish this. Staff are busy and stressed so they may perform their jobs with minimal concern for the patient as a person—not listening and not responding to make changes. Common barriers include inadequate staffing, lack of staff knowledge and understanding of patient-centered care, poor communication, fear that the patient will identify errors, view of patient-centered care as a nuisance, and failure to understand staff or patient roles in patient-centered care and CQI.

Strategies to Increase Engagement

The Institute of Health Improvement also strongly supports a patient-centered approach to health care. This healthcare improvement model integrates patient-centered care in five focus areas or drivers of CQI (Balik, Conway, Zipperer, & Watson, 2011, p. 8):

- *Leadership.* Governance and executive leaders demonstrate that everything in the culture is focused on patient- and family-centered care, practiced everywhere in the HCO—Patient-centered care needs to be a critical driver at the individual level, at the microsystem level (unit, department, service), and across the organization.
- *Hearts and minds.* The hearts and minds of staff are fully engaged through respectful partnerships with everyone in the organization and in a commitment to the shared values of patient- and family-centered care.
- *Respectful partnership.* Every care interaction is anchored in a respectful partnership, anticipating and responding to patient and family needs (e.g., physical, comfort, emotional, informational, cultural, spiritual, and learning needs).
- *Reliable care.* Healthcare systems deliver reliable, quality care when needed.
- *Evidence-based care.* The care team instills confidence by providing collaborative, evidence-based care.

HCOs are providing more patient educational materials to explain and motivate patients to engage in CQI. As Schwappach, Hochreutener, and Wernli (2010) explain, "We cannot just expect patients to participate in quality improvement without some information and support in doing so, nor can we require patients to participate. We can encourage and provide the information needed. Some patients will choose not to participate" (p. E85). As HCOs plan what information to share with patients to increase their engagement, HCOs should consider the following about patient-centered care and CQI (Finkelman & Kenner, 2016, p. 276):

- Provider–patient communication
- Patient educational materials about health concerns
- Self-management tools to help patients manage their illness or condition and make affirmed decisions
- Access to care (e.g., timely appointments, off-hour services) and use of information technology (e.g., automated patient reminders, patient access to electronic medical records)
- Continuity of care
- Post-hospital follow-up and support
- Access to reliable information about the quality of physicians and HCOs, with opportunity to give feedback

There are many other methods that HCOs use to integrate patient-centered care into practice and care delivery systems, including the following examples:

- *Patient participation in care planning.* The patient participates in care planning and agrees to the plan. Patient values, needs, preferences, and cultural factors should be part of the planning. If the patient agrees, family may participate.
- *Patient etiquette.* This may seem to be a strange topic, but it is very important. It relates directly to patient-centered care. All staff need to follow good etiquette, including the following practices: Knock when entering the patient's room; introduce yourself by name and identify your role; ask for the patient's permission to talk with the patient or to provide care; never call the patient by first name unless the patient agrees; recognize that patients and families need private time; and never assume that the family can be told anything about the patient unless the patient agrees, unless the patient's condition does not allow the patient to agree.
- *Care coordination.* Ensure that patient needs are met by coordinating providers, functions, activities, and sites over time. Coordination also implies patient involvement in care decisions and covers the continuum of care required by the patient—multiple providers and settings over time.

- *Self-management of care.* Self-management of care is an element of care that is recognized in the *Quality Chasm* reports as a critical component. Self-management programs include educative process and outcomes (McGowan, 2005). Today, with the growing number of patients with chronic illness, self-management is more important. Even though self-management is particularly important for chronic illness, it can apply to any type of patient. **Self-management** is "the systematic provision of education and supportive interventions to increase patients' skills and confidence in managing their health problems, including regular assessment of progress and problems, goal setting, and problem-solving approach" (IOM, 2003, p. 52). The patient accepts much of the responsibility for the care.

  The healthcare system is not set up to easily accommodate self-management, but this needs to change. A major step is to consider how the patient can assume more responsibility when it makes sense for the patient's needs and preferences. Today, more care takes place in the home, requiring more self-management even if the patient is receiving home healthcare services. Actively including the patient in planning sets the stage for a discussion about self-management. In many cases, an interprofessional team is used to ensure that the patient's complex, varied needs are met. There is also increasing use of electronic personal health records (EPHRs) to support the patient and self-management (Mitchell & Begoray, 2010). Use of EPHRs requires adequate patient health literacy, software, and technological support.

  Self-management is also a time of high risk, particularly if the patient does not have the preparation for self-management or support resources. The highest time of risk is when a patient who is actively involved in self-management requires professional intervention and may not realize it or deny the need for this action. Nurses need to work with the patient and, when the patient agrees, with the family to develop acceptable plans.

- *Patient education.* Patient education has long been part of health care; however, its effectiveness is not always so clear. Methods used to provide patient education need to be updated to consider different patient needs, changes in healthcare delivery, and health informatics. Patients in the acute care setting are sicker and are discharged sicker than in the past. This impacts the effectiveness of patient education. Is the patient really able to understand information enough to apply the information to his or her needs? In other settings, such as outpatient clinics, the patient may not be as sick, but healthcare providers have less time with patients, which is also true in acute care settings. The tendency is to rely on printed material and assume we have provided patient education; however, patients need time to discuss the information with healthcare providers. We are also not taking full advantage of informatics, such as smartphones, computers, the Internet, and other new technology that could be used to provide information when the patient really needs it. Providing patients with information that means something to them and their health emphasizes patient-centered care and patient advocacy.

- *Human resources and patient-centered care.* Human resources should also recognize cultural issues that can impact hiring, performance, and personnel policies and also patient-centered care. Is patient-centered care discussed with job applicants? Is patient-centered care commented on in position descriptions and performance evaluation? Staff meetings should include patient-centered care as staff discuss issues and problems at all levels in the HCO.

- *Health promotion and wellness and disease prevention.* Today, there is greater emphasis in healthcare delivery on health promotion and wellness and disease prevention. Many healthcare providers now incorporate screening of disease in their services. Community or public health services are particularly concerned with health promotion and wellness and disease prevention. Even within the community, healthcare providers must consider individual needs, health history, and so on, and these considerations apply, too, for the community at large.

    In the end, as with all health decisions, it really is the individual patient's choice. The 2010 healthcare reform legislation (ACA) established the National Prevention, Health Promotion, and Public Health Council within the HHS. In 2011, a National Prevention Strategy for the United States was published by this council, which identifies seven key goals to increase the number of Americans who are healthy at every stage of life. These goals are: (1) tobacco-free living, (2) prevention of drug abuse and excessive alcohol use, (3) healthy eating, (4) active living, (5) mental and emotional well-being, (6) reproductive and sexual health, and (7) injury- and violence-free living. These goals need to be supported by empowered people, healthy and safe community environments, clinical and community preventive services, and elimination of health disparities (HHS, 2011).

- *End-of-life.* End-of-life care, palliative care, and hospice care are all patient-centered approaches. The philosophy behind these services emphasizes the patient's individual needs and preferences.

- *Bedside rounds.* Some hospitals include patients and families (the latter with patient permission) in patient rounds, rather than just "doing rounds" and acting like the patient has a minimal role. Rounds are part of planning and evaluating care, and if patient-centered care considers the patient to be the most important part of care, then the patient's inclusion is critical. These rounds provide patients with more information and time for staff to listen to the patient's feedback. Rounds are also used to educate patients about current needs, treatment, and postdischarge treatment when in transition to another setting, including the home. Ensuring privacy and confidentiality during rounds can be difficult when the patient is not in a private room. Alternative arrangements need to be made if sharing of information needs to be private and there is no privacy in the typical room situation. Staff and healthcare profession students who participate in rounds need to understand the rounds procedure, integration of the patient (family), and all relevant privacy and confidentiality issues.

- *Discharge and transition planning.* Patients have shorter lengths of stay in acute care today, and as a consequence, they tend to go home sicker than in the past to continue recovery at home. Some go to other HCOs for either short-term or long-term care, such as rehabilitation and long-term care or home health care. Handoffs are times of increased risk of errors. Patients and their families need to be vigilant during these times and participate in identifying possible errors. Asking questions is a critical part of this process (patient to staff, staff to patients, and staff to staff). Patients should be involved in the planning. At all times, patients should be encouraged and asked, "Does this make sense to you in your situation?" If healthcare providers hear the patient say it does not make sense, if the patient asks questions that make the healthcare provider wonder if the plan will work, or if the healthcare provider thinks that the patient and/or family are not committed to the plan, then they should consider whether the planning needs to be reviewed and possibly revised. For the plan to have a chance of success, the patient and family must feel the plan is appropriate and commit to it. Discharge planning without the patient runs a high risk of problems and failure. With increasing concerns about the level of readmissions, using effective patient-centered discharge planning helps to reduce readmission.

- *Visiting policies and procedures.* Structuring visiting hours can limit patient and family interactions. Many hospitals are changing visiting hours to allow for more opportunities for visits. The patient needs to be able to say when visitors are a problem, but also staff need to be able to assess patient stress levels. If the patient is not able to set limits, then staff need to talk with the patient to plan effective visiting time. There have even been changes in intensive care, the service that has traditionally had the most rigid visiting policies. Having family visit in a reasonable number, such as one or two at a time, and more frequently may bring more comfort to the patient. In some cases, family members are even allowed to be present during codes, when the patient's life is at risk. There is also more flexibility now in the surgical arena, with some HCOs allowing families to stay with a patient longer prior to surgery and to see the patient sooner after surgery. Privacy of other patients must always be considered. The emergency department is another area where there may be more flexibility, if the patient wants family present and family members do not interfere with required treatment.

- *Patient- and family-centered facility design.* The design of any HCO should consider the needs of the patients and families who use the services. Consideration needs to be given to the physical layout. For example, does the layout facilitate ease of access, does the flow of services make sense in the design, does the environment appear clean and well lighted to reflect openness, are color tones welcoming and calming, is noise managed and are interventions used to reduce noise, is carpeting safe and easy to clean, is temperature regulated, are there appropriate waiting areas for visitors, are there general patient areas for sitting? More HCOs are now providing Wi-Fi so that patients, families, and visitors can use digital devices. Another issue today is facilities that make it easier for family members and significant others to stay overnight with the patient, which requires consideration of furniture (e.g., chairs) so that visitors can rest and be near the patient. The facility should be welcoming from the time the patient enters the HCO. Privacy should be part of all aspects of the facility. Patients and families should feel as comfortable as possible in the facility. The design should also support staff collaboration, providing private space for discussions and making it easier for staff to reach one another. Diversity should also be considered, such as clear signage that all visitors can understand, use of color codes to make it easy to get around the facility with minimal need to read signs, and information stations with staff prepared to assist regardless of language. Facilities for special populations, such as children, the elderly, and patients with mental health concerns, should reflect the needs and characteristics of these patients.

- *Staff preparation.* All staff need information and ongoing updates about patient-centered care—what it means and how to implement it. This information should be provided in orientation so that all new staff members understand the importance of patient-centered care. There should also be regular staff education for all staff on the topic. Staff should be asked to identify topics related to patient-centered care they think should be included in staff education. Including patient and family representatives in orientation to share their experiences and thoughts about patient-centered care is an effective tool to emphasize commitment to patient-centered care.

BOX 6-1 STRATEGIES TO HELP HEALTHCARE PROVIDERS ENCOURAGE PATIENT PARTICIPATION IN THE CRITICAL THINKING PROCESS

- Stay in the room. Don't talk to patients from the doorway.
- Pay attention to your body language and to the patient's body language.
- Sit down so that you are at eye level with the patient.
- Use open questions and comments, such as "Tell me about . . ." instead of closed questions that imply you expect a short answer.
- Touch patients, but be respectful of their space and cultural norms.
- Use collaborative thinking language, such as "We should think this through," "Let's look at some possible conclusions," and "Can we analyze this together?"
- Use phrases that let the patient know that the patient's situation is not so unusual that the patient cannot discuss it. For example, "Some people feel anxious when . . ."
- Address patients respectfully. Find out if they prefer Mr. or Mrs., Doctor, Professor, Reverend, and so on.
- Do not use affectionate terms to address the patient, such as "sweetheart", "dear" and so on.
- Do not look at your watch, no matter how busy you are.
- Be direct and honest. For example, tell patients when the schedule is backed up and why.
- If you feel like avoiding a patient, reflect on why you feel that way.

- *Teams.* Teams are also important in supporting patient-centered care, particularly interprofessional teams. There is greater emphasis today on interprofessional education to improve effectiveness of interprofessional teams (NAS/HMD, 2015). Teams should focus on the patient and engage the patient in the team process, increasing communication, coordination and collaboration, effective decision-making, and more. Additional information about teams and CQI are found in other chapters.

Box 6-1 highlights additional examples of strategies that might be used by healthcare providers to increase patient participation.

Stop and Consider #4

It is easy to assume patients do not understand CQI and that their engagement is not really an important part of patient-centered care.

Technology to Support Patient Engagement

Technology also impacts the caring process in patient-centered care, and in some situations it can get in the way of this process. If, however, nurses are vigilant and recognize the risk of reduced caring, then they are more able to ensure that as care is given active methods are used to ensure that technology and informatics do not become barriers but rather support patient-centered care. For example, if a nurse is using a laptop in the patient's room, the nurse needs to actively interact with the patient by looking at the patient and asking questions rather than just focusing on the screen. If a nurse is setting up infusion equipment, it is important to talk with the patient during the procedure, but still ensure that the equipment is used in a safe and effective manner.

Informatics is a part of all types of consumerism today, including health care. Patients now check the Internet for information, although they may not always know the most reliable sources or how to evaluate them. They can prepare themselves for medical appointments and hospitalization. By using the many benchmarking and report card methods available through the Internet, patients can get important information to help them compare healthcare providers and make knowledgeable decisions; however, as discussed in other chapters, these reports do not always reflect clear information about quality.

Patients use various types of technology (e.g., smartphones, tablet computers) to access the Internet and get health information and information about HCOs. Integrating all of this information puts the focus on the patient, who should be the decision maker. Some HCOs are using electronic methods to identify "decision windows" or times when a patient has a decision to make (Fowler et al., 2011). In this case, symptoms are tracked through an electronic rating scale. When certain symptoms occur or symptoms get worse, an alert is sent to the provider indicating that it may be time for a change in treatment and thus a patient decision, or it might alert the patient to contact the healthcare provider. This type of method integrates patient-centered care with informatics and healthcare providers.

There are more and more electronic methods used for patients to communicate with HCOs and healthcare providers, and vice versa. To date, there is not enough evidence supporting the positive impact of electronic methods on healthcare outcomes, but clearly, today many people are engaged in electronic communication and access information through these sources. As Carayon, Hoonakker, Cartmill, and Hassol (2015) report, this new arena of communication is promising:

> Some evidence indicates that these health IT applications may improve process measures, such as greater adherence, better self-care, improved patient–provider communication, and patient satisfaction. The results of this study support the findings in the literature that patients sharing their information with clinicians electronically can facilitate communication, improve the organization of work, reduce workload, and increase patient satisfaction. (p. ES-1)

Implementing and maintaining electronic methods are not simple to accomplish, and there are barriers to effective outcomes, such as the time commitment, interference with workflow, and increases in healthcare provider workload. Other issues that come up are patient access to their own medical records, patient self-reported data (i.e., accuracy and timeliness), secure messaging, and use of online reminders. As more emphasis is placed on digital communication methods, the healthcare system will see benefits and detriments, and there will be need for more strategies to make communication more secure, safe, accessible, and useful in healthcare delivery.

Stop and Consider #5

Technology can improve patient-centered care, but it also can act as a barrier to patient-centered care.

Monitoring and Measuring Patient Satisfaction and Patient-Centered Care

An HCO may proclaim itself to be patient-centered, but actually demonstrating this care approach daily is a much different matter. So, how do you know if an HCO demonstrates patient-centered care? A place to start is to determine how the HCO views patient-centered care. Does the HCO's culture and philosophy actually reflect patient-centered care (Institute for Patient- and Family-Centered Care, 2011)? There is no standard method to meet the goal, but there are some guidelines about the HCO that can be used in self-assessment. The following questions might guide an assessment of an HCO's commitment to patient-centered care:

- Are the concept and related principles found in the organization's written vision, mission, and goals?
- Does the organization's definition of quality health care include the patient and family?
- Has this priority been communicated to patients, families, and the community, and in what way?
- Is the care provided effective?
- Do the organization's policies, procedures, standards, programs, and other aspects of the organization consistently include patients and families as partners?
- Do all staff, clinical and nonclinical, understand and apply patient-centered care? How is this demonstrated?
- What is demonstrated in documentation? For example, do medical records indicate how the patient participates?
- Is the patient actively considered in collection of CQI data and root cause analysis? For example, are patient surveys used?
- Is patient-centered care demonstrated in the physical environment? If so, how?

Nurses have a major role in supporting patient-centered care, but if they are stressed and understaffed, these factors impact whether or not they are able to support patient-centeredness in daily practice. The self-assessment should include nurses.

The Planetree model is used by many HCOs to provide a framework to ensure that the HCO demonstrates patient-centeredness (Frampton & Guastello, 2010). HCOs that use this model consider organization structure and functions, including patient and family feedback; human interactions that focus on continuity, consistency, and accountability to personalize care; patient education and access to information; nutrition program with 24-hour access; healing environment both in architecture and interior design; arts program to offer therapeutic distractions; spirituality and diversity to meet these needs; healthy communities to improve community health; and measurement to determine satisfaction.

Patient Satisfaction Surveys

HCOs include patient satisfaction in their QI programs. Often HCOs use surveys developed and managed by external sources, such as Press Ganey®. The HCO pays for this service, and then it has access to a tested survey and often the ability to compare data with other similar HCOs.

It is important to get the data, but there are potential problems with the process and the data. A factor that has an impact on results of patient satisfaction surveys is concern about accepted definitions (Finkelman & Kenner, 2016). How a patient views quality care is often different from an HCO's view or an individual provider's view of quality care, meaning patients' responses to surveys may be difficult to interpret or not relevant to the provider's objectives. It is not uncommon for patients to complete satisfaction surveys and never hear anything from the HCO, though the patients may have noted negative experiences. This lack of response communicates that the feedback may not be important.

There are myths about patient satisfaction and data collected. The following list explores some of these myths and the realities of measuring patient satisfaction (Zimmerman, 2001, pp. 255–256).

- *Patient satisfaction is objective and straightforward.* Surveys are difficult to develop, and they are often poorly designed.
- *Patient satisfaction is easily measured.* Satisfaction is complex and not easily measured. Patient expectations play a major role in the process, and there are many factors that can affect patient responses that are not always easy to identify.
- *Patient satisfaction is accurately and precisely measured.* This is not possible at this time. Attitudes are being measured.

- *It is obvious who the customer is.* An HCO actually has many different types of customers beyond the patient, including families, physicians, insurers, and internal customers. (And to complicate matters, staff within the HCO are often customers to other staff; for example, the laboratory provides services to the units, and, thus, nursing staff on the units are the laboratory's customers.) A complete customer satisfaction analysis should include multiple types of HCO customers.

Monitoring Patient-Centered Care

In addition to monitoring patient satisfaction, monitoring patient-centered care should be part of HCO QI programs. One cannot assume that because it is written in the HCO's vision, mission, and goals and included in position descriptions, staff orientation, and staff education that patient-centered (family-centered) care is fully integrated in the HCO. In summary, the HCO needs to consider the following in its CQI data collection and analysis as part of its QI plans:

- Is there shared decision-making? If so, how is this objective accomplished?
- Is there coordination and continuity of care? If so, how is this objective accomplished?
- Do patients have access to care that meets their individual needs and in a timely manner?
- Do care documentation methods demonstrate patient-centered care?
- What do the patient satisfaction data indicate? Trends?
- What is the level of communication with the patient (content, with whom, timeliness)?
- How is the patient (and family) involved in the QI program?
- Are patients' emotional and physical comfort needs met? How?
- Are there disparities in the system, and what are they? How are they resolved?
- Is evidence-based practice used to meet the patient's individual needs?

CQI data collection should routinely include data on patient-centered care and should be reported in the HCO's CQI reports for discussion and development of improvement strategies. All aspects of CQI are important, and an HCO should not rely on just one particular method. An area that is often ignored is getting patient feedback on whether the patient participated in decision-making: How was the patient engaged, and were the patient's needs met?

Stop and Consider #6
Patient satisfaction data are not always reflective of quality care.

Examples of Patient-Centered Initiatives

Local, state, and federal government and nongovernment organizations have developed initiatives to support patient-centered care. The following discussion describes some of these initiatives, and the Connect to Current Information section at the end of the chapter provides links to other information on the Internet.

Collaboration and Care Coordination

An example of an initiative to increase patient engagement is the **collaborative care model**, which focuses on managing the health of a population rather than on treating a specific diagnosis. The goal is to reduce risks and cost of care through "use of a team-based, patient-centered approach and includes care coordination, and when needed self-management support" (HHS, AHRQ, 2015a, p. 2). Medicaid uses this model to integrate physical and mental health care. The AHRQ defines **coordination** as "care that is coordinated across all elements of the broader healthcare system" (HHS, AHRQ, 2015b). Coordination is one of the six National Quality Strategy priorities. As Craig, Eby, and Whittington (2011) explain, "Care coordination delivers health benefits to those with multiple needs, while improving their experience of the care system and driving down overall healthcare (and societal) costs" (p. 2).

The annual *National Healthcare Quality and Disparities Report* includes tracking and analysis of care coordination. With the passage of the ACA, several models of care that emphasize patient-centered care, coordination, collaboration, and interprofessional teams are now considered to be important for an effective healthcare delivery system. Examples of some of these models are accountable care organizations, medical homes, and nurse-managed health clinics. The *National Healthcare Quality and Disparities Report* notes the following:

> Conscious, patient-centered coordination of care improves the person's experience and leads to better long-term health outcomes, as demonstrated by fewer unnecessary hospitalizations, repeated tests, and conflicting prescriptions, as well as clearer discourse between providers and patients about the best course of treatment. (HHS, AHRQ, 2015c)

Consumer Assessment of Healthcare Providers and Systems

There is no federally required system for collecting patient satisfaction data and public reporting of the data. The Consumer Assessment of Healthcare Providers and Systems (CAHPS) is a system that does this, but it is not a required program. It was developed and is maintained by the HHS, specifically the Centers for Medicare and Medicaid Services (CMS) (HHS, AHRQ, 2016). Surveys and tools for collecting patient evaluation data are provided and accessible on the Internet. The AHRQ maintains the information, focusing on the principles of "identifying and supporting the consumer's or patient's information needs, conducting thorough scientific testing, ensuring comparability of data, maintaining an open development process, and keeping products in the public domain" (HHS, AHRQ, 2016). Multiple surveys are provided that focus on specific healthcare delivery settings and services: health plans, clinicians and groups, patient-centered medical homes, hospitals, and experience of care and health outcomes. The CAHPS database is a repository of the data collected from the surveys, providing detailed benchmark data per each type of survey.

Partnership for Patients Campaign

The Partnership for Patients campaign is composed of physicians, nurses, hospitals, employers, and patients and their advocates, and is maintained by the CMS (HHS, CMS, 2016). Its purposes are to make care safer and improve care transitions. The Partnership uses several initiatives to meet its purposes. The Hospital Engagement Network helps identify solutions to solving the problem of hospital-acquired conditions (HACs) across the country. The Community-Based Care Transitions Program identifies sites to participate in this program. The sites must meet criteria and use a collaborative approach, with a variety of HCOs and other agencies serving patient needs in the community. This program is particularly focused on reducing Medicare beneficiary 30-day unplanned readmissions. Other methods are used to improve patient and family engagement. Both the HAC initiative and the readmission initiative are discussed in more detail in other chapters.

Patient-Centered Outcomes Research Institute

The Patient-Centered Outcomes Research Institute (PCORI) is a nongovernmental, nonprofit organization in Washington, DC, that was authorized by Congress in 2010. The PCORI vision and mission are stated as follows (PCORI, 2015):

- *Vision.* Patients and the public have information they can use to make decisions that reflect their desired health outcomes.
- *Mission.* PCORI helps people make informed healthcare decisions and improves healthcare delivery and outcomes by producing and promoting high-integrity, evidence-based information that comes from research with decisions guided by patients, caregivers, and the broader healthcare community.

The focus is on evidence-based research using comparative effectiveness research (CER) to support decisions and recommendations. The national priorities in the PCORI research agenda are assessing prevention, diagnosis, and treatment options; improving healthcare systems; undertaking communication and dissemination research; addressing disparities; and accelerating PCORI and methodological research.

Quality Improvement Organization Program

According to the HHS, CMS (2011), complexity of health care drives the need for patient-centered care:

> Health care is personal. Every individual's experience with the health care system is different—influenced by preferences and values, family situation, cultural traditions, and lifestyle. Because these factors strongly affect health outcomes, patient-centered care is increasingly a top priority in every health care setting.

The Quality Improvement Organization (QIO) program focuses on better patient care, better individual and population health, and lower care costs through improvement (Triple Aim). It is supported by the National Quality Strategy (HHS, CMS, 2011). This is the largest federal program emphasizing improving healthcare quality at the community level. QIOs are located in all states and coordinate with the CMS. The CMS (2011) states, "Medicare beneficiaries, caregivers, and healthcare providers are encouraged to join in local and national initiatives to increase patient and family engagement. Beneficiaries and families also will have the opportunity to contribute to local QIO improvement initiatives." Collaborative initiatives provide opportunities to respond to concerns, increase communication with Medicare beneficiaries, and identify strategies to increase patient and family engagement emphasizing the CMS commitment to patient-centered care.

Speak Up™

Speak Up™ is a patient safety program developed by The Joint Commission, a nongovernmental organization, in 2002. The name Speak Up is an acronym for the following acts of patient advocacy (The Joint Commission, 2016):

- **S**peak up if you have questions or concerns.
- **P**ay attention to the care you get.
- **E**ducate yourself about your illness.
- **A**sk a trusted family member or friend to be your advocate (advisor or supporter).
- **K**now what medicines you take and why you take them.
- **U**se a healthcare organization that has been carefully checked out.
- **P**articipate in all decisions about your treatment.

The program offers free information in multiple forms, such as infographics, animated videos, brochures, and posters. The resources are offered in multiple languages and used globally. The focus of the program is on the patient and providing patients with information and tools to support patients to speak for themselves and empower patients as they interact with their healthcare system and healthcare providers. Examples of topics are anesthesia and surgery, the doctor's office, follow-up care, pain, prevention of medical errors, depression, at-home care, and antibiotics.

Stop and Consider #7

The federal government supports patient-centered care.

Conclusions

This chapter focused on patient-centered care as a critical element of effective care and healthcare systems. The patient is not only the center of care but also needs to actively participate in CQI. Patients, and when appropriate their families, can help to identify care concerns that need to be improved immediately or long-term. Staff and HCOs need to include them in their QI programs and plans and accept that this engagement is necessary for CQI.

Apply CQI

Chapter Highlights

- Patient-centered care is not a new approach, but it is now recognized as a critical element of an improved healthcare system.
- Patient rights and privacy are critical elements in ensuring patient-centered care. HIPAA supports this philosophy throughout the healthcare system.
- Disclosure of errors to patients is connected to ethics and legal issues but also demonstrates patient-centered care, as it emphasizes the right of the patient to know about the care process and outcomes and participate in decisions to improve care.
- Patients are concerned about the cost of care and reimbursement, and both are connected to CQI.
- The patient, and when appropriate the family, should assume an active role in CQI, and HCOs and healthcare providers need to communicate the importance of this role to patients and families.
- Many methods are used to engage the patient and family in CQI, such as asking patients to speak up when they have concerns about quality.
- Staff members need to respect patients and allow them to actively communicate during the care process. The patient makes the decisions about his or her care, unless the patient chooses not do so.
- Technology provides many opportunities to increase patient-centered care and patient inclusion in CQI.

- Government and nongovernment organizations now offer programs to HCOs, healthcare providers, and patients as consumers that support patient-centered care. Examples are care coordination and collaborative models, the Consumer Assessment of Healthcare Providers and Systems (CAHPS) surveys, the Partnership for Patients campaign, the Patient-Centered Outcomes Research Institute (PCORI), the Quality Improvement Organization (QIO) program, Speak Up™, and other efforts.

Critical Thinking and Clinical Reasoning and Judgment: Discussion Questions and Learning Activities

1. Review the article "A Trail of Medical Errors Ends in Grief, But No Answers," an account of one patient's experience (https://www.propublica.org/article/patient-safety-medical-error-hospital-no-answers?utm_source=Sailthru&utm_medium=email&utm_campaign=Newsletter). Provide a summary of errors and other experiences that should be noted for this patient. Discuss your results in a discussion group in the classroom or online. The group should select at least three of the incidents and develop strategies that an HCO might use to resolve these problems or prevent them from reoccurring.
2. Keep a log for one day of clinical. The log should have two columns. In one column, identify all the examples you observe or are involved in during the day that reflect positive patient-centered care. In the second column, identify examples that reflect negative patient-centered care. Share this information with a discussion group in the classroom or online, and compare and contrast examples. Next, identify solutions that might be used to prevent the negative examples.
3. For one week, keep a log of all CQI examples that you observe or are involved in during your clinical experiences. Identify how your examples are related to patient-centered care.

Connect to Current Information

- Information for reporting HIPAA violations
  http://www.hhs.gov/hipaa/filing-a-complaint/what-to-expect/index.html
- CMS: Patient and Family Engagement
  https://partnershipforpatients.cms.gov/p4p_resources/tsp-patientandfamilyengagement/tsppatient-and-family-engagement.html
- CAHPS: Surveys and Tools to Advance Patient-Centered Care
  https://cahps.ahrq.gov/

- United for Patient Safety
  http://www.unitedforpatientsafety.org/
- Planetree Organization
  http://planetree.org/
- Effective Health Care Program: Information on comparative effectiveness research
  http://effectivehealthcare.ahrq.gov/index.cfm/
      what-is-comparative-effectiveness-research1/
- Patient-Centered Outcomes Research Institute (PCORI)
  http://www.pcori.org/
- The Joint Commission: Speak Up™ Initiatives
  http://www.jointcommission.org/speakup.aspx
- CMS: Quality Improvement Organizations
  https://www.cms.gov/Medicare/Quality-Initiatives-Patient-Assessment-
      Instruments/QualityImprovementOrgs/index.html?redirect=/
      qualityimprovementorgs/

EBP, EBM, and Quality Improvement: Exemplar

Hughes, R. (2011). Overview and summary: Patient-centered care: Challenges and rewards. *Online Journal of Issues in Nursing, 16*(2). Retrieved from: http://www.nursingworld.org/MainMenuCategories/ANAMarketplace/ANAPeriodicals/OJIN/TableofContents/Vol-16-2011/No2-May-2011/Overview-and-Summary-Patient-Centered-Care.html
  This series of articles discusses nursing and patient-centered care.

Questions to Consider

1. What key points are addressed in the summary?
2. Select one of the articles in the series and determine how the content may relate to your practice.
3. Based on this series, what do we need to do to better achieve patient- and family-centered care, and what do the patient and family need to do?

Evolving Case Study

You have been working for 4 years on a medical unit with 20 beds. You serve as the unit's CQI representative, working with the nurse manager and the entire staff to improve care. During a meeting with the nurse manager, you are reviewing the data from the last 6-month patient satisfaction survey that you are routinely sent by the QI program. Both of you are concerned about a negative change of a drop of 10% in the area of patient satisfaction, particularly noting problems with patient education and staff sharing information with patients, such as lack of information about medications. This CQI information is shared in the next unit staff meeting. The staff decide to examine more data about the issue and to then determine strategies to improve. All staff agree to immediately focus more on sharing information with patients and families.

Case Questions:

1. What other data should be reviewed?
2. What specific measures/indicators should be used to track this problem?
3. What specific strategies should be used to engage the patients in their care?

References

American Nurses Association (ANA). (2015a). *Code of ethics for nurses with interpretive statements.* Silver Spring, MD: Author.

American Nurses Association (ANA). (2015b). *Nursing scope and standards of practice* (3rd ed.). Silver Spring, MD: Author.

Balik, B., Conway, J., Zipperer, L., & Watson, J. (2011). *Achieving an exceptional patient and family experience of inpatient hospital care.* IHI Innovation Series White Paper. Retrieved from https://kinwahlin.wordpress.com/2011/02/14/achieving-an-exceptional-patient-and-family-experience-of-inpatient-hospital-care-ihi-white-paper-2011/

Banja, J. (2005). *Medical errors and medical narcissism.* Sudbury, MA: Jones & Bartlett Publishers.

Banja, J., & Amori, G. (2005). The emphatic disclosure of medical error in *Medical errors and medical narcissism.* In J. Banja (Ed.), *Medical errors and medical narcissim* (pp. 173–192). Sudbury, MA: Jones & Bartlett Publishers.

Berwick, D. (2009). What "patient-centered" should mean: Confessions of an extremist. *Health Affairs, 28*(4), w555–w565.

Carayon, P., Hoonakker, P., Cartmill, R., & Hassol, A. (2015, May). Using health information technology (IT) in practice redesign: Impact of health IT on workflow. Patient-reported health information technology and workflow. (Prepared by ABT Associates under Contract No. 290-2010-00031I). AHRQ Publication No. 15-0043-EF. Rockville, MD: Agency for Healthcare Research and Quality.

Craig, C., Eby, D., & Whittington, J. (2011). Care coordination model: Better care at lower cost for people with multiple health and social needs. Institute for Health Improvement Innovation Series white paper. Cambridge, MA: Institute for Health Improvement. Retrieved from http://www.ihi.org/resources/Pages/IHIWhitePapers/IHICareCoordinationModelWhitePaper.aspx

Finkelman, A., & Kenner, C. (2016). *Professional nursing concepts: Competencies for quality leadership* (3rd ed.). Burlington, MA: Jones & Bartlett Learning.

Fowler, F., Levin, C., & Sepucha, K. (2011). Informing and involving patients to improve the quality of medical decisions. *Health Affairs, 30*(4), 699–706.

Frampton, S., & Guastello, S. (2010). Putting patients first: Patient-centered care; More than the sum of its parts. *AJN, 110*(9), 49–53.

Gallagher, T., Garbutt, J. M., Waterman, A. D., Flum, D. R., Larson, E. B., Waterman, B. M.,... Levinson, W. (2006). Choosing your words carefully: How physicians would disclose harmful medical errors to patients. *Archives of Internal Medicine, 166*, 1585–1593.

Gerteis, M., Edgman-Levitan, S., Daley, J., & Delbanco, T. (1993). Introduction: Medicine and health from the patient's perspective. In M. Gerteis, S. Edgman-Levitan, & J. Daley. (Eds.), *Through the patient's eyes: Understanding and promoting patient-centered care* (pp. 1–18). San Francisco, CA: Jossey-Bass.

Gruber, M. (2014). Diagnostic error: 10 things you could do tomorrow. Lists for physicians, healthcare organizations, and patients. *Inside Medical Liability*, (first quarter), 22–26, https://www.piaa.us/wcm/_News_Room/PI_Magazine.aspx

Institute of Medicine (IOM). (2001). *Crossing the quality chasm.* Washington, DC: The National Academies Press.

Institute of Medicine (IOM). (2003). *Health professions education: A bridge to quality.* Washington, DC: The National Academies Press.

Institute for Patient- and Family-Centered Care. (2010). HIPAA—Providing new opportunities for collaboration. Retrieved from http://www.ipfcc.org/tools/downloads.html

Institute for Patient- and Family-Centered Care. (2011). Partnering with patients and families to enhance safety and quality. A mini toolkit. Retrieved from http://www.ipfcc.org/tools/downloads.html

Johnson, B., Abraham, M., Conway, J., Simmons, L., Edgman-Levitan, S., Sodomka, P.,... Ford, D. (2008). *Partnering with patients and families to design a patient- and family-centered healthcare system.* Bethesda, MD: Institute of Family-Centered Care in collaboration with the Institute for Health Improvement.

McGowan, P. (2005). Self-management: A background paper. University of Victoria: Centre on aging. Retrieved from http://www.selfmanagementbc.ca/uploads/Support%20for%20Health%20 Professionals/Self-Management%20support%20a%20background%20paper%202005.pdf

Mitchell, B., & Begoray, D. (2010). Electronic personal health records that promote self-management in chronic illness. *OJIN, 15*(3). Retrieved from http://nursingworld.org/MainMenuCategories /ANAMarketplace/ANAPeriodicals/OJIN/TableofContents/Vol152010/No3-Sept-2010/Articles-Previously-Topic/Electronic-Personal-Health-Records-and-Chronic-Illness.aspx

National Academy of Sciences (NAS), Health and Medicine Division (HMD). (2015). *Measuring the impact of interprofessional education on collaborative practice and patient outcomes.* Washington, DC: The National Academies Press.

Patient-Centered Outcomes Research Institute (PCORI). (2015). About us. Retrieved from http://www.pcori.org/about-us

Schwappach, D., Hochreutener, M., & Wernli, M. (2010). Oncology nurses' perceptions about involving patients in the prevention of chemotherapy administration errors. *Oncology Nursing Forum, 37*(2), E84–E91.

Sofaer, S., & Schumann, M. (2013). Fostering successful patient and family engagement: Nursing's critical role. White paper for the Nursing Alliance for Quality Care. Retrieved from http://www.naqc.org/WhitePaper-PatientEngagement

The Joint Commission (2016). Speak Up™. Retrieved from https://www.jointcommission.org /facts_about_speak_up/

U.S. Department of Health and Human Services (HHS), Agency for Healthcare Research and Quality (AHRQ). (2015a). Care management issue brief. Care management: Implications for medical practice, health policy, and health services research. AHRQ Publication No. 15-0018-EF. Retrieved from https://pcmh.ahrq.gov/sites/default/files/attachments/Care-Mgmt-Issue-Brief-No-15-0018-EF.pdf

U.S. Department of Health and Human Services (HHS), Agency for Healthcare Research and Quality (AHRQ). (2015b). Coordinated care. Retrieved from https://pcmh.ahrq.gov/page/coordinated-care

U.S. Department of Health and Human Services (HHS), Agency for Healthcare Research and Quality (AHRQ). (2015c). Chartbook on care coordination. Retrieved from http://www.ahrq.gov/research/findings/nhqrdr/2014chartbooks/carecoordination/carecoord-care.html

U.S. Department of Health and Human Services (HHS), Agency for Healthcare Research and Quality (AHRQ). (2016). CAHPS: Surveys and tools to advance patient-centered care. Retrieved from https://cahps.ahrq.gov/

U.S. Department of Health and Human Services (HHS), Agency for Healthcare Research and Quality. (AHRQ), Patient Safety Network (PSNet). (2014, August). Error disclosure. Retrieved from https://psnet.ahrq.gov/primers/primer/2

U.S. Department of Health and Human Services (HHS), Agency for Healthcare Research and Quality (AHRQ), Patient Safety Network (PSNet). (March, 2015). The role of the patient in patient safety. Retrieved from https://psnet.ahrq.gov/primers/primer/17/the-role-of-the-patient-in-safety

U.S. Department of Health and Human Services (HHS), Centers for Medicare and Medicaid (CMS). (2011, October). Quality improvement organizations. Retrieved from www.cms.hhs.gov/qualityimprovementorgs

U.S. Department of Health and Human Services (HHS), Centers for Medicare and Medicaid (CMS). (2016). Welcome to the Partnership for Patients. Retrieved from https://partnership-forpatients.cms.gov/

U.S. Department of Health and Human Services (HHS), National Prevention, Health Promotion, and Public Health Council. (2011). National prevention strategy. Washington, DC: Retrieved from http://www.surgeongeneral.gov/priorities/prevention/strategy/index.html

Zimmerman, P. (2001). The problems with healthcare customer satisfaction surveys. In J. Dochterman & H. Grace (Eds.), *Current issues in nursing* (6th ed., pp. 255–260). St. Louis, MO: Mosby.

Quality and Safety: Basic Understanding

CHAPTER OBJECTIVES

At the conclusion of this chapter, the learner will be able to:

- Examine key models used to understand errors.
- Compare and contrast the common types of errors.
- Analyze the impact of staffing levels and workloads on outcomes.
- Examine frontline safety as an element of healthcare safety.
- Explain how human factors impact healthcare safety.
- Discuss workplace safety and implications for continuous quality improvement.

OUTLINE

KEY TERMS

Active error	Lapse	Physical fatigue
Adverse event	Latent conditions	Presenteeism
Bullying	Latent error	Red rules
Compassion fatigue	Lateral violence	Sentinel event
Errors of execution	Mental fatigue	Slip
Errors of planning	Missed care	Standardization
Frontline safety	Mistake	Stress
Frontline staff	Misuse	Swiss cheese model
Human error	Near miss	Technical failure
Human factors and ergonomics	Omission	Underuse
Human failure	Organizational failure	Workplace violence
Incivility	Overuse	

Introduction

According to Classen and colleagues (2011), "Identification and measurement of adverse medical events is central to patient safety, forming a foundation of accountability, prioritizing problems to work on, generating ideas for safer care, and testing which interventions work" (p. 581). The healthcare system has been undergoing major transformation to address the critical need to improve care. Are frontline nursing staff ready for this focus on continuous quality improvement (CQI)? In many cases, they are not. As noted in other chapters, nursing education must assume some of the responsibility to ensure that nurses are better prepared to engage in CQI. We need to recognize that good care should be based on good science (Larkin, Lorenz, Rack, & Shatzer, 2012). This insight applies to all the content in this text. Evidence-based practice is a critical theme and, when used, increases the opportunity to reach effective outcomes.

The landmark report *Keeping Patients Safe: Transforming the Work Environment for Nurses* (IOM, 2004) indicated that the work nurses do has a major impact on quality care, but the work environment needs to improve so that nurses can effectively meet patient outcomes. Hughes and Clancy (2005) state the following in response to this report:

> Caring for patients relies heavily on human decision-making and action. Nurses are vulnerable to being part of errors because the process of patient care leaves them exposed to the inevitable results of human fallibilities that occur throughout the entire process of care, the complexity of health care, or a combination thereof. (p. 289)

This chapter expands the discussion about CQI by examining errors and factors that impact the occurrence of errors. It is important to understand this content before examining CQI measurement and responses to quality problems and errors.

Understanding Errors

In 2012, the U.S. Department of Health and Human Services (HHS) Office of Inspector General (OIG) followed up on its 2010 report on adverse events in hospitals indicating that 27% of Medicare patients who were hospitalized in October 2008 experienced either a serious adverse event (resulting in prolonged hospitalization, permanent disability, life-sustaining intervention, or death) or temporary harm event (requiring intervention but not resulting in lasting harm). Another finding of this review was that only half of the hospitals had adverse event reporting systems. The 2012 report, which continued the review of the 2008 hospitals, states the following:

> We found that an estimated 60 percent of adverse and temporary harm events nationally occurred at hospitals in states with reporting systems, yet only

an estimated 12 percent of the events nationally met state requirements for reporting. We also found that hospitals reported only 1 percent of events. Most of the events that states required to be reported but that hospitals did not report were not identified by internal hospital incident reporting systems. This suggests that low reporting to state systems is more likely the result of hospital failure to identify events than of hospitals' neglecting to report known events. (HHS, OIG, 2012)

These findings indicate that there continues to be need for better understanding of errors and application of this understanding to respond to and prevent errors. An error itself is not bad, but the consequence or outcome may be. Since we cannot eliminate risk of errors, we focus on adverse consequences (Reason, 2002).

Models Used to Understand Errors

There are many models that healthcare organizations (HCOs) and the government might apply to understanding errors. The following discussion focuses on three of the more commonly used models.

The Swiss Cheese Model

Reason's work on errors is a model that is frequently used (Reason, 2000). This model is called the **Swiss cheese model**. It focuses on system failure and recognizes that there is potential for an error in any process. Reason compared this situation to a stack of slices of Swiss cheese. The holes are opportunities for errors, and all processes have them, just like all slices of Swiss cheese have holes. The slices represent defenses to prevent errors. Sometimes an error goes through a hole, yet there is no serious problem or harm because the next slice prevents the error from passing further, thus avoiding a major problem or error. When the holes are aligned, an error may go straight through consecutive slices, and a major error occurs. The Agency for Healthcare Research and Quality (AHRQ) describes the model as follows:

> [The model] illustrates how analyses of major accidents and catastrophic systems failures tend to reveal multiple, smaller failures leading up to the actual hazard.... For example, if the hazard was wrong-site surgery, slices of the cheese might include conventions for identifying sidedness on radiology tests, a protocol for signing the correct site when the surgeon and patient first meet, and a second protocol for reviewing the medical record and checking the previously marked site in the operating room. Many more layers exist. The point is that no single barrier is foolproof. (HHS, AHRQ, PSNet, 2015c)

In health care it is recognized that some errors are not acceptable, such as operating on the wrong site or wrong person. Such incidents represent times when the holes align, which is infrequent. As discussed elsewhere in this text, an emphasis on the system is of growing concern to CQI. Reason and others have also noted the importance of systems problems, as the AHRQ articulates:

> Many of the systems problems discussed by Reason and others—poorly designed work schedules, lack of teamwork, variations in the design of important equipment between and even within institutions—are sufficiently common that many of the slices of cheese already have their holes aligned. In such cases, one slice of cheese may be all that is left between the patient and significant hazard. (HHS, AHRQ, PSNet, 2015c)

The Connect to Current Information section at the end of the chapter provides a link to figures that illustrate the Swiss cheese model.

Enthoven Classification of Causes of Errors

Another example of a model for understanding and responding to errors such as near misses is the Enthoven model. This model focuses on three sources of errors and is described in **Figure 7-1** (Henneman & Gawlinski, 2004; Henneman et al., 2010):

1. **Technical failure** *or active error, a system failure.* Examples of related factors are physical equipment not available or not working adequately and computer and software availability.

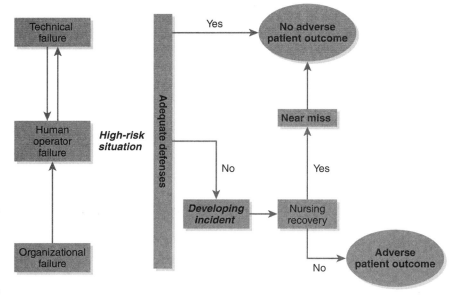

Figure 7-1. Near-Miss Model
Reproduced from Henneman, E., & Gawlinski, A. (2004). A "near-miss" model for describing the nurse's role in the recovery of medical errors. *Journal of Professional Nursing, 20*(3), 196–201. Copyright 2004, with permission from Elsevier.

2. **Organizational failure** *or latent error, a system failure.* Examples of related factors are staff orientation and training, policies, procedures, and use of clinical pathways or protocols. Enthoven also combined technical and organizational error and referred to these dynamics as latent error or condition.

3. **Human failure** *or individual failure.* Examples of related factors are staff knowledge and competencies. This source of error is also referred to as an active failure.

Enthoven also included a category he called "other" for errors that did not fall into his major error categories.

An effective CQI system provides defenses to respond when a risk situation occurs that could result in an error. If the defense works, then there is no error; however, if the defense does not work, then an error may be in process. It is at this time that nursing recovery may stop the error and thus a near miss may occur, in which case there is no adverse patient outcome. What this means is the nurse involved in direct care identifies, interrupts, and corrects the error. This intervention on the part of the nurse is a critical aspect in improving care, and one that each nurse needs to apply in practice.

Generic Error-Modeling System

Reason developed the generic error-modeling system (GEMS) to pinpoint the key concerns when examining errors. He notes that there seem to be several common types of errors. **Human error** is "a generic term to encompass all those occasions in which a planned sequence of mental or physical activities fails to achieve its intended outcome, and when these failures cannot be attributed to the intervention of some chance agency" (Reason, 1990, p. 7). The following error types are identified in the GEMS model (Van Metre, Slovensky, & McLaughlin, 2013):

- *Skill-based performance* is directed by the individual's education and expertise.
- *Rule-based performance* occurs when there are "familiar problems in which solutions are governed by stored rules of the 'if-then' type. These rules are based on previous experiences and are called into play when a trigger event or situation occurs" (p. 317). An example would be a cardiac arrest procedure that is not applied correctly.
- *Knowledge-based performance* occurs in situations that require the provider to think about what needs to be done and how best to do it. In this case, planning errors may occur.

Classification of an error begins with determining if the error results from action or inaction. If inaction, then there is little if any physical evidence and often the event is not viewed as an error and thus not reported as one. Inaction errors may be of two types: Knowledge-based and rule-based. If the error is an action error, then one has to determine if it is related to planning, execution, or intention. Most errors fall into the area of execution. For both planning and execution errors, the GEMS type of performance error is identified. Intention may also be a concern and is related to violations, such as staff not following a procedure in order to reduce their work time. Individual accountability is important in this category; even though systems are emphasized, there are circumstances in which accountability and blame are important to consider.

Stop and Consider #1

The major models used to understand errors recognize that errors cannot be totally eliminated.

Types of Errors

There are many different types of errors. As noted in other chapters, an error is "the failure of a planned action to be completed as intended or the use of wrong plan to achieve an aim" (IOM, 1999, p. 28). Broadly, errors can be described as **errors of planning** (e.g., You included the wrong intervention in a plan for a patient.). This may also be referred to as an error of judgment. Care begins with the patient, and the provider uses knowledge and expertise along with clinical judgment and reasoning to plan care and implement that plan. Anywhere in the process errors can occur and are referred to as **errors of execution** (e.g., You use an intervention at the wrong time.). The most frequent error is leaving a step out of a planned sequence of activities (Gawande, 2009; Reason, 2002). **Latent conditions**, or less apparent organization failures that contribute to errors, are important factors influencing the occurrence of errors. An example is the failure of a drug alert. In this situation, the threats are not immediately clear, and this typically relates to system problems (ISMP, 2011).

HCO management and staff may focus so much on avoiding failure or errors that they become preoccupied with this step rather than considering the full picture and developing effective response strategies (Clark & Bramble, 2013). It is not uncommon for managers and staff to ignore the smaller errors and even to view them as disruptions and nothing more. This scenario then is a lost opportunity to learn more about potential errors. For example, a nurse takes the wrong intravenous fluids to the patient's room and realizes she has the wrong fluids, requiring a search for the correct fluids. Even as the nurse is complaining about how long this is taking, she is ignoring that this was a near miss that should be analyzed to determine why the wrong fluids were selected. Was the order not

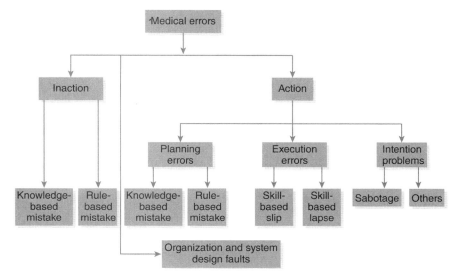

Figure 7-2. Potential Classification of Human Medical Errors
Reproduced from Van Metre, J., Slovensky, D., & McLaughlin, C. (2013). Classification of medical errors. In *McLaughlin & Kaluzny's Continuous quality improvement in health care,* (4th ed., pp. 312–334). Burlington, MA: Jones & Bartlett Learning.

clear? Was the label on the fluid wrong or difficult to read? Was the storage area confusing, making it easy to pick the wrong item? Did the nurse read or interpret the order incorrectly because she is at the end of a long shift and exhausted? Was the nurse interrupted and distracted from what she was doing? Finally, what made the nurse stop and realize the wrong fluids had been selected?

Figure 7-2 shows some of the types of medical errors.

Underuse, Overuse, Misuse

Three common types of errors are underuse, overuse, and misuse, and all are found in a variety of HCO settings and may involve a variety of staff (Finkelman & Kenner, 2016, p. 382):

- **Underuse**. This error is a failure to provide a service that would have produced a favorable outcome for the patient. It may be due to lack of access to needed services or resources that are recognized as important in meeting the outcomes (Sadeghi, Barzi, Mikhail, & Shabot, 2013). Example: The patient is not able to get a specialty service needed for cancer treatment because of distance from resources, or the patient's insurer will not cover a medication for arthritis that could make the patient more mobile.
- **Misuse**. This error is an avoidable event that prevents patients from receiving full potential benefit of a service. Misuse may relate to incorrect diagnoses, medical errors, or avoidable complications (Sadeghi et al., 2013).

Example: The patient receives a medication that is not prescribed and conflicts with the patient's allergies; the patient experiences anaphylaxis.

- **Overuse.** This error occurs when the potential for harm from the provision of a service exceeds the possible benefit. In this situation, risks outweigh benefits (Sadeghi et al., 2013). Example: An elderly patient is on multiple medications, and the patient's multiple healthcare providers do not know the medications that have been prescribed by different specialists. Overuse can result in several negative outcomes. The most obvious is cost. If we provide more services than needed, healthcare costs may add up. Other examples of possible problems are overtesting, overdiagnosis, and overtreatment, all of which may increase risk for patient harm such as more risk for complications and more opportunities for errors (Gawande, 2015).

Active Errors

An **active error** is an error that results from noncompliance with a procedure that involves a frontline worker (i.e., direct care worker). Another term that refers to this type of error is *error at the sharp end*. *Sharp end* refers to staff or parts of the system that come in direct contact with the patient, while the *blunt end* refers to factors that impact the sharp end. Active errors are what we think of as errors that are obvious, or sharp end.

Latent Errors

Latent errors are associated with errors that are caused by system problems that then impact a frontline worker. Latent conditions are not immediately apparent (Finkelman & Kenner, 2012). An example might be when staff have not been informed about a change in a procedure. Staff then do not follow the new procedure, and an error occurs.

Latent errors are less apparent failures. There are two types: slips and mistakes (HHS, AHRQ, PSNet, 2015a). A **slip** happens when you are not clear. For example, you may write down the wrong date and time because you are not focused on what you are doing, or you may have lapses in concentration, often due to sensory or emotional distractions, fatigue, or stress. A **lapse** happens when you fail to check something that is part of the procedure, something that you should be monitoring as you implement the procedure. **Mistakes** relate to wrong decisions, often related to inexperience, inadequate training, or even negligence. For example, we practice and learn how to do a procedure, and we might then experience a lapse or a slip. Factors that may lead to latent errors are identified in **Table 7-1.**

TABLE 7-1 Factors That May Lead to Latent Errors	
Type of Factor	**Example**
Institutional/regulatory	The hospital was under regulatory pressure to improve pneumococcal vaccination rates.
Organizational/ management	A nurse detected a medication error, but the physician discouraged her from reporting it.
Work environment	Lacking the appropriate equipment to perform hysteroscopy, operating room staff improvised using equipment from other sets. During the procedure, the patient suffered an air embolism.
Team environment	A surgeon completed an operation despite being informed by a nurse and the anesthesiologist that the suction catheter tip was missing. The tip was subsequently found inside the patient, requiring additional surgery.
Staffing	An overworked nurse mistakenly administered insulin instead of an antinausea medication, resulting in hypoglycemic coma.
Task-related	An intern incorrectly calculated the equivalent dose of long-acting MS Contin for a patient who had been receiving Vicodin. The patient experienced an opiate overdose and aspiration pneumonia, resulting in a prolonged intensive care unit care.
Patient characteristics	The parents of a young boy misread the instructions on a bottle of acetaminophen, causing their child to experience liver damage.

Reproduced with permission from AHRQ Patient Safety Network, Ranji, S., Wachter, R.M., & Hartman, E.E. (August 2014). Patient safety primer: Root cause analysis. Retrieved from https://psnet.ahrq.gov/primers/primer/10.

Near Misses

A **near miss** occurs when an error almost happened, but staff caught it before it became an error. Near misses should not be ignored, as much can be learned from them. This is a weak area of monitoring, with many HCOs not tracking near misses, staff not reporting them, or staff and management not even knowing they occurred. Near misses occur 300 times more often than do adverse events (Barach & Small, 2000).

Adverse Events

An **adverse event** is an injury resulting from a medical intervention, not from the patient's underlying condition. It is an untoward, undesirable event, usually not expected, and it may have a long-term effect. This event may be due to errors or be preventable. Adverse events can be classified according to type and causes (WHO Collaborating Center for Patient Safety Solutions, 2008). They are typically related to the following situations and factors:

- Anesthesia
- Environmental factors
- Equipment factors
- Infection
- Medication errors
- Medical events
- Pediatric events
- Surgical events
- Transfer or discharge
- Unanticipated events

Though the situations/factors listed here are the most common, adverse events can happen during any number of other situations. Causes of adverse events are also broad, and the following areas have greater potential for causing adverse events:

- Care planning
- Communication
- Continuum of care
- Coordination and collaboration
- Human factors
- Information management
- Organization culture
- Patient assessment
- Patient identification
- Patient involvement and education
- Inadequate physical resources

Root cause analysis, discussed in other chapters, is often used to identify and understand causes and may result in identifying multiple causes.

If the adverse event is related to drugs or medical equipment and the event is serious, it should be reported to Food and Drug Administration when the patient outcome is any of the following (HHS, FDA, 2014):

- *Death.* Report if you suspect that the death was an outcome of an adverse event, and if known, include the date of the event.

■ *Life threatening.* Report if it is suspected the patient was at substantial risk of dying at the time of the adverse event, or report if use or continued use of a device or other medical product might have resulted in the death of the patient.

■ *Hospitalization (initial or prolonged).* Report if admission to the hospital or prolongation of hospitalization was a result of an adverse event. Emergency room visits that do not result in admission to the hospital should also be evaluated for one of the other serious outcomes (e.g., life threatening, required intervention to prevent permanent impairment or damage, other serious medically important event).

■ *Disability or permanent damage.* Report if an adverse event resulted in substantial disruption of a person's ability to conduct normal life functions (e.g., a significant, persistent or permanent change, impairment, damage, or disruption in the patient's body function/structure, physical activities, and/ or quality of life).

■ *Congenital anomaly/birth defect.* Report if you suspect that exposure to a medical product prior to conception or during pregnancy may have resulted in an adverse outcome in the child.

■ *Required intervention to prevent permanent impairment or damage (devices).* Report if you believe that a medical or surgical intervention was necessary to preclude permanent impairment of a body function or prevent permanent damage to a body structure; report if either situation is suspected to be due to the use of a medical product.

■ *Other serious outcome (important medical events).* Report when the event does not fit the other outcomes, but the event may jeopardize the patient and may require medical or surgical intervention (treatment) to prevent one of the other outcomes. Examples include allergic bronchospasm requiring treatment in an emergency department, serious blood dyscrasias, seizures/convulsions that do not result in hospitalization, or the development of drug dependence.

Table 7-2 provides additional examples of serious reportable events as identified by the National Quality Forum.

Sentinel Events and Alerts

Sentinel events are unexpected events that happen to patients resulting in major negative outcomes, such as an unexpected death or a critical physical or psychological complication that can lead to major alteration in the patient's health. The term "sentinel" is used for these events because the events indicate the need for immediate response and analysis (The Joint Commission, 2014). Examples of sentinel events are suicide, wrong-site surgery, and serious operative and post-operative complications. These events may be quite unique and unexpected. For

TABLE 7-2 List of National Quality Forum Serious Reportable Events

Event	Additional Specifications
1. Surgical events	
A. Surgery performed on the wrong body part	Defined as any surgery performed on a body part that is not consistent with the documented informed consent for that patient. Excludes emergent situations that occur in the course of surgery and/or whose exigency precludes obtaining informed consent.
B. Surgery performed on the wrong patient	Defined as any surgery on a patient that is not consistent with the documented informed consent for that patient.
C. Wrong surgical procedure performed on a patient	Defined as any procedure performed on a patient that is not consistent with the documented informed consent for that patient. Excludes emergent situations that occur in the course of surgery and/or whose exigency precludes obtaining informed consent. Surgery includes endoscopies and other invasive procedures.
D. Retention of a foreign object in a patient after surgery or other procedure	Excludes objects intentionally implanted as part of a planned intervention and objects present prior to surgery that were intentionally retained.
E. Intraoperative or immediately postoperative death in an <u>American Society of Anesthesiologists</u> (ASA) Class I patient	Includes ASA Class I patient deaths in situations where anesthesia was administered; the planned surgical procedure may or may not have been carried out. Immediately postoperative means within 24 hours after induction of anesthesia (if surgery not completed), surgery, or other invasive procedure was completed.
2. Product or device events	
A. Patient death or serious disability associated with the use of contaminated drugs, devices, or biologics provided by the healthcare facility	Includes generally detectable contaminants in drugs, devices, or biologics regardless of the source of contamination and/or product.

B. Patient death or serious disability associated with the use or function of a device in patient care, in which the device is used for functions other than as intended	Includes, but is not limited to, catheters, drains and other specialized tubes, infusion pumps, and ventilators.
C. Patient death or serious disability associated with intravascular air embolism that occurs while being cared for in a healthcare facility	Excludes deaths associated with neurosurgical procedures known to be a high risk of intravascular air embolism.
3. Patient protection events	
A. Infant discharged to the wrong person	
B. Patient death or serious disability associated with patient elopement (disappearance) for more than 4 hours	Excludes events involving competent adults.
C. Patient suicide, or attempted suicide resulting in serious disability, while being cared for in a healthcare facility	Defined as events that result from patient actions after admission to a healthcare facility. Excludes deaths resulting from self-inflicted injuries that were the reason for admission to the healthcare facility.
4. Care management events	
A. Patient death or serious disability associated with a medication error (e.g., errors involving the wrong drug, wrong dose, wrong patient, wrong time, wrong rate, wrong preparation, or wrong route of administration)	Excludes reasonable differences in clinical judgment on drug selection and dose.
B. Patient death or serious disability associated with a hemolytic reaction due to the administration of ABO-incompatible blood or blood products	

(Continued)

TABLE 7–2 List of National Quality Forum Serious Reportable Events (Continued)	
Event	**Additional Specifications**
C. Maternal death or serious disability associated with labor or delivery in a low-risk pregnancy while being cared for in a healthcare facility	Includes events that occur within 42 days post delivery. Excludes deaths from pulmonary or amniotic fluid embolism, acute fatty liver of pregnancy, and cardiomyopathy.
D. Patient death or serious disability associated with hypoglycemia, the onset of which occurs while the patient is being cared for in a healthcare facility	
E. Death or serious disability (kernicterus) associated with failure to identify and treat hyperbilirubinemia in neonates	Hyperbilirubinemia is defined as bilirubin levels >30 mg/dL. Neonates refers to the first 38 days of life.
F. Stage 3 or 4 pressure ulcers acquired after admission to a healthcare facility	Excludes progression from Stage 2 to Stage 3 if Stage 2 was recognized upon admission.
G. Patient death or serious disability due to spinal manipulative therapy	
5. Environmental events	
A. Patient death or serious disability associated with an electric shock while being cared for in a healthcare facility	Excludes events involving planned treatments such as electric countershocks.
B. Any incident in which a line designated for oxygen or other gas to be delivered to a patient contains the wrong gas or is contaminated by toxic substances	

C. Patient death or serious disability associated with a burn incurred from any source while being cared for in a healthcare facility	
D. Patient death associated with a fall while being cared for in a healthcare facility	
E. Patient death or serious disability associated with the use of restraints or bedrails while being cared for in a healthcare facility	
6. Criminal events	
A. Any instance of care ordered by or provided by someone impersonating a physician, nurse, pharmacist, or other licensed healthcare provider	
B. Abduction of a patient of any age	
C. Sexual assault on a patient within or on the grounds of the healthcare facility	
D. Death or significant injury of a patient or staff member resulting from a physical assault (i.e., battery) that occurs within or on the grounds of the healthcare facility	

Reproduced from Kizer, K.W. & Stegun, M.B. (October 2014). Serious reportable adverse events in health care. In Agency for Healthcare Research and Quality (AHRQ), *Advances in patient safety*. Rockville, MD: Author. Retrieved from http://www .ahrq.gov/professionals/quality-patient-safety/patient-safety-resources/resources/advances-in-patient-safety/index.html

example, in 2016 in a pediatric hospital, parents of a hospitalized baby took heroin in their baby's hospital room. One parent died in the room, and the other required medical treatment. The father had a gun in his pocket (Seelye, 2016). This is not a typical event, and it put the parents at risk and also their baby, other patients and their families, and the staff. This type of event requires immediate response and analysis to ensure safety of all and long-term response to prevent similar occurrences. Factors that should be assessed in the analysis include the status of the patient admission assessment, including the parents, and the presence of active surveillance so that changes in behavior might have been noticed. Guns in hospitals are a major risk, although most hospitals in the United States do not have security that would identify when guns are brought into the hospital. Psychiatric hospitals are usually more alert to weapons and consider bringing weapons into a hospital a sentinel event.

Not all errors are sentinel events, but when errors are sentinel events, they should not be ignored. It is also important that staff involved in a sentinel event get support. It can be extremely traumatic and lead to staff physiological and psychological problems (The Joint Commission, 2015).

The Joint Commission distributes sentinel alerts to its accredited HCOs and identifies them on its website. The alerts are classified based on their healthcare site and information provided to The Joint Commission for review. When HCOs report these events, information should include a plan identifying action(s) the HCO will take, responsibility, timelines, and strategies for evaluation and sustaining the change. The plan is, of course, useful to the individual HCO, but it also provides important data that can be used to alert other HCOs about potential risks and possible responses (Sorbello, 2008). Root cause analysis, discussed elsewhere in this text, is used to analyze sentinel events to provide understanding of the event and steps that might be taken to respond to and prevent these events. All of these efforts provide opportunities for HCOs, healthcare providers, and healthcare professions to learn more about the trajectory of care. HCOs benefit from self-reporting to The Joint Commission in the following ways (The Joint Commission, 2014):

- Reporting allows The Joint Commission to provide support and expertise during the review of a sentinel event.
- Reporting enables collaboration with a patient safety expert in The Joint Commission's Sentinel Event Unit of the Office of Quality and Patient Safety.
- Reporting raises the level of transparency in the organization and promotes a culture of safety.
- Reporting conveys the HCO's message to the public that it is doing everything possible, proactively, to prevent similar patient safety events in the future.

Omissions and Missed Care

Errors may also be classified as **omissions**. This type of error occurs when assessment, planning, and interventions are not provided, and it may lead to problems for the patient and interfere with reaching expected outcomes. Nurses care for many patients and have many responsibilities, all of which can lead even the best practice to errors of omission (Kalisch, 2015). Research indicates that some of the common reasons for omissions are communication problems, difficulties getting material resources such as supplies or equipment that are not available when needed, unavailability of needed drugs, equipment not working effectively, and inadequate staffing (Kalisch, Landstrom, & Williams, 2008).

Missed care should also be considered an error and is a type of omission. Nursing care that is delayed, partially completed, or not completed is missed care (HHS, AHRQ, PSNet, 2015b). This event is associated with higher rates of adverse events and lower patient satisfaction (Jones, Hamilton, & Murray, 2015). Missed care is primarily identified by staff self-report and patient report. The AHRQ reports that in a review of 42 studies, 55% to 95% of nurse respondents reported missed care for one or more items (HHS, AHRQ, PSNet, 2015b). Factors that increase risk for missed nursing care are ineffective culture of safety; high nursing workload, such as high patient-to-nurse ratio; resource inadequacy; and overall problems with work environment (Ball, Murrells, Rafferty, Morrow, & Griffiths, 2014). Ineffective teamwork between nurses may also lead to missed nursing care (Kalisch & Lee, 2010). In summary, the AHRQ notes that there are several predictors of missed care (HHS, AHRQ, PSNet, 2015b):

- Missed nursing care is primarily a problem of time pressure, competing demands, and adequate nurse staffing needed to prevent it.
- Organizational and unit culture influence missed nursing care.
- The organization of nursing work and the organization of the supply chain that supports nursing work may contribute to preventing missed care.

With concern about missed nursing care, some nurse experts have developed a model of missed nursing care that is based on the structure-process-outcome framework (also described by others as "unfinished nursing care" and "care left undone") (HHS, AHRQ, PSNet, 2015b; Kalisch, 2015; Kalisch et al., 2008; Kalisch, Xie, & Dabney, 2014). In this model, the following factors are associated with structure, process, and outcome and missed care. When assessing missed nursing care, structure factors to examine are labor resources (e.g., number and types of nursing staff, competence level of nursing staff, staff education and experience), material resources (e.g., availability of necessary medications, supplies, and equipment), and teamwork and communication (e.g., among patient care team members, between nurses and physicians, between nurses and support staff). The model suggests that when one or more of these resources is missing in an organization or during a work period, nurses need to prioritize their care activities, and this then may lead to delayed or omitted nursing care activities. When a nurse experiences limited resources, the common response is for the nurse to identify priorities; the nurse may then decide to delay care, which may result in omission of care. This decision process is influenced by four individual-level factors (HHS, AHRQ, PSNet, 2015c; Kalisch, Xie, & Dabney, 2014; Kalisch et al., 2008):

1. The nurse's perceptions of team or group norms
2. The nurse's judgment about the importance of various aspects of care relative to the conditions of multiple patients the nurse may be responsible for
3. The nurse's values, attitudes, and beliefs
4. The nurse's usual practice.

As stated by the AHRQ, "The outcome of the clinical prioritization process in the face of resource or time scarcity is missed nursing care" (HHS, AHRQ, PSNet, 2015c).

Risk of Errors

Due to the *Quality Chasm* reports on quality, there has been more attention placed on risk of errors in order to better understand reasons for errors and also when possible to develop strategies to prevent errors. Communication dysfunction is the number one risk factor. Poor communication can occur between the healthcare provider and patient, among staff members, between staff and management, or more generally from an organization perspective. Verbal and written communication that is not clear or timely may lead to error risk. Problems with the flow of information—someone left out of the communication process, for example—increases risk.

Another risk factor is staff preparation. This relates directly to the *Quality Chasm* report, *Health Professions Education* (IOM, 2003) that examined professional education and identified the five healthcare professions core competencies. HCOs need to have competent healthcare providers applying for positions. On the other end, HCOs need to focus on effective orientation for new staff and knowledge transfer and continuing staff education for all levels of staff. Improved knowledge and competence reduce risk of errors. HCO standards, policies, and procedures provide consistency, effective communication, and greater ability to measure care outcomes based on the criteria identified in these documents. These efforts decrease risk.

As health care becomes more technical, risk is increasing—not only in the use of informatics but also in the use of complex equipment needed for complex patient care. This equipment needs to be as new as possible and maintained. When working with equipment, staff and patients can be injured. Staff need to recognize when equipment is not functioning at the level required or when it might cause harm. HCOs need to have experienced staff knowledgeable in the use of medical equipment and provide staff training in the equipment's use. Maintenance of equipment, both routine and following unexpected malfunctions, is also critical.

Staff need access to this assistance in a timely manner. Another technology-related issue of increasing relevance is use of passwords, which are sometimes required for equipment use, particularly if associated with computers. Staff need access to current passwords and methods to get passwords in emergencies to avoid errors and inability to provide care when needed.

Figure 7-3 describes five drivers and related elements that influence clinical quality and patient safety.

Stop and Consider #2

There are many types of errors, such as missed care, which many staff may not recognize as an error.

Staffing Levels, Workloads, and Outcomes

Staffing levels have long been a concern. HCOs need the right staff with the right preparation and experience in positions and need the number of staff required to provide care effectively. Human factors are also important to consider in the staffing process. Many HCOs have problems with staffing levels, overscheduling of staff, use of temporary staff, and other staffing challenges that impact knowledge of the situation, consistency, communication, and teamwork. These staffing dynamics all impact the risk of errors.

Staffing is an important topic in this chapter because it has an impact on quality, including patient and staff safety. A bill introduced in the House of Representatives

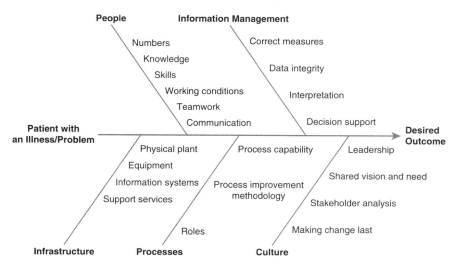

Figure 7-3. Five Drivers of Clinical Quality and Patient Safety
Reproduced from Ettenberg, W. (2006). Basic tools for quality improvement. In D. Nash & N. Goldfarb, *The quality solution*, (pp. 115–132). Burlington, MA: Jones & Bartlett Learning.

on April 29, 2015 (H.R. 2083, S. 1132, Registered Nurse Safe Staffing) demonstrates that staffing has become a national concern (U.S. Congress, House of Representatives, 2015). This is not the first time this bill has been introduced, and when introduced in 2015, seven states had passed state legislation using a similar model as the federal legislation. The bill, however, in 2016 had not moved forward despite the need for greater regulation, as noted by the American Nurses Association (ANA). The ANA participated in the development of this bill and strongly supported it, noting that registered nurses help to reduce deaths and errors. This requires unit-by-unit nurse staffing plans, and the ANA bases this on its *Principles for Nurse Staffing* (ANA, 2012a). The principles focus on three aspects of staffing: patient care unit (patient-specific and unit-specific factors), nursing staff (experience and expertise), and organizations (policies and practices).

Some nursing staff and leaders have questioned whether it is best to legislate mandatory staffing levels. For example, Massachusetts decided to take a different approach that did not include mandatory ratios but rather provided flexibility, recognizing that HCOs and units within HCOs vary (Gale & Noga, 2013). This approach is called *PatientCareLink*, which uses a dashboard to describe required staff skills, staffing per shift, staffing levels, and nurse management and support staff requirements along with the characteristics of the HCO and the unit. HCO participation is voluntary, but it has been very high. This information is now available to the public for comparison along with online quality data. Over time, quality has improved. Along with this type of statewide initiative, there is greater emphasis now on entry-level nursing education that supports the recommendations of *The Future of Nursing* report (IOM, 2010).

Nursing research has examined the impact of staffing on patient outcomes, but much more is needed. Several experts note that it is important to examine the influence of the intensity of patient needs and required nursing care (Aiken et al., 2010; Domrose, 2010; Rogers, Hwang, Scott, Aiken, & Dinges, 2004; Welton, 2007). These factors need to be considered for mandatory staffing levels or any type of staffing that might be used. Who should provide care is important and should also be part of effective delegation decisions.

Other studies have examined work schedules (Trinkoff et al., 2010). What is it about work schedules and errors that we should be concerned about? Work schedules identify hours worked per day, hours worked per week, weekends worked per month, number of breaks lasting 10 minutes or more, including meals during a workday, and shift rotation (Trinkoff et al., 2010). The work schedule element that is most commonly related to patient mortality is lack of nurse recovery time or time away from work, which often results in staff fatigue and injury. The researchers for this study also comment that HCOs should examine the impact of 12-hour shifts, as this might not be the best schedule given the need for recovery time after working long hours.

The Aiken et al. (2010) study examined the association between lower patient-to-nurse ratios and inpatient mortality to find that when the number of patients decreased, mortality rates decreased, as did failure to rescue. These hospitals also had effective work environments, but if the work environment was not effective, reducing the ratio did not decrease mortality. This finding indicates that staffing may not be the only important factor.

Another study examined the relationship between nurse staffing in general and intensive care units and patient outcomes (Blegen, Goode, Spetz, Vaughn, & Park, 2011). This study also compared safety-net and non-safety-net hospitals. A safety-net hospital is "a hospital receiving adjustment payments to provide care to a significantly disproportionate share of low-income patients who are not paid by other payers, such as Medicare, Medicaid, the Children's Health Insurance Program, or other health insurance" (Blegen et al., 2011, p. 407). In one study, it was thought that safety-net hospitals have higher rates of errors and greater need to improve quality of care because their patients are more complex (VanDeusen et al., 2015). The conclusion from the sample of 54 hospitals is there is an association between higher staffing and lower hospital-acquired infections, lower failure to rescue events, lower mortality, and reduced hospital stay. The safety-net hospitals did experience higher rates of congestive heart failure, failure to rescue events, and decubitus ulcers, but the average staffing levels were not much different from non-safety-net hospitals. There was no specific explanation for this, but it could be related to the long-term concern that the safety-net hospital patients are more complex and generally have poorer health status. There can be many other reasons, including how staffing is done and the quality improvement programs in these HCOs.

Other studies also address staff turnover and patient outcomes (Bae, Mark, & Fried, 2009). Why is staff turnover a factor? When units lose staff familiar with the unit and HCO, they are losing expertise and consistency. Teams are also affected when members leave. Some units may have to use temporary staff until new staff are hired, and temporary staff usually are not familiar with the unit, patients, policies, and other workplace dynamics and may not have the best level of expertise and practice. Teams are affected, as a temporary member may not be as welcomed, and this may impact communication, collaboration, and decision-making. When new staff are hired, there also is an orientation period, new team members need time to integrate, and other adjustments must be made. All of these changes are costly for the HCO. Bae and colleagues (2009) describe the situation as follows:

> Workgroup processes mediate the nursing unit turnover–patient outcomes relationship. Nursing turnover leads to changes in workgroup processes such as decreased member attraction to the nursing unit, ineffective coordination, and inaccurate communication. Such inefficient workgroup processes in turn negatively affect patient outcomes. (p. 42)

In addition to the importance of staffing levels or patient-to-nurse ratios, the following factors related to staff have an impact on care quality: nurse burnout, job satisfaction, teamwork, nurse turnover, nursing leadership, and the nurse practice environment (HHS, AHRQ, 2013). Burnout is a frequent topic in the nursing profession. An important element of burnout is "emotional exhaustion, which is associated with emotional and cognitive detachment from work as a way to cope with work demands" (Cimiotti, Aiken, Sloane, & Wu, 2012, p. 486; Maslach, 2003). For example, a nursing study that examined the impact of burnout on nurse staffing and specifically on hospital patient infections proposed and concluded that there is an association between these factors (Cimiotti et al., 2012). When nurse burnout combines with high patient-to-nurse ratios, job dissatisfaction results, which has an impact on quality of care. The AHRQ describes clinician burnout as follows:

> The burned out clinician may develop a sense of cynical detachment from work and view people, especially patients, as objects. Fatigue, exhaustion, and detachment coalesce such that clinicians no longer feel effective at work because they have lost a sense of their ability to contribute meaningfully. (HHS, AHRQ, 2016)

Another factor that requires further examination is the use of non–registered nurse (RN) staff and the impact this practice has on patient outcomes. For example, does the use of non-RN staff to do routine tasks give the RN more time for monitoring patients and providing more complex nursing care? This study had a small sample, but its results are supported by other studies with similar results; staffing levels and mix (e.g., types of staff) make a difference in a variety of patient outcomes.

Stop and Consider #3
Staffing and workload are factors that should be part of error analysis.

Frontline Safety

Frontline staff are direct care staff, who often get lost in the big picture. However, in the end, it is the frontline staff who make the biggest difference in CQI, regardless of the type or size of the HCO. During direct care, **frontline safety** occurs when staff consider patient safety and quality in their daily work. Nurses are represented in large numbers in the frontline staff, and to make an impact, they need to assume leadership and engagement in CQI.

Impact on CQI

A study published in 2012 indicated that the safety culture is associated not only with patient and staff injuries, but also with working conditions that increase risk, such as nursing hours per patient day and staff turnover (Taylor et al., 2012). This study describes safety as the perception of HCO commitment to safety and team-work. Another critical factor is perception of the quality of collaboration. The study concludes by suggesting the following:

> Patient and nurse safety may constitute linked outcomes rather than distinct silos. Traditionally, the fields of occupational and patient safety have been addressed separately, but regarding them as related components of an organization's safety culture might be more apt. Future healthcare safety research and intervention efforts should consider a new paradigm integrating lessons learnt from both disciplines to more comprehensively and efficiently reduce preventable injuries to both workers and patients. (Taylor et al., 2012, p. 109)

Staff that are energized and healthy are more productive and provide more effective quality care.

Red Rules: Do They Help?

Some HCOs have identified **red rules**, which are rules that must be followed to ensure CQI. This approach is used in other industries. A red rule must not be violated, and if one is, staff must stop work (e.g., procedure, treatment). The goal is to empower staff to intervene; however, there is concern that this system can cause staff to fear that they will get in trouble. Red rules can also be problematic if they are used for situations that may at times make it difficult to follow the rules (Griffith, 2007; ISMP, 2008; Scharf, 2007). For example, a red rule may require that bar coding always be used before medications are given, yet there may be situations when they cannot be applied. Red rules represent situations in which nurses can directly influence quality. The Institute for Safe Medication Practice recommends the following criteria for red rules (ISMP, 2008).

- It must be possible and desirable for everyone to follow a red rule every time in a process under all circumstances (i.e., red rules should not contain verbiage such as "except when..." or "each breach will be assessed for appropriateness").
- Anyone who notices that the red rule has been breached has the authority and responsibility to stop further progress of the patient care associated with the red rule while protecting the patient or employee from harm.
- Managers and other leaders (including the board of trustees) always support the work stoppage and immediately begin rectifying the problem and addressing the underlying reason for breaking the rule.
- The people who breached the red rule are given an opportunity to support their behavioral choices and then judged fairly based on the reasons for breaking the rule, regardless of rank and experience.
- The red rules are few, well understood, and memorable.

Examples of common red rules in health care are the following: Staff behavior related to patient abuse, sexual abuse, or practicing while under the influence of drugs or alcohol is unacceptable. Practice examples are reconciling sponges in surgery and taking time-outs before an invasive procedure.

Standardizing

Safety, as described by Barach and Johnson (2013), is a "property of the clinical microsystem that can be achieved only through systematic application of a broad array of process, equipment, organization, supervision, training, simulation and teamwork changes" (p. 258). Systems will experience errors; there are methods that might reduce this risk, but they will not eliminate it (Reason, 2000; Sadeghi et al., 2013). Risk of adverse events can be controlled to some extent or totally eliminated by process improvement, standardization, and better understanding of safety in systems (Bernstein, 1996). **Standardization** focuses on making work consistent by regulating procedures, equipment, supplies, and so on "to increase reliability, improve information flow, and minimize cross training needs. Standardizing equipment across clinical settings... is one basic example, but standardized processes are increasingly being implemented as safety measures" (HHS, AHRQ, PSNet, 2015a).

Staff do best with routines that can be learned, and risk for problems goes up as we do things that are less routine to us. However, there is a negative side to using routines. If routines lead to automatic responses, with staff not using effective thinking and problem solving, then routines such as procedures may lead to errors (Galt, Fuji, Gleason, & McQuillan, 2011). We may not be focused enough on details or catch things we should notice. Most human errors are difficult to stop; however, HCOs can develop systems that might decrease the risk of errors. On the one hand, we have a high rate of system errors, and on the other hand, it is recommended that systems might help to identify when errors might occur and steps to take to respond and improve. Other chapters discuss some of the methods used to help staff, but here it is important to know that health care is complex and that human and system errors are related.

Stop and Consider #4

Red rules indicate situations in which you must stop work and investigate what is happening; any staff should be able to stop work for a red rule violation.

Human Factors and Quality

Human factors and ergonomics are physical, cognitive, and organizational factors that can have an impact on errors. More attention has been given to staff, their work environment, and their relationship to errors and CQI.

Importance of Human Factors

Human factors have a major impact on the quality of care. It is important for all staff to understand this impact, as it applies to all staff. The first step is for staff to recognize the factors in order to prevent problems or take steps to stop problems. **Presenteeism** refers to staff who are at work but not functioning at their fullest, often due to a medical problem, physical or psychological. This reduced functioning then impacts the quality of work. A Robert Wood Johnson Foundation, Nursing Research Network, summary of some studies on this topic notes that nurses who reported a high level of presenteeism were less likely to report high levels of quality on their units and reported higher levels of medication errors and patient falls during their work hours (Letvak, Ruhm, & Gupta, 2013). Assessing human factors has become a more important aspect of CQI. The process recognizes that the nature of human fallibility is universal; errors will occur, and changes in the workplace may reduce errors and their consequences (WHO, 2011).

Types of Human Factors That Impact Quality Care

Human factors that impact care can be categorized as (1) environmental, (2) organizational and job, and (3) human and individual. Common examples of human factors that are of concern include the following:

- *Fatigue.* This factor impacts all the work that staff do and can lead to staff injuries. Staff may experience mental fatigue, physical fatigue, or both. **Mental fatigue** is "a state that arises in response to increasing mental task demands and stresses (mental workload), and results in a perceived sense of weariness, reduced motivation, reduced alertness, and reduced mental performance in workers" (Pasupathy, & Barker, 2011, p. 22). **Physical fatigue** is "a state that develops throughout the body in response to increasing physical task demands and stresses (physical workload), as well as expectancy of work demands, and can lead to physical discomfort and a decreased capacity to generate force or power" (Pasupathy & Barker, 2011, p. 22). There are data to support that as fatigue increases, staff experience decreased perceived performance. They have less ability to recognize that a change is occurring as they experience acute and chronic fatigue. When staff can reduce acute fatigue, this does make a difference in reducing risk to performance.
- *Stress, hunger, and illness.* These factors interfere with work productivity due to decreasing energy and also impact effective thinking.
- *Unfamiliarity with task.* Not knowing how to complete a task can lead to errors, and a person may put off doing the task in a timely fashion or may not do the task at all; both approaches impact quality.
- *Inexperience.* New, inexperienced staff are at high risk for all types of errors and may not feel comfortable asking for help.

- *Shortage of time.* If staff do not have enough time to complete an activity as it should be done and they feel rushed, patient care is compromised and patients often feel dissatisfied. The staff member who does not have time to talk to patients may miss important information or observations.
- *Inadequate checking.* This factor can impact any staff who need to check orders, patient documentation, steps in a procedure, or patient identification.
- *Interruptions and noise.* This factor can affect, for example, a nurse who is preparing medications, a pharmacist preparing medications for a unit, or dietary staff identifying special diets.
- *Poor procedures to follow.* Policies and procedures need to be clear and accessible when staff need them.
- *Limited memory capacity.* Situations that rely on memory increase the risk of errors, so efforts should be made to reduce reliance on memory by providing easy access to information or using methods to improve memory such as checklists.
- *Unwillingness or inability to ask for help.* No one can know everything, but it is difficult for many staff to admit this and ask for help. Going ahead and doing something that one does not know how to do or understand is very risky.
- *Language and culture factors.* Diversity in staff and patients is a recognized fact; however, language and cultural differences can interfere with clear communication, leading to errors.

The AHRQ identifies additional examples of human factors and ergonomics (HHS, AHRQ, 2013, p. 326):

- Physical dimensions of tools that do not fit physical characteristics of users (e.g., font size too small on computer screen), inappropriately designed physical environments (e.g., lighting too bright and creating glare, noisy and distracting environment), and physical layout that does not support clinician work (e.g., monitoring patients from the central nursing station).
- Cognitive issues include interactions between people and the rest of the system such as perception, memory, attention, mental workload, and support for decision-making.
- Organizational level factors are communication and coordination, teamwork, job design, sociotechnical system, system design, and change (e.g., participatory ergonomics).

Factors that are most difficult to predict and control in order to reduce errors are transitory mental states such as momentary inattention, distraction, preoccupation, and forgetting (Barach & Johnson, 2013; Hollnagel, Woods, & Leveson, 2006).

The system and its processes need methods for responding to prevent errors when these human factors arise. Anything that interferes with effective performance needs to be considered in the CQI plan to reduce risk of errors due to human factors and ergonomics. HCO systems need to be resilient and alert to factors that may lead to errors. This includes an understanding of how errors can be detected, mitigated, and resolved. These efforts are discussed in other chapters in more detail.

A 2014 study examined the relationship between sleep deprivation and occupational and patient care errors among staff nurses who worked the night shift (Johnson, Jung, & Brown, 2014). Night shift is not uncommon in nursing. Sometimes the same staff work this shift permanently, and sometimes staff have to rotate in and out of the night shift or cover for staff on a periodic basis. Working the night shift increases the risk of sleep deprivation. The results indicated that more than half of the 289 nurses who participated in this study were sleep deprived, and as hours of sleep decreased, errors increased. The study concluded that sleep deprivation should also be considered one of the factors that impacts errors; however, collecting data about this topic is not always easy, as it requires staff to admit to sleep concerns and to report errors and near misses. Staff may not be open about this information out of concern for how their employer may view them.

With staff working longer shifts, such as 10 and 12 hours, and often not getting off work as scheduled, errors and staff injuries are more likely to occur. Occupational errors may seem insignificant to staff, but they may have significant implications, warning of fatigue and sleep deprivation. Failure of staff to get the amount of sleep they need to feel rested impacts both the personal and professional aspects of their lives. Examples are an increase in car accidents to and from work place, infections and other illnesses, musculoskeletal injuries such as when lifting patients, and exposure to bloodborne pathogens. The ANA addresses staffing and fatigue, emphasizing the need for healthy work hours and avoiding working when fatigued, as described in The Connect to Current Information section at the end of the chapter. Working when fatigued is an ethical issue, requiring decisions about whether a person is able to work safely and effectively. In 2011, The Joint Commission issued a sentinel event alert asking hospitals to increase efforts to address risk of fatigue caused by extended shifts. Stimpfel, Sloane, and Aiken (2012) note the following:

> Working longer for fewer shifts may also attract nurses who work a second job. However, the strain of those three long work days and the rest and re-covery time needed may offset any perceived benefit, if our survey results are any indication. When a three-day week turns into more days or additional, unplanned-for overtime, nurses' satisfaction appears to decrease. (p. 2507)

As is true for most of the studies about staffing, work environment, and patient outcomes, the studies are difficult to conduct, but more research is needed to better understand this problem. In addition, research results may mean that HCOs, staff, and healthcare professions will need to make difficult decisions. Some of these changes may relate to 12-hour shifts, such as decreasing hours per shift, changing staffing levels to avoid overscheduling existing staff, and budgeting to allow for any increased costs to the HCO.

The Joint Commission's sentinel event alert on staff fatigue, which is based on evidence supported by a study reported in 2004, identifies the following factors that impact performance (Hughes & Rogers, 2004; The Joint Commission, 2011):

- Lapses in attention and inability to stay focused
- Reduced motivation
- Compromised problem solving
- Confusion
- Irritability
- Memory lapses
- Impaired communication
- Slowed or faulty information processing and judgment
- Diminished reaction time
- Indifference and loss of empathy

Consider how each of these factors might impact a nurse's thinking and practice.

Staff Stress

Stress, as defined by Kuntz, Mennicken, and Scholtes (2014), "results from an imbalance between demands and resources, occurring when demand pressure exceeds an individual's perceived ability to cope" (p. 754). The biological response to stress is elevated hormone levels, particularly cortisol, and this impacts cognitive abilities such as memory, attention, and decision-making (Dickerson & Kemeny, 2004; Sonnentag & Fritz, 2006). In some cases, posttraumatic stress disorder may occur. Stress in some staff may be contagious; for example, when staff complain to one another that their workload is too heavy and work cannot be done safely, other staff may then complain about the stress of their own workload. The common reasons for stress among nurses are the following (HHS, CDC, NIOSH, 2008, pp. 2–3):

- Work overload
- Time pressure
- Lack of social support at work (especially from supervisors, nurse managers, and higher management)
- Staff incivility
- Exposure to infectious diseases
- Risk of needlestick injuries
- Exposure to work-related violence or threats

- Sleep deprivation
- Role ambiguity and conflict
- Understaffing
- Career development issues
- Dealing with difficult or seriously ill patients

We need to know much more about how the system load impacts quality, as reported by a study done by Kuntz and colleagues (2014). This study indicates that clinical unit occupancy does not impact mortality rate until it reaches a "tipping point." Typical responses to changes in occupancy are to request more staff, such as from temporary staff pools; ask staff to work longer hours in overtime; admit to other units; or delay admissions from emergency department. As staff workload increases, staff may ration access to care—less time to do everything. This hurried care leads to increased staff and unit stress and patient dissatisfaction.

Compassion fatigue is an "intense drain on the body, emotions, and spirit, and it adds to nurse stress" (Carpenter, 2011, p. 34). Today, there is more attention on this problem. As mentioned earlier, working long hours increases staff fatigue, but fatigue is also increased because of stress in the workplace. Staff are worn out and stressed when they leave work; as a result, they get less rest when off and then return reluctantly, still tired and stressed.

The National Occupational Institute for Occupational Safety and Health (NIOSH) recommends the following strategies/interventions to assist HCOs in reducing staff stress (HHS, CDC, NIOSH, 2008, pp. 4–5). These strategies/interventions address many of the common causes of stress in nurses:

- Ensure that the workload is in line with workers' capabilities and resources.
- Clearly define workers' roles and responsibilities.
- Give workers opportunities to participate in decisions and actions affecting their jobs.
- Improve communication.
- Reduce uncertainty about career development and future employment prospects.
- Provide opportunities for social interaction among workers.

In addition to these strategies/interventions, HCOs are increasing their use of team processes and interprofessional teams. To be effective, the HCO needs to include staff in the development, implementation, and evaluation of strategies/interventions used to reduce staff stress. Stress management is also employed in some HCOs. Methods might include learning coping strategies such as progressive relaxation and biofeedback, improving time management, and expanding interpersonal skills. Some HCOs provide the opportunity for exercise, yoga, gym memberships, on-site child care, and other such perks. Reducing stress improves care quality and productivity and helps reduce incivility in the workplace.

Staff: At-Risk Attitudes and Behaviors

Disruptive behavior and incivility are a growing concern in health care. One might wonder why this topic is related to CQI. When this type of negative behavior occurs, communication is broken. Broken communication may be defined by unclear and confusing or mixed messages. Emotions may limit the ability to communicate, or there may be no communication at all. Ineffective communication is the most common type of problem that can increase risk of errors. When staff have difficulties with one another and do not communicate effectively, teamwork is compromised, negatively impacting care. Improving staff communication has been one of The Joint Commission's annual patient safety goals. There is a clear relationship between communication and near misses, errors, and quality care.

Incivility may include rude and discourteous behavior, gossiping and spreading rumors, or refusing to help others in the work situation. **Bullying**, as defined by the ANA (2015a), is "repeated, unwanted harmful actions intended to humiliate, offend, and cause distress in the recipient" (p. 2). Bullying may happen between peers as well as with staff from top to bottom or bottom to top within the HCO. Workplace mobbing may also occur when staff groups use bullying against a staff member. In addition to incivility and other related behavior, there has been an increase in violence that may be initiated by staff, family members, or external sources. NIOSH defines **workplace violence** as "physically and/or psychologically damaging actions that occur in the workplace or while on duty" (DOL, NIOSH, 2006).

Nurse–physician interaction or communication that is inappropriate and disruptive needs to be stopped. As is true for any behavior that interferes with effective work, it is important to understand why it is happening and to respond in a positive manner using "I" language—for example, "I think" or "I observe" (Gessler, Rosenstein, & Ferron, 2012). If the behavior cannot be stopped, then staff need to use the HCO procedure for reporting problems, and management needs to respond. **Lateral violence,**—which refers to acts between coworkers (e.g., nurse to nurse)—bullying, hostility, reprisals for speaking out, and so on, have increased in HCOs (Daley, 2012).

Zero-tolerance of incivility has become the norm in many HCOs and is supported by the ANA (2015a). These HCOs have clear policies that describe a code of conduct and acceptable behaviors. This topic is often part of orientation and staff education for managers and staff. Diversity issues (e.g., biases, differences in cultures, and differences in communication) must be handled with care, but all must follow the policy. Tracking these incidents helps to better understand the level of the problem and typical concerns that arise. Armed with this information, the HCO can better assess the culture, determine outcomes, and identify and implement strategies that will be used to prevent or respond to incivility.

Problems of incivility, bullying, and workplace violence are recognized by the ANA as critical concerns for the nursing profession and healthcare delivery. Such problems impact not just nurses, but also patients and families and the overall quality of care delivered. This recognition led to the development of a position statement on the problems (ANA, 2015b) and also a position statement on zero tolerance (ANA, 2015a). The incivility statement notes that these problems are not just problems for the nursing profession or for nurses to solve, but rather employers must also be involved and use an interprofessional perspective. The ANA's *Nursing: Scope and Standards of Practice* also relates to the need for a healthy workplace (ANA, 2015c). Creating a healthy workplace requires a culture of respect. The ANA's *Code of Ethics* requires that nurses work to establish an ethical environment and culture of civility, which is connected to a culture of safety. This culture should consider kindness and treating colleagues, coworkers, employees, students, and others with dignity and respect (ANA, 2015a, 2015c). The *Code of Ethics* provides the basis for our understanding of the meaning of civility and its relevance to the nursing profession.

Many HCO settings experience problems with staff incivility and workplace violence, and some are at greater risk, such as emergency departments, psychiatric hospitals, nursing homes, long-term care facilities, and acute care settings. These settings may also experience problems with security, weapons, drugs, and other threats. There is increased risk within the HCO; for example, employees who float from one unit to another experience assault three times more often than do permanent employees (ANA, 2015a; Hodgson et al., 2004).

Strategies to Improve: Eliminate or Reduce Problems With Human Factors

The best approach to reduce inappropriate behavior is prevention. The most effective prevention interventions are developing interpersonal relationships and teams; dealing with problems before they get out of control; engaging staff in decision-making; developing clear communication; and offering training on communication, procedures, delegation, teamwork, conflict and conflict resolution, and other group dynamics. These interventions are the responsibility of the HCO and the staff. The employer has obligations to provide leadership, support, resources, and education and to develop plans and strategies to prevent and, if necessary, respond to incivility and workplace violence. Staff who commit to respecting others make the difference in the HCO. When incivility, bullying, or workplace violence occur, staff need to feel comfortable confronting the situation in a respectful manner. The HCO needs to respond in a timely manner, clarify the situation, speak respectfully with involved staff, and support staff to reach a positive resolution.

It is not easy to speak up about a situation in which you have experienced or observed incivility or lateral violence. Many staff fear retaliation or even loss of job. What can you do to respond in a professional and direct manner? Developing your self-awareness is critical, and the following tips are helpful in managing your own emotions (Gessler et al., 2012, p. 42):

- Communicate your concerns.
- Refuse to dwell on negative thoughts or emotions.
- Avoid negative behaviors.
- Admit to mistakes.
- Accept and act on valid feedback.

Taking care of self gives you more energy to deal with negative situations without turning them into a negative reaction for yourself.

Supportive practice environments assist in nursing quality care (Flynn, Liang, Dickson, Xie, & Suh, 2012). There is recognition today that when staff are involved in errors, they may become the second victims due to the experience, the response from others, and their own personal response. It is estimated that one in seven patients experience adverse events and at least half of all providers/clinicians are involved. This prevalence of adverse events represents a major problem (HHS, AHRQ, PSNet, 2015d). In order to improve performance and view errors as opportunities to learn and not blame, HCOs need to make more efforts to support staff and help them cope when they experience stress. Professional and personal self-esteem are factors that influence staff and their ability to cope in the work environment. What do clinicians consider to be supportive and helpful? The AHRQ reports the following:

> A survey of 898 clinicians at the University of Missouri found that clinicians wanted a unit- or department-based support system that could relieve them of immediate patient care duties for a brief period; provide one-on-one peer support, professional review, and collegial feedback, as well as access to patient safety experts and risk managers; and offer of crisis support and external referral when needed. (HHS, AHRQ, PSNet, 2015d)

Programs to reduce stress and burnout have been developed, and some have been tested. In one study, nurses were surveyed via a questionnaire to assess health-related consequences of stress and also related costs of absenteeism and turnover (Sallon, Katz-Eisner, Yaffe, & Bdolah-Abram, 2015). A program called Caring for the Caregivers used an 8-month course on stress reduction as an intervention. The course included multiple methods to reduce staff stress. Several reliable and valid rating scales, such as the Maslach Burnout Inventory, were used in the study. Ninety-seven participants improved, compared to 67 participants in the control group; for example, participants experienced less respiratory infections, doctor visits, and stress symptoms. The intervention was effective, although the length of the course may be problematic for many HCOs and their staff. This study does, however, indicate that organized strategies can assist staff.

The "I'M SAFE" checklist is one method that is taught to staff as a self-assessment tool to ensure safety. Staff determine if they have problems in any of the following areas, which may then limit their performance (HHS, AHRQ, 2014):

- Illness
- Medication
- Stress
- Alcohol and drugs
- Fatigue
- Eating and elimination

Mutual support among team members assists the team in working toward their goals together. As they work together, team member feedback should be respectful, timely, specific, directed toward improvement, and considerate.

Stop and Consider #5
Managing your own stress has an impact on quality care.

Workplace Safety

It is common to emphasize safety for patients, but there is another aspect of safety— safety for staff in the workplace. HCOs are settings where there is risk for staff everyday, such as the examples mentioned in the previous discussion on fatigue, incivility, violence, and stress. Workplace safety is, however, concerned with many other factors that may lead to staff harm as they work.

Importance of Maintaining Workplace Safety

Why is workplace safety so important? When the HCO makes workplace safety an important goal, it may experience reduced costs; safer care for patients, who may be injured when staff are injured or not able to function to full capacity when recovering from harm; consistent care; and decrease staff stress (Finkelman & Kenner, 2012). If staff are unhealthy or injured while working, this may impact patient care. For example, if a staff member is using patient lift equipment in an unsafe manner or the equipment is not functioning correctly, both the staff member and the patient may be injured. Staff who miss work due to illness or injury cost the HCO money for paid sick time, disability payments (when appropriate), and the cost of finding coverage for the staff member, which may be more costly than paying the employee (i.e., temporary staff may get more pay). Error risk is also increased, as new staff or temporary staff may not be prepared for the position or may miss critical communication, and consistency might be affected.

HCOs are concerned about all of these considerations and thus often have staff health services or occupational health services on-site to assist in ensuring that staff can function fully. Other issues that would be managed through this service are required immunizations, staff education related to health and safety, and referrals to other health services as needed. The ANA website on workplace safety provides information on the major concerns of safe patient handling, needlestick injury prevention, staff drug and alcohol use, workplace violence, and environmental health.

OSHA and NIOSH: Standards for Workplace Safety

NIOSH and the Occupational Safety and Health Administration (OSHA) provide important services to better ensure safe labor practices and a healthy workforce. HCOs must pay attention to the requirements from these two federal agencies, particularly to legislative mandates.

NIOSH's mission is "to develop new knowledge in the field of occupational safety and health and to transfer that knowledge into practice" (HHS, CDC, NIOSH, 2016). Its goals are: (1) Conduct research to reduce worker illness and injury and to advance worker well-being, (2) promote safe and healthy workers through intervention, recommendations, and capacity building, and (3) enhance international worker safety and health through global collaborations.

This agency is part of the HHS, Centers for Disease Control and Prevention. Some of the programs NIOSH leads are Prevention Through Design, which looks at how physical design impacts equipment and processes; improving total worker health; and health hazard evaluation in the workplace. The NIOSH website provides extensive information on many workplace health and safety topics. The Connect to Current Information section at the end of the chapter provides a link to this site.

OSHA is part of the U.S. Department of Labor, so it is under different control than NIOSH. This agency "assures safe and healthful working conditions for working men and women by setting and enforcing standards and by providing training, outreach, education, and assistance" (DOL, OSHA, 2012a). Federal law assures that OSHA mandates on worker rights be enforced. One of these rights is that workers are entitled to working conditions that do not pose a risk of serious harm (DOL, OSHA, 2012b). To help ensure a safe and healthful workplace, OSHA also provides workers with the right to the following (DOL, OSHA, 2012a):

- Receive information and training about hazards, methods to prevent harm, and the OSHA standards that apply to their workplace. The training must be in a language that workers can understand.
- Get copies of test results used to identify workplace hazards.

- Review records of work-related injuries and illnesses.
- Get copies of their medical records.
- Ask OSHA to inspect their workplace.
- Use their rights under the law, free from retaliation and discrimination.

An employer cannot deny these rights to a worker, and if the employer attempts to do so, employees can complain to OSHA. Violating an OSHA mandate would be a serious situation for the HCO, as this would be breaking federal law. So not only must care be as safe as possible and of the best quality, staff are protected in the workplace to ensure their health and safety.

Common Healthcare Workplace Concerns

Healthcare staff work in a variety of settings and circumstances that can increase their risks. Examples of common staff healthcare workplace safety concerns are the following (ANA, 2012b; Finkelman & Kenner, 2012):

- *Infections.* Some infections are common, and some, such as Ebola, are not so common.
- *Bloodborne infections.* Needlesticks may expose nurses to bloodborne infections, such as HIV, hepatitis B, and hepatitis C. This risk has been addressed by the use of safe needle devices, but also there is need to ensure there are human resources (staffing levels), equipment and supplies, policies and procedures, and training to ensure that staff are safe. These precautions improve care and safety of patients (Daley, 2012). The ANA has position statements on these concerns on its website. The Needlestick Safety and Prevention Act of 2000 requires that employers do the following:
  - Identify, evaluate, and implement safer medical devices.
  - Maintain a sharps injury log.
  - Involve healthcare workers in device selection.
  - Implement engineering controls for sharps disposal containers, self-sheathing needles, safer medical devices, and use of engineering controls to eliminate or reduce employee exposure to pathogens.
  - Train employees in proper use of engineering and work practice controls.
- *Ergonomics and safe patient handling.* Addressing this concern may reduce injuries due to ergonomics. Nurses have to move patients, help them with mobility, and perform other activities, often using equipment that can lead to injuries and often without supportive equipment. Neck, shoulder, and back injuries are common. Factors that impact injury risk are staff age, height and weight, strength, health status, and knowledge and availability and use of safe ergonomics and assistive equipment. Patient factors are weight, strength to assist, age, medical problem, and needs. Handle With Care® is a program that "seeks to educate, advocate,

and facilitate change from traditional practices of manual patient handling to emerging, technology-oriented methods" (ANA, 2016). The Connect to Current Information section at the end of the chapter provides a link to the ANA website on safe handling and its resources and training materials. Schools of nursing and HCOs use this information to prepare students and staff.

- *Exposure to chemicals.* Chemicals that nurses should be concerned about include housekeeping chemicals, mercury-containing devices, latex, anesthetic gases, antiretroviral medications, chemotherapeutic agents, and some sterilization and disinfectant agents. Nurses need to know what chemicals are used in their area of practice and how to protect themselves. They should also protect against radiation exposure. When needed, the HCO should also provide training and protective equipment/supplies.

There are many causes of staff injuries, and settings and staff roles influence risk to staff. Common causes of staff injuries include the following (Gerwig, 2014, p. 335):

- Lack of consistent, timely, and positive feedback for performance improvement
- Lack of employee engagement and empowerment
- Unresponsive systems (hazards go uncorrected)
- Miscommunication
- Information deficits
- Conflict between immediate and long-term goals (e.g., performance standards such as operating room turnover may conflict with adequate time to perform required tasks safely)
- Misaligned or conflicting goals among departments
- Lack of contingency planning and response
- Unclear allocation of responsibility
- Breakdown in coordination
- Lack of teamwork
- Inadequate training
- Poor supervision
- Inflexible policies
- Poor labor relations
- Cumbersome technology
- Undue time pressure
- Understaffing/overtasking
- Interruptions/distractions
- Inadequate policies and procedures

- "Drift" or noncompliance with policies and procedures
- Difficulty in speaking up when another staff member is doing something that is unsafe
- Lack of leadership engagement and sponsorship

Stop and Consider #6
Workplace safety is a concern not only of HCOs but also of the federal and state governments.

Conclusions

In this chapter, we began the second section of this text with an examination of quality health care by introducing safety and errors. Safety is not separate from quality; rather, it is a critical component of quality. In an integrative review of literature that included 20 studies focused on patient safety in nursing curricula, several key concerns are identified that nurses need to consider as they become active participants in the CQI process (Tella et al., 2014). These concerns are learning from errors, responsible individual and interprofessional teamwork, anticipatory action in complex environments, and patient safety-centered nursing. Understanding basic factors influencing errors and terminology is required before you can appreciate CQI planning, measurement, analysis, and development of strategies to improve care. In summary, when examining events, there are three factors to remember that impact errors (Barach & Johnson, 2013; Perrow, 1984):

- All human beings, regardless of their skills, abilities, and specialist training, make fallible decisions and commit unsafe acts.
- All man-made systems possess latent (unseen) failures to some degree.
- All human endeavors involve some measure of risk.

Apply CQI
Chapter Highlights

- There are multiple models for understanding errors, including the Swiss cheese model, the Enthoven model, and the generic error-modeling system (GEMS). The Swiss cheese model is more commonly used by HCOs and some government initiatives.
- There are multiple types of errors that require tracking and analysis to improve care.

- Underuse, overuse, and misuse are common types of errors found in a variety of HCOs and involve a variety of staff.
- Active errors are associated with direct care providers.
- System factors impact latent errors, which are often not as apparent to staff.
- Near misses occur when staff almost make an error but no actual error occurs. Staff may do something consciously or unconsciously to block the error.
- Adverse events are injuries resulting from medical interventions, not from the patient's underlying condition. They are untoward, undesirable events, usually not expected, and may or may not have a long-term effect.
- Sentinel events are critical patient-related events that require a response; examples include a suicide, wrong-site surgery, and serious operative and postoperative complications.
- The Joint Commission issues sentinel alerts to share information about reported sentinel events to help HCOs learn from these events.
- Frontline safety focuses on direct care staff and their impact on quality improvement.
- Red rules are used to identify events that the HCO does not consider to be acceptable performance. A red rule must not be violated, and if one is, staff must stop work (e.g., procedure, treatment). The goal is to empower all staff to intervene.
- Standardizing care can reduce risk of quality problems; however, this cannot be done for all situations. Standards, policies, and procedures assist in ensuring greater standardization while still meeting individual needs.
- Human factors and ergonomics are physical, cognitive, and organizational factors that can have an impact on errors.
- Staff stress negatively impacts care quality, interfering with staff performance.
- Workplace safety focuses on direct care staff and their safety in the workplace.
- OSHA and NIOSH standards are important in supporting staff safety to ensure more effective quality improvement.

Critical Thinking and Clinical Reasoning and Judgment: Discussion Questions and Learning Activities

1. Using the three error models described in this chapter, create a visual (e.g., poster, PowerPoint slide, graphic) that highlights their key points. Compare your visual to those of your classmates.
2. What is your opinion of the use of red rules in frontline safety initiatives? Provide your opinion in one paragraph.
3. In a small group, compare and contrast the types of errors, and when possible, provide examples from clinical experiences. Summarize your discussion.

4. In a small group, discuss examples from your own clinical experiences relating to human factors and errors (or possible errors). Summarize your discussion.
5. Assess your own response to stress. Write down your assessment. How might your typical responses to stress impact your clinical practice? Provide examples of how your responses have affected your clinical practice as a student. How might you better cope with stress?

Connect to Current Information

- Multiple graphics of the Swiss cheese model
  http://www.bing.com/images/search?q=swiss+cheese+model+health+care
- NIOSH: Workplace Safety Resources
  http://www.cdc.gov/niosh/topics/default.html
- OSHA: Workplace Safety Resources
  https://www.osha-safetytraining.
     net/?gclid=CPqZmd_bxs4CFQKNaQodxZkNuA
- OSHA: Healthcare Wide Hazards
  https://www.osha.gov/SLTC/etools/hospital/hazards/hazards.html
- AHRQ: Patient Safety Primers
  http://psnet.ahrq.gov/primerHome.aspx
- ANA: Nursing Practice and Work Environment
  http://www.nursingworld.org/MainMenuCategories/WorkplaceSafety
- ANA: Safe Patient Handling and Mobility
  http://www.nursingworld.org/MainMenuCategories/WorkplaceSafety
     /SafePatient
- ANA: Nursing fatigue
  http://www.nursingworld.org/fatigue

EBP, EBM, and Quality Improvement: Exemplar

Dang, D., Bae, S., Karlowicz, K., & Kim, M. (2015). Do clinician disruptive behaviors make an unsafe environment for patients? *Journal of Nursing Care Quality, 31*(2), 115–123.

This article describes a study that focuses on staff behavior and its impact on patients and quality care.

Questions to Consider:

1. What is the design used for this study, including research question(s), sample, interventions, data collection, and analysis?
2. What are the results of the study?
3. How might you apply these results to a clinical setting or your practice to improve care?

Evolving Case Study

In the unit's monthly staff meeting, staff stress is brought up as a growing problem. Staff complain that they are overworked and there is not enough staff. They are also tired of orienting new staff, and temporary staff members are not effective. Two nurses mention they have personally experienced more near misses when administering medications. The unit experienced three sentinel events that resulted in complications for patients and extended their length of stay. One of the errors was due to overdose of medications that was not recognized before major complications occurred. The nurse manager tells the staff that he recognizes from the discussion that there is a lot of tension and this is a concern. The manager leaves the meeting, and in his office he begins to consider how he and the unit should respond to the problems.

Case Questions:

1. You, as the nurse manager, arrange to have a staff meeting to increase staff knowledge of stress and stress responses. What will the presentation include? How will you engage the staff in the process to improve stress management?

2. You want to better understand the impact of stress, workload, staffing, and quality care problems on your unit. How will you accomplish this?

3. What strategies might you use to decrease stress and improve care? Be specific.

References

Aiken, L., Sloane, D. M., Cimiotti, J. P., Clarke, S. P., Flynn, L., Seago, J. A., ... Smith, H. (2010). Implications of the California nurse staffing mandate for other states. *Health Services Research, 45*(4), 904–921.

American Nurses Association (ANA). (2012a). *Principles for nurse staffing* (2nd ed.). Silver Spring, MD: Author.

American Nurses Association (ANA). (2012b). Nursing practice and work environment. Retrieved from http://nursingworld.org/MainMenuCategories/WorkplaceSafety

American Nurses Association (ANA). (2015a). ANA sets "zero tolerance" policy for workplace violence, bullying. ANA position statement. Retrieved from http://nursingworld.org/MainMenuCategories/WorkplaceSafety/Healthy-Nurse/bullyingworkplaceviolence/ANA-Sets-Zero-Tolerance-Policy-for-Workplace-Violence-Bullying.html

American Nurses Association (ANA). (2015b). Position statement: Incivility, bullying, and workplace violence. Retrieved from http://www.nursingworld.org/Bullying-Workplace-Violence

American Nurses Association (ANA). (2015c). *Nursing: Scope and standards of practice* (3rd ed.). Silver Spring, MD: Author.

American Nurses Association. (ANA). (2016). Handle with Care® fact sheet. Retrieved from http://www.nursingworld.org/MainMenuCategories/ANAMarketplace/Factsheets-and-Toolkits/FactSheet.html

Bae, S., Mark, B., & Fried, B. (2009). Impact of nursing unit turnover on patient outcomes in hospitals. *Journal of Nursing Scholarship, 42*(1), 40–49.

Ball, J., Murrells, T., Rafferty, A., Morrow, E., & Griffiths, P. (2014). Care left undone during nursing shifts: Associations with workload and perceived quality of care. *BMJ Quality Safety, 23*(2), 116–125.

Barach, P., & Johnson, J. (2013). Assessing risk and harm in the clinical microsystem. In W. Sollecito & J. Johnson (Eds.), *McLaughlin and Kaluzny's continuous quality improvement in health care* (4th ed., pp. 249–274). Burlington, MA: Jones & Bartlett Learning.

Barach, P., & Small, S. (2000). Reporting and preventing medical mishaps: Lessons from non-medical near miss reporting systems. *BMJ, 320*, 759–763.

Bernstein, P. (1996). *Against the gods: The remarkable story of risk*. New York, NY: Wiley.

Blegen, M., Goode, C., Spetz, J., Vaughn, T., & Park, S. (2011). Nurse staffing effects on patient outcomes: Safety-net and non-safety-net hospitals. *Medical Care, 49*(4), 406–414.

Carpenter, H. (2011). Environment, health, and safety. *American Nurse Today, 6*(11), 34–35.

Cimiotti, J., Aiken, L., Sloane, D., & Wu, E. (2012). Nurse staffing, burnout, and health care-associated infection. *American Journal of Infection Control, 40*, 486–490.

Clark, B., & Bramble, J. (2013). Safety improvement is achieved within organizations. In K. Galt & K. Paschal (Eds.), *Foundations in patient safety for health professionals* (pp. 71–78). Burlington, MA: Jones & Bartlett Learning.

Classen, D., Resar, R., Griffin, F., Federico, F., Frankel, T., Kimmel, N.,... James, B. (2011). "Global trigger tool" shows that adverse events in hospitals may be ten times greater than previously measured. *Health Affairs, 30*(4), 581–580.

Daley, K. (2012). Let's put an end to bullying and lateral violence. *American Nurse Today, 7*(3), 18.

Dickerson, S., & Kemeny, M. (2004). Acute stressors and cortisol responses: A theoretical integration and synthesis of laboratory research. *Psychology Bulletin, 130*(3), 355–391.

Domrose, C. (2010). States consider merits of mandated staffing rations. Retrieved from https://news.nurse.com/2010/02/10/states-consider-merits-of-mandated-staffing-ratios/

Finkelman, A., & Kenner, C. (2012). *Teaching IOM: Implications of the IOM reports for nursing education* (3rd ed., Vol. I). Silver Spring, MD: American Nurses Association.

Finkelman, A., & Kenner, C. (2016). *Professional nursing concepts: Competencies for quality leadership* (3rd ed.). Burlington, MA: Jones & Bartlett Learning.

Flynn, L., Liang, Y., Dickson, G., Xie, M., & Suh, D. (2012). Nurses' practice environments, error interception practices, and inpatient medication errors. *Journal of Nursing Scholarship, 44*(2), 180–186.

Gale, S., & Noga, P. (2013). Creating a transparent and dynamic view of staffing as a foundation for improving quality and efficiency. *Nursing Administration Quarterly, 37*(3), 129–135.

Galt, K., Fuji, K., Gleason, J., & McQuillan, R. (2011). Why things go wrong. In K. Galt & K. Paschal (Eds.), *Foundations in patient safety for health professionals* (pp. 107–120). Burlington, MA: Jones & Bartlett Learning.

Gawande, A. (2009). *The checklist manifesto: How to get things done right*. New York, NY: Metropolitan Books.

Gawande, A. (2015, May 11). Overkill: An avalanche of unnecessary medical care is harming patients physically and financially. What can we do about it? *New Yorker*. Retrieved from http://www.newyorker.com/magazine/2015/05/11/overkill-atul-gawande

Gerwig, K. (2013). When employees are safe, patients are safer. In B. Youngberg (Ed.), *Patient safety handbook* (2nd ed., pp. 333–346). Burlington, MA: Jones & Bartlett Learning.

Gessler, R., Rosenstein, A., & Ferron, L. (2012). How to handle disruptive physician behaviors. Find out the best way to respond if you're the target. *American Nurse Today, 7*(11), 8–10.

Griffith, S. (2007). An examination of red rules in a just culture. The Just Culture Community administered by Outcome Engineering, LLC. Retrieved from http://legacy.justculture.org /newsletters.aspx?id=8

Henneman, E., & Gawlinski, A. (2004). A near-miss model for describing the nurse's role in the recovery of medical errors. *Journal of Professional Nursing, 20*(3), 196–201.

Henneman, E., Gawlinski, A., Blank, F., Henneman, P., Jordan, D., & McKenzie, J. (2010). Strategies used by critical care nurses to identify, interrupt, and correct medical errors. *American Journal of Critical Care, 19*(6), 500–509.

Hodgson, M., Reed, R., Craig, T., Murphy, F., Lehmann, L., Belton, L., Warren, N. (2004). Violence in healthcare facilities: Lessons from the Veterans Health Administration. *Journal of Occupational Environmental Medicine, 46*, 1158–1165.

Hollnagel, E., Woods, D., & Leveson, D. (Eds.). (2006). *Resilience engineering: Concepts and precepts.* Aldershot, UK: Ashgate.

Hughes, R., & Clancy, C. (2005). Working conditions that support patient safety. *Journal Nursing Care Quality, 20*(4), 289–292.

Hughes, R., & Rogers, A. (2004). Are you tired? Sleep deprivation compromises health—and jeopardizes patients. *American Journal of Nursing, 104*(3), 15.

Institute of Medicine (IOM). (1999). *To err is human.* Washington, DC: The National Academies Press.

Institute of Medicine (IOM). (2003). *Health professions education.* Washington, DC: The National Academies Press.

Institute of Medicine (IOM). (2004). *Keeping patients safe: Transforming the work environment of nurses.* Washington, DC: The National Academies Press.

Institute of Medicine (IOM). (2010). *The future of nursing: Leading change, advancing health.* Washington, DC: The National Academies Press.

Institute for Safe Medication Practice (ISMP). (2008). Some red rules shouldn't rule in hospitals. Retrieved from https://webcache.googleusercontent.com/search?q=cache:d4F6pCKT7i4J: https://www.ismp.org/newsletters/acutecare/articles/20080424.asp+&cd=1&hl=en&ct= clnk&gl=us

Institute for Safe Medication Practice (ISMP). (2011, May 5). Multiple latent failures align to allow a serious drug interaction to harm a patient. Retrieved from http://www.ismp.org/newsletters /acutecare/articles/20110505.asp

Johnson, A., Jung, L., & Brown, K. (2014). Sleep deprivation and error in nurses who work the night shift. *Journal of Nursing Administration, 44*(10), 17–22.

Jones, T., Hamilton, P., & Murray, N. (2015). Unfinished nursing care, missed care, and implicitly rationed care: State of the science review. *International Journal of Nursing Studies, 52*, 1121–1137.

Kalisch, B. (2015). *Errors of omission: How missed nursing care imperils patients.* Chevy Chase, MD: American Nurses Association.

Kalisch, B., Landstrom, G., & Williams, R. (2008). Missed nursing care: Errors of omission. *Nursing Outlook, 57*(1), 3–9.

Kalisch, B., & Lee, K. (2010). The impact of teamwork on missed nursing care. *Nursing Outlook, 58*, 233–241.

Kalisch, B., Xie, B., & Dabney, B. (2014). Patient-reported missed nursing care correlated with adverse events. *American Journal Medical Quality, 29*, 415–422.

Kuntz, L., Mennicken, R., & Scholtes, S. (2014). Stress on the ward: Evidence of safety tipping points in hospitals. *Management Science, 64*(4), 754–771.

Larkin, J., Lorenz, H., Rack, L., & Shatzer, M. (2012). Good care, good science: Leveraging frontline staff for quality. *Nursing Administrative Quarterly, 36*(3), 188–193.

Letvak, S., Ruhm, C., & Gupta, S. (2013, August 1). The effects of nurse presenteeism on quality of care and patient safety. Robert Wood Johnson Foundation, Nursing Research Network. Research Brief. Retrieved from http://www.rwjf.org/content/dam/farm/reports/issue_briefs/2013/rwjf407337

Maslach, C. (2003). Job burnout: New directions in research and interventions. *Current Directions Psychological Science, 12*, 189–192.

Pasupathy, K., & Barker, L. (2011). Impact of fatigue on performance in registered nurses: Data mining and implications for practice. *Journal for Healthcare Quality, 34*(5), 22–30.

Perrow, C. (1984). *Normal accidents, living with the high-risk technologies.* New York: NY: Basic Books.

Reason, J. (1990). *Human error.* Cambridge, UK: Cambridge University Press.

Reason, J. (2000). Human error: Models and management. *British Medical Journal, 320* (March), 768–770.

Reason, J. (2002). Combating omission errors through task analysis and good reminders. *Quality Safety Health Care, 11*, 40–44.

Rogers, A., Hwang, W., Scott, L., Aiken, L., & Dinges, D. (2004). The working hours of hospital staff nurses and patient safety. *Health Affairs, 23*(4), 202–212.

Sadeghi, S., Barzi, A., Mikhail, O., & Shabot, M. (2013). *Integrating quality and strategy in healthcare organizations.* Burlington, MA: Jones & Bartlett Learning.

Sallon, S., Katz-Eisner, D., Yaffe, H., & Bdolah-Abram, T. (2015). Caring for the caregivers: Results of an extended, five-component stress-reduction intervention for hospital staff. *Behavioral Medicine, November*, 1–15.

Scharf, W. (2007). Red rules: An error-reduction strategy in the culture of safety. *Focus on Patient Safety, 10*(1), 1–2.

Seelye, K. (2016, March 7). Use of heroin in public view across the U.S. *New York Times*, p. A1.

Sonnentag, S., & Fritz, C. (2006). Endocrinological processes associated with job stress: Catecholamine and cortisol response to acute and chronic stressors. In P. Perrewé & D. Ganster (Eds.), *Employee health, coping, and methodologies* (pp. 1–59). Bingley, United Kingdom: Emerald.

Sorbello, B. (2008). Responding to a sentinel event. *American Nurse Today, 3*(10). Retrieved from http://www.americannursetoday.com/responding-to-a-sentinel-event/

Stimpfel, A., Sloane, D., & Aiken, L. (2012). The longer the shifts for hospital nurses, the higher the levels of burnout and patient dissatisfaction. *Health Affairs, 31*(11), 2501–2509.

Taylor, J. Dominici, F., Agnew, J., Gerwin, D., Morlock, L., & Miller, M. R. (2012). Do nurse and patient injuries share common antecedents? An analysis of associations with safety climate and working conditions. *BMJ Quality Safety, 22*(2), 101–111.

Tella, S. Liukka, M., Jamookeeah, D., Smith. N., Partanen, P., & Turunen, H. (2014). What do students learn about patient safety? *Journal of Nursing Education, 53*(1), 7–13.

The Joint Commission. (2011). Sentinel alert issue 48: Healthcare worker fatigue and patient safety. Retrieved from http://www.jointcommission.org/sea_issue_48/

The Joint Commission. (2014). Sentinel events policy and procedures. Retrieved from http://www.jointcommission.org/Sentinel_Event_Policy_and_Procedures/

The Joint Commission. (2015). *Compliance accreditation manual for hospitals.* Retrieved from http://www.jointcommission.org/assets/1/6/CAMH_24_SE_all_CURRENT.pdf

Trinkoff, A., Johantgen, M., Storr, C. L., Gurses, A. P., Liang, Y., Han, K. (2010). Nurses' work schedule characteristics, nurse staffing, and patient mortality. *Nursing Research, 60*(1), 1–8.

U.S. Congress, House of Representatives. (2015). Nurse Staffing Standards for Patient Safety and Quality Care Act of 2015 (Introduced in House) H.R. 1602. Retrieved from https://www .govtrack.us/congress/bills/114/hr1602/text/ih

U.S. Department of Health and Human Services (HHS), Agency for Healthcare Research and Quality (AHRQ). (2013). Making health care safer II: An updated critical analysis of the evidence for patient safety practices. Comparative Effectiveness Review No. 211. (Prepared by the Southern California-RAND Evidence-Based Practice Center under Contract No. 290-2007-10062-I.) AHRQ Publication No. 13-E001-EF. Retrieved from www.ahrq.gov/research /findings/evidence-based-reports/ptsafetyuptp.html

U.S. Department of Health and Human Services (HHS), Agency for Healthcare Research and Quality (AHRQ). (2014, March). TeamSTEPPS® Fundamentals Course: Module 1. Introduction. Retrieved from http://www.ahrq.gov/professionals/education/curriculum-tools/teamstepps /instructor/fundamentals/module1/slintro.html

U.S. Department of Health and Human Services (HHS), Agency for Healthcare Research and Quality (AHRQ). (2016, February). Burnout among health professionals and its effect on patient safety. Retrieved from https://psnet.ahrq.gov/perspectives/perspective/190

U.S. Department of Health and Human Services (HHS), Agency for Healthcare Research and Quality (AHRQ), Patient Safety Network (PSNet). (2015a, March). Human factors engineering. Retrieved from https://psnet.ahrq.gov/primers/primer/20

U.S. Department of Health and Human Services (HHS), Agency for Healthcare Research and Quality (AHRQ), Patient Safety Network (PSNet). (2015b). Patient safety primer: Missed nursing care. Retrieved from http://psnet.ahrq.gov/primer.aspx?primerID=29

U.S. Department of Health and Human Services (HHS), Agency for Healthcare Research and Quality (AHRQ), Patient Safety Network (PSNet). (2015c). PSNet Glossary: Swiss cheese. Retrieved from https://psnet.ahrq.gov/glossary/s

U.S. Department of Health and Human Services (HHS), Agency for Healthcare Research and Quality (AHRQ), Patient Safety Network (PSNet). (2015d, July). Support for clinicians involved in errors and adverse events (second victims). Retrieved from https://psnet.ahrq.gov/primers /primer/30/support-for-clinicians-involved-in-errors-and-adverse-events-second-victims

U.S. Department of Health and Human Services (HHS). Centers for Disease Control and Prevention (CDC). National Institute for Occupational Health and Safety (NIOSH). (2016). About NIOSH. Retrieved from http://www.cdc.gov/niosh/about/default.html

U.S. Department of Health and Human Services (HHS), Centers for Disease Control and Prevention (CDC), National Institute for Occupational Safety and Health (NIOSH). (2008). *Exposure to stress: Occupational hazards in hospitals.* HHS (NIOSH) Publication No. 2008-136. Retrieved from https://www.cdc.gov/niosh/docs/2008-136/pdfs/2008-136.pdf

U.S. Department of Health and Human Services (HHS), Food and Drug Administration (FDA). (2014). What is a serious adverse event? Retrieved from http://www.fda.gov/safety/medwatch /howtoreport/ucm053087.htm

U.S. Department of Health and Human Services (HHS), Office of Inspector General (OIG). (2012, July 19). Few adverse events in hospitals were reported to state adverse event reporting systems. Retrieved from http://oig.hhs.gov/oei/reports/oei-06-09-00092.asp

U.S. Department of Labor (DOL), National Institute for Occupational Safety and Health (NIOSH). (2006). Workplace violence prevention strategies and research needs. NIOSH Publication No. 2006-144. Cincinnati, OH: NIOSH Publication Dissemination.

U.S. Department of Labor (DOL), Occupational Health and Safety Administration (OSHA). (2012a). About OSHA. Retrieved from http://www.osha.gov/about.html

U.S. Department of Labor (DOL), Occupational Health and Safety Administration (OSHA). (2012b). Frequently asked questions. Retrieved from http://www.osha.gov/OSHA_FAQs.html

Van Metre, J., Slovensky, D., & McLaughlin, C. (2013). Classification and reduction of medical errors. In W. Sollecito & J. Johnson (Eds.), *McLaughlin and Kaluzny's continuous quality improvement in health care* (4th ed., pp. 311–334). Burlington, MA: Jones & Bartlett Learning.

VanDeusen, L., Holmes, S., Koppelman, E., Charns, M., Frigand, C., Gupte, G., & Neal, N. (2015). System redesign responses to challenges in safety-net systems: Summary of field study research. Rockville, MD: Agency for Healthcare Research and Quality. AHRQ Pub. No. 15-0053-EF.

Welton, J. (2007). Mandatory hospital nurse to patient staffing ratios: Time to take a different approach. *The Online Journal of Nursing, 12*(3). Retrieved from http://www.nursingworld.org/MainMenuCategories/ANAMarketplace/ANAPeriodicals/OJIN/TableofContents/Volume122007/No3Sept07/MandatoryNursetoPatientRatios.html

World Health Organization (WHO). (2011). WHO patient safety curriculum guide. Retrieved from http://www.who.int/patientsafety/education/curriculum/en/index.html

World Health Organization (WHO), Collaborating Center for Patient Safety Solutions. (2008). Adverse events. Retrieved from http://www.ccforpatientsafety.org

Setting the Stage for Quality Improvement

CHAPTER OBJECTIVES

At the conclusion of this chapter, the learner will be able to:

- Analyze the impact of fragmentation and variation in care.
- Examine the value of surveillance for nursing and continuous quality improvement.
- Compare and contrast examples of high-risk situations for errors and reduced quality care.
- Critique examples of two major national initiatives focused on response to potential risk of inadequate quality care: hospital-acquired conditions and 30-day unplanned readmissions.

OUTLINE

KEY TERMS

Alarm/alert fatigue	Harm	Point of care
Diagnostic error	High-risk	Surveillance
Failure to rescue	Hospital-acquired condition (HAC)	30-day unplanned readmission
Handoff	Medication error	Workaround

Introduction

This chapter examines the specific environment in which continuous quality improvement (CQI) is applied. Healthcare organizations (HCOs) and healthcare providers need to understand the care process and particularly the impact of fragmentation and variation in care. These are important factors that drive errors and difficulties in effectively meeting expected outcomes. Surveillance and measures/indicators are elements that impact the CQI environment and process. Consideration of these factors sets the stage for effective CQI initiatives. Two current major federal government initiatives that have a major impact on healthcare delivery and costs are described in this chapter. Understanding how the stage is set for effective CQI will assist in your examination of the specific elements of CQI and how they may be applied in individual HCOs by healthcare providers and in macro-CQI initiatives on the state and federal levels.

Impact of Fragmentation of Care and Variation in Care

As we continue to examine healthcare quality and how HCOs pursue the goal of improved care, it is important to recognize how the healthcare environment and care process impact CQI. HCOs need to understand their own healthcare environment and care processes to better appreciate their strengths, weaknesses, and improvement needs. Some care process concerns commonly found in HCOs are point of care, fragmentation, and variation.

Point of Care

Point of care refers to direct care experiences when the healthcare provider and patient intersect for care, such as for assessment and intervention. Ideally, this is the key place for CQI, as staff work toward effectively meeting the patient's needs and expected outcomes. At the point of care, staff can identify near misses and stop an action that might lead to error or interfere with expected care outcomes. It is important that the quality improvement (QI) program and its plans emphasize the importance of CQI at the point of care. In doing so, there is greater chance not only to identify problems early but also to increase direct care staff engagement in CQI. Direct care staff include physicians, nurses, nursing assistants, laboratory staff, radiology staff, transportation staff who take patients to other locations, and dietary staff.

Fragmentation of Care

The *Quality Chasm* reports noted that there were major problems in the healthcare systems, describing them as dysfunctional (IOM, 1999, 2001). Gaps in the continuum of care can have a negative impact on quality care. For example, medication reconciliation, which is discussed in this chapter, is a method to address potential gaps in care related to problems with communication about medication needs and orders. Ineffective communication during transfer of care or handoff is another example that may lead to gaps in care. Gap analysis is a critical part of CQI and measurement, as discussed in more detail in other sections of this text. Here in this chapter, we recognize that fragmentation needs to be considered in the QI program and its plans. There is concern today about patient flow and emergency department crowding, both of which contribute to fragmentation of care, ineffective communication, handoff errors and workarounds, and reduced quality of care and patient satisfaction. Noting the importance of fragmentation in care, the Agency for Healthcare Research and Quality (AHRQ) developed a guide for hospitals to improve these important problems (HHS, AHRQ, 2014c).

Variation of Care

Care varies from one patient to another (even if they have the same diagnosis), from one individual healthcare provider to another, and from one HCO to another; to complicate matters, geographic areas may have different care practices and quality. A QI program needs to be aware of the factors that may impact this variation—factors that are more than just individual patient differences. Variation in care impacts performance comparisons or benchmarking (discussed in more detail in other areas of this text). It also impacts care planning. Furthermore, variation in care has implications for care interventions, which may result in different outcomes even when it appears the outcomes should be the same or similar. When such instances arise, HCOs are left to wonder, was the best intervention chosen? Was it possible to really identify and control factors that led to the variation? It is not always easy to make such determinations prospectively, but learning from retrospective results may assist in understanding variation in care and its influence on quality. Nurses should be actively involved in this analysis, as they work closely with patients and must respond to these variations daily. HCOs also need to consider whether variation in patients, providers, use of treatment, resource variability, access to care, influence these differences, or whether there are other factors at play.

Do transient working conditions just prior to an adverse event or during the shift in which the event occurred affect occurrence rates (Grayson et al., 2014)? This is another type of variation in care. A study examined this question and potential triggers that were present when an adverse event occurred compared with a time when an adverse event did not occur. The results indicated that there is variation within a shift and across shifts for specific risk factors. Variation does impact event occurrence. An example is occurrence of unexpected, time-consuming events that then disrupt nurses from their tasks and increase workload. This study indicated that errors increase on busier, more demanding shifts and at times when information sharing is incomplete.

Unit variations related to nurse workforce characteristics, workload, and specific practices influence predicting outcomes in acute care. The Robert Wood Johnson Foundation, Nursing Research Network, developed a research brief on this subject. The brief provides examples that illustrate how variations may impact care and practice and the role of nurses (RWJF, INQRI, 2012):

- Nursing intervention to facilitate patient activation for improved pain self-management
- Empowering home care nurses to efficiently resolve medication discrepancies
- Impact of medical-surgical acute care microsystem nurse characteristics and practices on patient outcomes
- Implementation of a risk specific fall prevention bundle to reduce falls in hospitals
- Implementation and dissemination of an interdicsiplinary nurse-led plan to manage delirium in critically ill adults
- Rural hospital quality collaborative on evidence-based nursing
- SPEACS 2: Improving patient communication and quality outcomes in the ICU
- A diabetes prevention program in the community
- Quality of pediatric nursing care from the children's perspective.

These examples illustrate the complexity of variations in care and also recognize the key element of nursing and nurses in understanding variations and their impact on care quality.

Stop and Consider #1

Care is complex, and its complexity has a major impact on CQI.

Surveillance

The report *Keeping Patients Safe* identifies the need for monitoring patient status or **surveillance** as one of the six major concerns related to direct care quality. The goal is "early identification and prevention of potential problems, which requires behavioral and cognitive skills" (IOM, 2004, p. 91). Assessment is typically done at one point in time, and surveillance is ongoing. Effective surveillance depends on staff competence, staffing levels, skill mix, communication, interprofessional issues and effective teamwork, limiting staff stress level and staff fatigue, use of evidence-based practice (EBP), equipment and supplies, health informatics, and leadership (Finkelman & Kenner, 2012). If surveillance is not effective, then failure to rescue may occur, resulting in possible complications.

Surveillance is considered to be a critical performance measure, primarily focused on nurses and nursing care. Recognition of this process, data collection, identification of problems, and strategies to resolve should be integrated into the QI plan. Surveillance has an impact on when care is received, particularly identifying times of risk such as variations in care and gaps in care. Effective surveillance systems should meet the following objectives (Keroack & Rhinehart, 2013, p. 128):

- Determine the overall magnitude of the problem relative to others.
- Decide whether it is increasing or decreasing in incidence.
- Identify which patient groups or care areas are most affected and therefore most in need of resources.
- Decide whether efforts to improve are succeeding.

Stop and Consider #2

Nurses have the primary responsibility for surveillance.

Examples of High-Risk Situations for Errors and Reduced Quality Care

Risk is the chance that something will happen. An HCO cannot focus on all of its problems and must prioritize its CQI activities. A place to begin in identifying CQI focus areas is with **high-risk** concerns. The term *high risk* applies to situations in which there is greater chance of near misses and errors occurring. In addition, there are barriers to reaching expected outcomes, reducing care quality. Today, there is more concern about diversity and health literacy as factors that impact risk for errors and reduce quality care.

High-risk situations are described as times when quality care may be compromised, or there is increased chance of reduced quality. Recognizing the possibility of such outcomes means the HCO and healthcare providers need to consider the possible consequences and then identify interventions. As Barach and Johnson (2013), state, "There is substantial evidence that the majority of harm caused by health care is avoidable and the result of systemic problems rather than poor performance or negligence by individual providers" (p. 250). With the growing concerns about errors, we know we have to continue improving care, and what has been done to date is not making a significant difference.

Working in Silos

Working in silos means staff are focused exclusively on their specific work area and concerns; they cannot see beyond their own work concerns. It is easy for this mentality to develop in health care, as there is a tendency to focus on specialties and even subspecialties. For example, a women's health department may be divided into gynecology and maternal–child (obstetrics) services. Gynecology may then be subdivided into gynecology units, maybe oncology gynecology, and outpatient clinics; and maternal–child services may be subdivided into pregnancy support (usually through clinics), labor and delivery, neonatal and maybe neonatal intensive care, and postpartum care. In addition, there may be a variety of clinics within the women's health department.

Nurses typically work in one specific unit or clinic. They often forget that there are staff in other areas, and they may not feel connected to the department and the HCO. Nurses are also part of the nursing organization (department, service) within the HCO, which adds another level to their responsibilities. Working in silos may lead to problems such as misunderstanding the trajectory of care, ineffective communication, inadequate coordination, lack of consistency, and lack of commitment to the broader vision and goals. Staff may have fewer relationships and communication with staff outside the "silo" area. All of these factors impact reaching outcomes, risk of errors, and CQI. For example, handoffs occur across silos, but when there is little routine connection and communication, communication and coordination may be limited.

Another factor that is important to consider when identifying risk is the opposite of working in silos. Today, with the increased use of teams, there is much more change even within work teams, such as team members coming and going, and these changes increase risk (Wachter, 2008). HCOs need to use strategies to increase communication and ensure that when people work alone they are communicating effectively with others, and when the team changes, clear communication continues.

Annual Joint Commission National Patient Safety Goals: Identification of High Risk

After the publication of several of the *Quality Chasm* reports, The Joint Commission began an initiative that now has a major impact on quality care. Annually, The Joint Commission identifies key safety goals (The Joint Commission, 2016a). These goals are identified from the information The Joint Commission receives from its accredited HCOs. The goals are identified per specific type of HCO (e.g., for acute care hospitals, for ambulatory care). The 2016 goals focus on patient identification, staff communication, medication safety, safe use of false alarms, prevention of infection, identification of patient safety risks (suicide focus), and prevention of mistakes in surgery (The Joint Commission, 2016b). Current goals may be accessed through The Joint Commission link identified in Connect to Current Information section at the end of the chapter.

HCOs accredited by The Joint Commission must now use the National Patient Safety Goals as one of their critical CQI guides. The goals provide information and alert staff to these high-risk concerns. Data about the goals are collected by individual

HCOs, submitted to The Joint Commission, described in aggregate form to assess progress in meeting the annual goals, and then shared with HCOs and others. The goals apply to anyone who works in the HCO, including all healthcare professions students. Schools of nursing must stay up to date with the current goals, discuss them with students, expect students to be alert about the high-risk concerns, and initiate any interventions that the HCO requires to meet the goals.

Care Transitions and Handoffs

Handoffs are times when patients are transitioned from one form of care to another, such as from one clinical site (e.g., unit, department, HCO) to another, from one provider to another, or from a clinical site back to the patient's home (HHS, AHRQ, PSNet, 2014b). HCOs and the government recognize these times as high risk. The Joint Commission requires that their accredited HCOs develop structured communication methods to address concern about the risk for errors during care transitions or handoffs. The Centers for Medicare and Medicaid Services (CMS) readmission program, which is discussed later in this chapter, focuses on increased risk with care transition during discharge. The electronic medical record/electronic health record (EMR/EHR) also assists in providing information during handoffs, particularly if there is an opportunity to share communication between care providers (e.g., from hospital to hospital, among individual providers, from hospital to a long-term care facility). Providing information across providers, such as hospitals or individual providers, is critical and a weak area. We now have a number of structured communication methods to assist staff during this transition. Multiple methods are discussed in this text, but more needs to be done to improve understanding of handoffs and communication during this time. For example, there is need to have more information to better identify high-risk patients, identify best time to intervene and best strategies/interventions, track outcomes, and then use this information to continue improvement (Sehgal, 2014).

Common barriers to effective handoffs are ineffective communication or no communication; lack of or misuse of time; stressful work environment; inconsistent information; environmental issues, such as interruptions; distractions, such as noise; multitasking; lack of standardization, such as standardized communication methods; problems sharing digital information; health informatics technology (HIT) equipment problems; leadership and management concerns, such as unclear policies and procedures; limited staff support and inadequate resources; lack of staff preparation and understanding of the transition process; inadequate staffing levels; and equipment problems (Risenberg, Leitzsch, & Cunningham, 2010; Welsh, Flanagan, & Ebright, 2010). Identification of the barriers should then guide effective development of strategies/interventions to prevent or respond to handoff problems and should be used to prepare staff for this experience.

Nursing shift change is a time of handoffs, the handoff of all the patients on the unit to different nursing staff, typically done two to three times per 24 hours (Mayor, Bangerter, & Aribot, 2012). There are some units where staff may change multiple times, with staff working individualized schedules. This approach increases the risk of problems during handoffs. Various types of reports may be used such as a unit report, team reports, bedside rounds, written or tape-recorded report, or a combination of methods. The purpose is to ensure greater communication and coordination of care. The type and amount of information shared varies from unit to unit. Management and staff influence how these methods are used. Patient condition also impacts how the handoff report is done and information included; for example, in a situation when staff are overworked and in a hurry to get on with other tasks, there is higher risk of providing incomplete or incorrect information.

As mentioned in this text, some experts, including The Joint Commission, recommend that shift handoff require more structured and standardized methods. For example, the standard might be to use the situation-background-assessment-recommendation (SBAR) approach discussed in other chapters. Although it makes sense that these methods would improve communication, there is no strong evidence to indicate they make a difference in quality of shift handoffs (Mayor et al., 2012; Perry, Wears, & Patterson, 2008). In a study that examined shift handoffs, researchers hypothesized that uncertainty or variation drives the topics and communication during a shift change (Mayor et al., 2012). This means when patients are unstable and/or in critical condition, there is more uncertainty and handoff duration increases. In this study, the most common topics that did vary from different types of units and amount of uncertainty were the treatment, care process, and organization of work. Recommendations indicate that management needs to consider uncertainty and shift handoff to ensure that the units have resources to provide the information necessary for efficient handoffs. More research is needed to better understand the importance of handoffss, something that occurs routinely throughout the healthcare delivery system every day, and a critical component of nursing care.

Bedside reports may improve effectiveness, efficiency, patient safety, and patient satisfaction, thus impacting CQI (Hagman, Oman, Kleiner, Johnson, & Nordhagen, 2013). A study that examined the implementation of bedside reports notes difficulties with using this method. Typically, reports are an opportunity for staff not only to discuss patients, but also to interact with one another and build relationships, which is an important part of a work environment and provides time to discuss general work issues (Hagman et al., 2013). This type of interaction and sharing is not typically part of a bedside report. Some staff also do not feel comfortable sharing all information in front of patients, even with the increased emphasis on patient-centered care. This study found other barriers that need to be considered: frequent patient requests during the bedside report, concern for sleeping patients, patients in isolation, non-English speaking patients, and lack of privacy in a semiprivate room. Staff were generally satisfied, but barriers do need to be addressed. Staff need training to use this method of shift handoff. Problems with communication such as missing information require interventions focused on using more concise and accessible communication; for example, computer-generated summaries and standardized formats may facilitate more timely exchange of critical patient information (Kripalani et al., 2007).

Handoff information should be timely and correctly dated. It should include clear information about diagnosis, testing, treatment, and communication with the patient and family (as appropriate), and outcomes. The following strategies might be used to provide more effective handoff coordination and communication (Patterson et al., 2004).

- Use face-to-face verbal updates with interactive questioning.
- Provide additional updates relevant to other providers in addition to the major provider.
- Limit interruptions during updates.
- Incoming and outgoing staff should initiate topics for discussion or clarification.
- Discussion includes outgoing staff views about changes in plans.
- Information is read back to ensure it was accurately received.
- Outgoing staff writes summary before handoff completed.
- Incoming staff assesses current status.
- Information is updated in the same order every time to ensure all critical information is covered.
- Incoming staff scans historical data before update from outgoing staff.
- Incoming staff receives primary access to the most up-to-date information.
- Incoming staff receives paperwork that includes handwritten annotations.
- It is made clear to others at a glance which staff are responsible for which duties at a time.
- The transfer of responsibility is delayed when there is concern about the status or stability of the process; such concerns should be clearly addressed as part of routine information during handoffs.

Staff need to ask questions and clarify information received, both written and verbal information. This process should not be rushed or viewed as just another task. How it is done and the content make a difference in patient care, outcomes, and CQI.

Examples of barriers to effective handoffs are highlighted in **Table 8-1**.

Table 8-1 Examples of Barriers in the Handoff Process

Technological Factors
- Patient rosters (e.g., whiteboards)
- Electronic health records

Team Factors
- Shift schedules
- Physician compensation methods
- Peer relationships and power balances
- Failure to recognize importance of handoff
- Ambiguous moment during transfer of care

Task Factors
- Too much noise in background to hear communication
- Salience versus completeness
- Varied clinical volume, presentations, complexity
- Lack of standard approach
- Absence of "red flags"

Patient Factors
- Alertness
- Education
- Pain
- Language barrier
- Knowledge of own illness
- Unclear diagnosis

Local and Institutional Environmental Factors
- Location: loud, chaotic, lacking privacy
- Competing demands for time and attention
- Inpatient boarding
- Long emergency department lengths of stay

Caregiver Factors
- Fatigue, stress
- Inattention
- Poor memory
- Inexperience
- Knowledge deficit
- Cognitive bias
- Personal agendas after shift change

Data from Cheung, D.S., Kelly, J.J., Beach, C., Berkeley, R.P., Bitterman, R.A., Broida, R.I., . . . American College of Emergency Physicians Section of Quality Improvement and Patient Safety. (2009). Improving handoffs in the emergency department. *Annals of Emergency Medicine, 55*(2), 171–180.

Failure to Rescue

Failure to rescue is "missing an opportunity to prevent complications" (Finkelman & Kenner, 2016, p. 404). Active surveillance is required to limit incidents of failure to rescue. These are times of high risk for patients, impacting potential for errors and limiting reaching expected outcomes. One of the common steps taken when failure to rescue occurs is to use rapid response teams, discussed in other chapters as a CQI strategy. The purpose of the failure to rescue measure is to determine "the hospital's ability to rescue patients that have developed a serious complication" (Manojlovich & Talsma, 2007, p. 304). What constitutes a failure to rescue situation is not universally accepted. The lack of a universal definition impacts collecting data about the event and comparing data with other HCOs. Even within one HCO, there can be different views of when failure to rescue occurs.

To understand these events and then to initiate interventions to prevent them, HCOs need to analyze the events to examine causes and staff responses. The following are examples of common causes (Jones, DeVita, & Bellomo, 2011, p. 141):

- Monitoring technology is used only in the intensive care unit or step-down units.
- Hospital unit monitoring is only intermittent (e.g., vital sign measurements).
- Intervals between measurements may be 8 hours or longer.
- Regular visits by a hospital unit nurse vary in frequency and duration.
- Visits by a unit doctor may occur only once a day.
- When vital signs are measured, they are sometimes incomplete.
- When vital signs are abnormal, there may be no specific criteria for activating a higher-level intervention.
- Individual judgment is applied to a crucial decision.
- Individual judgment varies in accuracy according to training, experience, professional attitude, working environment, hierarchical position, and previous responses to alerts.
- If an alert is issued, the activation process goes through a long chain of command (e.g., nurse to charge nurse, charge nurse to intern, intern to resident, resident to fellow, fellow to attending physician). Each step in the chain is associated with individual judgment, delays, and possible miscommunication.
- In surgical units, doctors are sometimes physically unavailable because they are performing operations.
- Modern hospitals provide care for patients with complex disorders and coexisting conditions, and unexpected clinical deterioration may occur while nurses and doctors are busy with other tasks.

Diagnosis and Errors

The report *Improving Diagnosis in Health Care* focuses on quickly identifying, resolving, and reducing the incidence of diagnostic errors (NAS/HMD, 2015). Most people will experience at least one diagnostic error in their lifetime. These errors may occur in all types of care. They are often related to malpractice claims, factoring into approximately 10% of patient deaths and between 6% and 17% of hospital adverse events (Kronick, 2013). National data indicate that diagnostic error is one of the most common errors and impacts an estimated 12 million patients each year, although HCOs do not commonly focus on this type of error (Singh, 2015). Diagnosis is a complex process that involves multiple providers and the patient, as described by Singh (2014) **diagnostic error** is "a missed opportunity to make a correct or timely diagnosis based on the available evidence, regardless of patient harm" (p. 99). The report addresses an important problem and identifies possible causes of diagnostic errors, such as ineffective collaboration and communication (healthcare providers/clinicians, patients, and families), healthcare system that is not supportive of an effective diagnosis process, need for greater feedback about performance related to diagnosis, and an HCO culture that does not support transparency and disclosure of these errors (NAS/HMD, 2015).

Ineffective patient-centered care has an impact on diagnostic errors (Kaplan, 2016). Patients may be reluctant to be open about their diagnosis and their concerns. Physicians may make assumptions and then not be able to consider other aspects of diagnosis. Past experience has an impact on how physicians view current patient problems and can interfere with objectivity. Physicians may also think they have the complete diagnosis and consider diagnostic errors to be rare situations. During the diagnosis process, it is best to take a diagnostic time-out to stop and reflect for at least a few minutes. Time may be needed to seek advice or a second opinion and discuss tests and radiology results with experts and others, all of which may expand on information that was in written reports (Society to Improve Diagnosis in Medicine, 2016).

This examination of diagnostic errors also discusses possible strategies to prevent these errors, such as greater teamwork to improve collaboration and communication, use of AHRQ resources such as the Patient and Family Engagement Guide, toolkits on various topics to help HCOs (inpatient and ambulatory care) be more effective, and use of interventions to measure and better understand these errors. Despite this extensive report, it is still difficult to fully understand the extent of the problem. The report describes the Safer Diagnosis Framework, which can be used to improve strategies to prevent and respond to this type of error (NAS/HMD, 2015). This framework, accessible in the report *Improving Diagnosis in Health Care*, focuses on the patient and four diagnostic dimensions, which interact with one another: Encounter with the patient and healthcare provider and the initial diagnostic assessment, diagnostic testing and interpretation, consultations and referrals, and follow-up and monitoring of diagnostic information. When diagnostic errors are measured consideration should be given to reliability, validity, and retrospective and prospective views. Safer diagnosis should lead to improved value of health care and improved patient outcomes.

Patients should also participate in reducing these errors; for example, they may inform healthcare providers of errors providers may not know about such as diagnosis problems from an emergency visit, ask for second opinions, keep track of their personal health information, ask about laboratory and other test results, and speak up—asking questions, requesting further information to understand the diagnosis, and stating when there is concern that care may not be effective (Graber, 2014).

In regard to the nurse's role in monitoring and responding to diagnostic errors, Graber (2014) recommends the following: "Empower nurses to become involved in improving diagnosis. Monitor for new or resolving symptoms, [and] facilitate communication between patients and providers" (p. 26). Other recommended strategies include use of morbidity and mortality conferences to better understand care provided and outcomes; use autopsies to learn more about diagnoses, although this is done less and less; get second opinions; provide best possible expertise for radiology and clinical laboratory testing; send laboratory test results to patients; monitor how many critical test results (including radiology) are acted upon within 30 days; empower patients to participate and speak up; and actively use root cause analysis, requiring clinicians to participate in the process (Graber, 2014). Many of these strategies should involve nurses.

Medication Administration

Medication administration is a high-risk event for possible errors. A **medication error** is defined by the U.S. Department of Health and Human Services (HHS), Food and Drug Administration(FDA) (2015) as a "preventable event that may cause or lead to inappropriate medication use or patient harm while the medication is in control of the healthcare professional, patient, or consumer." The FDA notes that these errors are related to factors such as professional practice, healthcare products, and procedures and systems, including prescribing, communication of medication order, product labeling, packaging, and nomenclature, compounding, dispensing, distribution, and administration of the medication. Staff education and monitoring of the process are also critical factors.

Medication Administration: A Process and Its Implications

Medication administration is a complex process. The Institute for Safe Medication Practices (ISMP) identifies the following as key interrelated elements that affect the entire medication use system (ISMP's Key Elements of the Medication Use System™; ISMP, 2015):

1. *Patient information.* Obtaining the patient's pertinent demographic (age, weight) and clinical (diagnoses, allergies, lab results) information will assist practitioners in selecting the appropriate medications, doses, and routes of administration. Having essential patient information at the time

of medication prescribing, dispensing, and administration will result in a significant decrease in preventable adverse drug events (ADEs).

2. *Drug information.* Providing accurate and usable drug information to all healthcare practitioners involved in the process reduces the amount of preventable ADEs. Not only should drug information be readily accessible to the staff through many sources (e.g., drug references, formulary, protocols, HCO-prepared information, dosing scales), it must be up to date and accurate.

3. *Communication of drug information.* Miscommunication between physicians, pharmacists, and nurses is a common cause of medication errors. To minimize the amount of medication errors caused by miscommunication, it is always important to verify drug information and eliminate communication barriers.

4. *Drug labeling, packaging, and nomenclature.* Drug names that look alike or sound alike, as well as products that have confusing drug labeling and nondistinct drug packaging, significantly contribute to medication errors. The incidence of medication errors is reduced with the use of proper labeling and the use of unit dose systems within hospitals.

5. *Drug storage, stock, standardization, and distribution.* Standardizing drug administration times, regulating drug concentrations, and limiting the dose concentration of drugs available in patient care areas reduce the risk of medication errors or minimize their consequences should an error occur.

6. *Drug device acquisition, use, and monitoring.* Appropriate safety assessment of drug delivery devices should be made both prior to their purchase and during their use. Also, a system of independent double-checks should be used within the HCO to prevent device-related errors, such as selecting the wrong drug or drug concentration, setting the rate improperly, or mistaking the infusion line for another line.

7. *Environmental factors.* Having a well-designed system offers the best chance of preventing errors; however, sometimes the environment in which we work contributes to medication errors. Environmental factors that often contribute to medication errors include poor lighting, noise, interruptions, and a significant workload.

8. *Staff competence and education.* Staff education should focus on priority topics, such as new medications used in the hospital, high-alert medications, medication errors that have occurred both internally and externally, and protocols, policies, and procedures related to medication use. Staff education can be an important error prevention strategy when combined with the other key elements for medication safety.

9. *Patient education.* Patients must receive ongoing education from physicians, pharmacists, and the nursing staff about the brand and generic names of medications they are receiving, their indications, usual and actual doses, expected and possible adverse effects, drug or food interactions, and how to protect themselves from errors. Patients have a vital role in preventing

Table 8-2 Common Sources of Medication Errors	
Ambiguous orders	Incorrect drug selected
Drug device use	Incorrect patient
Environmental stress	Insufficient drug information
Errors in communication or miscommunication of drug orders	Insufficient information about other drugs patient is on (therapeutic duplication)
Error-prone abbreviation	Insufficient laboratory information
Illegible handwriting	Known allergy
Improper dose	Limited patient education
Incomplete orders	Limited staff education
Incomplete or insufficient monitoring	Look-alike or sound-alike drugs
Incomplete patient information or unavailable patient information	Poor communication

Reproduced from Youngberg, B. (2013). Patient safety handbook (2nd ed.). Burlington, MA: Jones & Bartlett Learning.

medication errors and should be encouraged to ask questions and seek answers about their medications before drugs are administered in an HCO, prescribed by a healthcare provider, or dispensed at a pharmacy.

10. *Quality processes and risk management.* The way to prevent errors is to redesign the systems and processes that lead to errors, rather than focus on correcting the individuals who make errors. Effective strategies for reducing errors include making it difficult for staff to make an error and promoting the detection and correction of errors before they reach a patient and cause harm.[1]

Examples of common sources of medication errors are identified in **Table 8-2**.

The National Coordinating Council for Medication Error Reporting and Prevention (NCCMERP), a collaboration of 27 national organizations, recognized the need for a standardized categorization of errors and compared preventable ADEs with nonpreventable ADEs, as describe in **Figure 8-1**. The following are some of the key types of errors (NCCMERP, 2015):

- A *preventable ADE* is harm caused by the use of a drug as a result of an error (e.g., patient given a normal dose of drug, but the drug was contraindicated for this patient). These events require examination by the provider to determine why they happened.
- A *nonpreventable ADE* is drug-induced harm occurring during appropriate use of medication (e.g., anaphylaxis from penicillin in a patient who had no previous history of an allergic reaction). While these events are currently nonpreventable, future studies may reveal ways to prevent them.

---

[1] © ISMP. Used with permission.

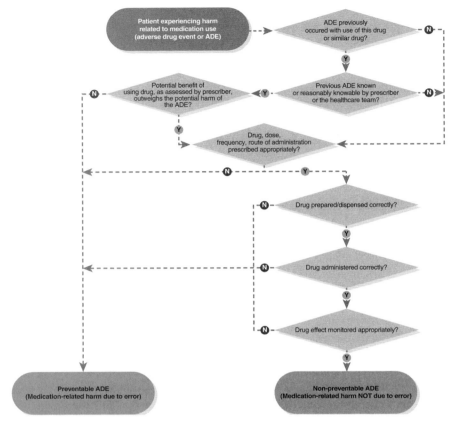

Figure 8-1. Comparing Preventable Adverse Drug Event with Non-preventable Adverse Drug Event

Reproduced from National Coordinating Council for Medication Error Reporting and Prevention. (2015). Contemporary view of medication-related harm. A new paradigm. Retrieved from http://www.nccmerp.org/sites /default/files/nccmerp_fact _sheet_2015-02-v91.pdf

- An *adverse drug reaction (ADR)* is any response to a drug that is noxious and unintended and occurs at doses normally used for prophylaxis or diagnosis or for the modification of a physiological function.

Figure 8-2 compares preventable ADEs and nonpreventable ADEs. Both the NCCMERP and the FDA provide online methods to report medication errors and concerns, identified in the Connect to Current Information section at the end of the chapter. These resources will help expand nurses' knowledge about medications and errors.

The five rights (right patient, right drug, right dosage, right time, right route) have long been the standard for nursing care. Applying these rights helps to reduce errors and keeps nurses alert to common medication risk areas. Other rights that are also important are right documentation, right to refuse medication, and right to evaluation and monitoring (Anderson & Townsend, 2010). Two other rights have been recommended given the need for improvement: identify the right indication or reason for the medication, and ensure the right documentation (Walton, 2014).

HCOs and CQI initiatives tend to emphasize reliance on medication error rates; however, not all experts agree with the value of these rates. In 2002, the NCCMERP reported that it did not consider it helpful to rely on incidence rates for medication errors, and in 2008 it restated its belief (NCCMERP, 2008). Focusing on numbers is not enough, as there is need to gain better understanding of errors beyond numbers. The NCCMERP gives the following reasons for not overrelying on incidence rates when comparing results with other HCOs (ISMP, 2015):

- *Differences in culture* among HCOs can lead to significant differences in the level of reporting of medication errors.
- *Differences in the definition* of a medication error among HCOs can lead to significant differences in the reporting and classification of medication errors.
- *Differences in the patient populations* served by various HCOs can lead to significant differences in the number and severity of medication errors occurring among organizations.
- *Differences in the type(s) of reporting and detection systems* for medication errors among HCOs can lead to significant differences in the number of medication errors recorded.

The goal of every HCO should be to focus on CQI processes to prevent harm to patients due to medication errors (ISMP, 2015). Achieving this goal requires monitoring of actual and potential medication errors that occur within the HCO. NCCMERP recommends that each HCO work to improve and prevent harm to patients within the organization. It defines **harm** as "impairment of the physical, emotional, or psychological function or structure of the body and pain or injury resulting therefrom" (NCCMERP, 2001). Focusing on the prevention of harm allows the HCO to identify limitations in its medication systems and identify opportunities to learn from the experience. This should be done by using root cause analysis, as discussed in other chapters, to further understand medication errors and make changes as need, recognizing that the number of errors is less important than the quality of the data.

Nursing Education and Medication Administration

Nursing education has a major role in reducing medication errors. Nurse educators need to consider the topic of medication administration a critical part of content and experience, emphasizing with students that medication administration is a time in the care process when they must be engaged in CQI, both as students and after graduation. The most common student nurse medication errors are related to failure to follow administration rights, system issues, and lack of knowledge and understanding about medications (Cooper, 2014). These situations should be considered red flags for students, putting them on alert to be more careful.

The focus of this text is primarily on CQI within HCOs, although the content does include the need to recognize core competencies that should be demonstrated not only by nurses in practice but also by those entering practice. Nursing students are involved in a variety of near misses and errors when they are in their clinical rotations. Simulated experiences provide a safe environment in which students can not only practice medication administration but also learn about medication administration risks, strategies to prevent errors, and how to respond and track near misses and errors. In a study conducted from 2011 to 2013 funded by the National Council of State Boards of Nursing (NCSBN), the researchers collected and analyzed information about school of nursing practices and policies for student near misses and errors (Disch & Barnsteiner, 2014). A web-based survey was sent to 1,667 schools, and 557 (33%) responded. Of the responding schools, 86 (16%) had a tool or policy focused on student errors. This is a very small percentage, indicating the need for schools of nursing to examine CQI and how the schools handle student near misses and errors. There should be clear school of nursing policies and procedures related to these situations, and schools should also review and consider clinical agency policies and procedures. Schools of nursing need to coordinate and share information with their clinical agencies so that there is effective CQI implemented within schools of nursing and there is collaboration with clinical agencies and their QI programs. It should be clear that when an error occurs in which a student and/ or faculty is involved, there are procedures to follow at the clinical agency and at the school of nursing to ensure effective information sharing. Just as HCOs should avoid a blame environment, so should schools of nursing.

Following the first phase of the NCSBN-funded school of nursing study, a pilot was conducted in 10 schools of nursing. Using the survey form provided by the study, the sample submitted 70 error or near-miss reports in this period. The survey form identified the following types of incidents that would then be tracked in a new national database (Disch & Barnsteiner, 2014, p. 7):

- Medication error
- Needlestick
- Inadequate preparation for providing patient care
- Blood/pathogen exposure
- Fall event
- Outside scope of practice
- Injury to body
- Change in patient condition
- Deviation in protocols
- Equipment or medical device malfunction
- Environmental safety for self, patient, and others
- Inappropriate or inadequate communication by faculty, preceptor, other student, healthcare team, patient, or visitor
- Breach of confidentiality

This survey includes not only data underlying the type of incident, but also data about the recipient of the unsafe event, event demographics, event description in narrative form, location of the event, and follow-up action. The long-term goal of this study is to establish a web-based national data repository with anonymous reporting by students, faculty, or both to reduce student incidents. The repository is called Generating Reports about Safe Student Practice (GRaSSP) Network. Membership in the network allows members (schools of nursing) to access the data and track data for their students, and it provides opportunities to identify trends and additional information to better understand student learning needs related to safe medication administration.

This major study and the development of a national database support the need for schools of nursing to examine medication and medication administration content and learning experiences to ensure they are in line with current CQI information and recommendations for effective medication administration. Competence in this content has a major impact on CQI. It is also important for students to appreciate the implications of effective and safe medication use for all patients in all settings; that is, in all situations, students should understand their role and responsibilities.

Strategies to Reduce Medication Errors

It is vital that HCOs consider how their QI program and related CQI activities can reduce medication error risk. Examples of critical guidelines for safe medication administration include the following (Anderson & Townsend, 2010, p. 3):

- Reading back and verifying medication orders given verbally or over the phone
- Asking a colleague to double-check medications when giving high-alert drugs
- Using an oral syringe to administer oral or nasogastric medications
- Assessing patients for drug allergies before giving medications
- Becoming familiar with the facility's "do not use" list of abbreviations

It is common to use abbreviations in documentation and orders; however, there are risks associated with this practice. The objective here is not to eliminate use of abbreviations, but to caution staff to be careful. HCOs should have an approved list of abbreviations, and staff must use only abbreviations that are on the list. Staff orientation and education include this information, and when changes are made, staff need to be informed. Electronic documentation programs provide more opportunities to alert staff to incorrect use of abbreviations and should be set up to block their use.

There is now greater use of unit-based dispensing cabinets that include storage and unit-dose and some multiple-dose options (decentralized automated dispensing devices). These systems are often connected in real time to the pharmacy so that staff can get assistance when needed, allowing for timely administration of medication with a safer dose method (Ehlert & Rough, 2013). The devices have also altered methods used for management of controlled substances, reducing time for staff to complete this more complex medication administration procedure, and providing a more effective, secure procedure.

Since the 1980s and 1990s, the dispensing systems have helped nurses during medication administration, reducing time and in some cases errors; however, there are potential problems with these systems that need to be considered in QI programs. HCOs need to have the right equipment, maintained so that it functions correctly, and enough dispensing cabinets to cover workload and care needs. Problems with the equipment can lead to risk of errors and also increase staff frustration, requiring more work when time is limited. However, using these devices does not ensure an error-free procedure. When a nurse opens a patient's container or drawer, there is still the risk of selecting the wrong drug and administering it; for example, the nurse may assume that all drugs in the container are correct according to the patients' orders without confirming. The HCO system must be consistent so that the same drugs and equipment are kept in the same place, eliminating the possibility that the nurse may be on autopilot and grab something that is misplaced. Policies and procedures related to a decentralized automated dispensing device should be routinely reviewed, including staff feedback, and when changes are made, they should be shared with staff. New staff must be oriented to the system and supervised on initial use until the supervisor and the nurse feel comfortable with correct use, policies and procedures are followed, and the nurse has an understanding of the system.

Medication near misses have an impact on nurses' workload. When nurses experience a near miss, they need to double-check orders and may need additional communication with the provider who ordered the medication. This process has an impact on other patients, too, as time is taken away from other care as staff are distracted. In the end, this situation increases risk for other problems and possibly results in worse than a near miss—an outright error (Anderson & Townsend, 2010).

High-alert medications are drugs that have high potential to cause patient harm when misused (Ehlert & Rough, 2013). HCOs should develop a list of these medications. Examples are chemotherapy, heparin, and insulin. These drugs require double-checking with another licensed professional whenever the drug is taken from a multidose vial. Staff education should include information about these drugs, related policy and procedure, and also testing to ensure competency in administration of the drugs. If an automated dispensing system is used, there should be clear labels and other methods to indicate these drugs are included. The pharmacy must also use high-alert labels for the drugs; for example, when these drugs are used in infusion pumps specific labeling should be used. Intravenous infusions with these drugs should be handled carefully, such as reporting on their use at point of handoffs and at shift change and resetting the amount infused at each shift. The HCO should have a policy and procedure on this care issue. In a recent study, it was identified that 60% of the sample experienced one or more errors—for example, labeling error, bypassing of the smart pump (workaround), and violation of HCO policy (Schnock et al., 2016). Despite this high percentage, harm to patients was minimal. This type of result, however, should not be ignored, as it demonstrates that errors occur at a high rate and could be harmful.

Some changes to improve care may be viewed negatively and may lead to controversy. Not all changes are the right ones, and some may add complexity that makes work more difficult for staff and negatively impacts care. For example, a policy that medications should be administered within 30 minutes of the time ordered was supported by the CMS. This led to concerns that failure to meet this policy would be classified as an error (Cipriano, 2011). The ISMP is not in favor of this policy (ISMP, 2010). What is the potential problem with this policy? If an order is written to administer a medication at 10:00 a.m. and the nurse is busy with an emergency or took longer with a procedure and does not administer the medication until 10:15 a.m., then the policy has not been met. But has an error occurred? Staff frequently use workarounds, increasing risk of errors, and this 30-minute policy creates just the scenario in which a nurse might use a workaround. Those who disagree with overemphasizing the 30-minute rule think it does not recognize that nurses should be able to use clinical reasoning and judgment. For example, does a 15-minute delay make a real difference in the effect of a specific drug or in the condition of an individual patient? As a result of data that ISMP collected about increased risk of using workarounds during these situations, in 2011, the CMS rescinded its support of the 30-minute policy (HHS, CMS, 2011). This is an example of how data can make an impact when collected in a structured manner and analyzed to determine outcomes. Now hospitals must identify specific time-critical scheduled medications rather than having a rule that applies to all medications.

The most commonly identified incidents in anesthesia are drug administration errors. Medication administration has received a lot of attention, and many methods are used to prevent and respond to events, such as use of safety checks, active pharmacy participation, and multiple nursing checks during medication administration. These efforts, however, are not extended to perioperative care. There is also a great difference in stress levels between the operating room (OR) and other units. Both are stressful, but the OR may be much more stressful. This has an impact on work and staff responses. Most of the data about the OR are self-reported, and this is not the most reliable method for studies. Although nonoperative areas have seen a decrease in medication errors, this is not the case in the OR. In a study conducted in a large medical center with 40,000 operations annually in 64 ORs, it was concluded that approximately 1 in 20 perioperative medication administrations resulted in a medication error and/or adverse event (Nanji, Patel, Shaikh, Seger, & Bates, 2016). This was a prospective observational study, and when compared with other retrospective studies, the rate of these events was higher in this study. Of the 193 events identified in the study, 153 (79.3%) were thought to be preventable and 20.7% nonpreventable. None of the events were life threatening; the majority of the events were serious (68.9%) or significant (29.5%). Fifty-three percent of the events occurred during induction (first 20 minutes of anesthesia process). Problems that were identified with the events were: labeling errors, wrong dose, omitted medication or failure to act, delay or failure to treat an adverse event, and error in monitoring. Longer procedures (more than 6 hours) and procedures with 13 or more medication administrations experienced more events. The researchers recommend greater use of point-of-care bar coding anesthesia documentation systems and examination of the timing of documentation (e.g., using the bar coding to identify potential problems before drugs are administered and documented). Most drugs used in the

OR are documented at some time after they are administered and in some cases at the conclusion of the surgery. Areas in which improvements are needed include decreasing opportunities for workarounds, connecting infusions to the most proximal intravenous port, and carefully selecting equipment and provision of training on use of equipment.

When preparing and administering medications, disruptions are a major concern and increase the risk of errors. Nurses use multitasking all the time, and when they do this, they often experience interruptions, distractions, lack of focus, and task switching (Clark & Flanders, 2012). Error recovery is something that nurses are involved in, and it can make a difference in the quality of care. Examples of error recovery strategies include knowing the plan of care, who is involved, and patient information; applying relevant policies and procedures; double-checking information and questioning; actively using surveillance; and using expected systematic processes (Henneman et al., 2010).

Clinical reasoning and judgment are important, but the nurse should be aware that interruptions and distractions might affect reasoning (Dickson & Flynn, 2012). In a study of nursing interruptions in the emergency department, it was noted that interruptions during patient care can come from other staff and may also be associated with the patient and the family (Cole, Stefanus, Gardner, Levy, & Klein, 2015). This study recommended that future research consider the impact of interruptions that are urgent versus routine or unnecessary. Better understanding of the nature of interruptions should guide nurses in determining their best response choice.

Admission is a time of increased risk for medication errors (Gleason et al., 2010). It is at this time that the patient's medication history should be obtained, and there may be barriers to getting accurate and complete information. Examples of these barriers include the following:

- Older patients may not have good recall of medications they take.
- The patient's condition may make it difficult to get information.
- Look-alike or sound-alike medications may cause problems.
- Patients may have limited health literacy, may have language problems, may be poor historians, and/or may withhold information.

To complicate matters, staff may be busy with multiple admissions and other required work, leading to distractions and disruptions. Handoffs, as mentioned earlier, increase risk, and an admission may be a transfer—for example, a patient moving from the emergency department to inpatient services or from the hospital to a long-term care facility. Errors at the time of admission are influenced by factors that may impact obtaining an accurate medication history.

Medication administration is an important part of home care that has risks for errors. Most patients in home care are older adults, and this patient population has a higher risk for ADEs and ADRs, which might be due to under- or overprescribing

(Anathhanam, Powis, Cracknell, & Robson, 2012). In the home environment, older adults are at risk for taking too much or too little medication and/or using the wrong medication. These medication errors may then lead to incidents such as sedation, falling, medical complications, and unintended overdose. In some cases, ADEs may lead to confusion of medication side effects with symptoms, impacting diagnosis, and may then lead to problems that require hospitalization. LeBlanc and Choi (2015) propose that the following strategies be considered to make the home a safe environment (p. 317):

1. Increase the ability of patients to self-manage medications.
2. Identify and make necessary medication changes.
3. Create an accurate, up-to-date medication list to be available in the home.
4. Provide communication between the primary care provider, patient, and case manager.

Medication assessment should be completed prior to developing the care or treatment plan after discharge to ensure medication safety when the patient is discharged home. The GerontoNet ADR Risk Score can be used to identify hospitalized elderly patients who are at risk for ADEs (Onder et al., 2010). Having this assessment can then help the clinical team use interventions to prevent ADEs. The following factors are important to consider (Anathhanam et al., 2012):

- Identify prescribing omissions (underprescribing).
- Identify inappropriately prescribed medications.
- Develop methods for safer use of high-risk medications such as antipsychotic medications, anticoagulation for atrial fibrillation, and opioids.
- Improve safety in healthcare settings and across care transitions.

The ISMP provides guidelines and alerts for staff about medications; see the Connect to Current Information section at the end of the chapter for a link to this site. Practicing nurses should use this source to keep up to date with high-risk situations that may lead to medication error. In summary, the following is a list of suggested strategies that may assist in decreasing risk of medication errors (Walton, 2014, p. 14; Wachter, 2008, p. 48). Notes are included to help HCOs identify potential CQI measures that will improve monitoring of medication administration:

- Recognize and report errors.
- Review patient medication orders, considering patient outcomes, duplications, and drug interactions.
- Verify and ensure orders are complete.
- Verify the five (preferably the seven) rights of medication administration.
- If there are any questions about the order, confirm before giving the medication, even if it means medication administration may be late.
- Double-check dosage and flow rate calculations with another staff member, especially if standard dose concentration or dosage charts are not available.

- Double-check orders with another staff member, such as when administering blood or for special drugs identified by the pharmacy or high-risk/alert or error-prone medications. HCOs may require that certain drugs be checked with a second nurse.
- Do not circumvent (work around) the medication delivery system by "borrowing" medications from one patient and administering to another even if the label indicates the same drug and dosage.
- If there is a question about a large dose, check this with prescriber.
- If using an infusion pump, know how to use it, monitor the equipment, and make sure any previously administered drugs are not in the tubing.
- Talk with the patient to determine if the patient understands prescribed medications and indications. If the patient questions a medication, then check the order.
- Consider your fatigue and stress levels and how these factors impact safe practice.
- Use acceptable abbreviations, and be particularly alert for abbreviations prone to causing errors; do not use any tailing zeros when transcribing dosages.
- Document administration immediately after giving medication.
- Follow HCO policies and procedures and keep up to date with changes.
- Do not guess on an order; double-check if in doubt.
- Be on alert when using look-alike and sound-alike medications.
- Use bar coding as required, following the procedure.
- Collaborate with the pharmacy to ensure stock medications are available; use the pharmacist as a source of information; ask about potential risk of medication error.
- Use the medication dispensing equipment correctly, and if you do not know how to use it or have questions, get assistance.
- Identify allergies and apply allergy alert system.
- Do not leave medication with the patient to take.
- Remind the patient of safety issues (e.g., call for help to get out of bed or chair), tell the patient to report if pain does not decrease, and otherwise encourage measures of patient self-advocacy.
- Listen to the patient, who may alert you to problems with a medication.
- Complete medication reconciliation at time of admission and discharge, or when needed, such as for home care services.
- Provide patient education about medications; include family, with permission of the patient (permission is not required if the family is legal guardian).
- Understand how computerized physician order entry (CPOE) works—if it is available.
- Maintain and increase knowledge about medications; this requires that nurses recognize when they do not know about a drug and need to get further

information such as from the pharmacy or other resources. Some HCOs assign clinical pharmacists to provide direct consultation to unit clinical staff.

- Use sterile technique when required for administering drugs and infusions.
- Wash hands before preparing medications and before and after administering.
- Recognize and apply guidelines for medications that require monitoring of data before administering (e.g., temperature, blood pressure, lab results).

Alarm/Alert Fatigue

The problem of alarm/alert fatigue has increased so much that The Joint Commission issued a sentinel event alert for medical device alarm safety in hospitals (The Joint Commission, 2013). There are a number of devices that are relevant to alarm safety, such as bedside physiologic monitors that include electrocardiogram machines, pulse oximetry devices, and monitors of blood pressure and other parameters; bedside telemetry; central station monitors; infusion pumps; and ventilators (HHS, AHRQ, PSNet, 2015). In some cases, on a single unit there can be several hundred alarms per patient in a day. If you multiply this number by the number of patients on a unit, it is easy to see how these alarms can over time stress staff, and added to this is the problem that between 85% and 99% of the alarms are false, requiring no clinical intervention (The Joint Commission, 2013). The persistence of these (often false) alarms may lead to staff experiencing **alarm/alert fatigue**, which may mean staff respond by ignoring alarms or not rushing to respond. The following factors commonly impact alarm/alert sentinel events (The Joint Commission, 2013, p. 2):

- Alarm fatigue—the most common contributing factor
- Alarm settings that are not customized to the individual patient or patient population
- Inadequate staff training on the proper use and functioning of the equipment (e.g., inconsistent team training, response, and interpretation of alarm signals)
- Inadequate staffing to support or respond to alarm signals
- Alarm conditions and settings that are not integrated with other medical devices
- Equipment malfunctions and failures

Three years after the these recommendations were made, the problem continued. The Joint Commission 2014 Patient Safety Goals required that by 2016 HCOs accredited by The Joint Commission must do the following: designate alarm management as a patient safety priority, understand clinical alarm hazards, create an action plan, implement the plan, and identify best practices (The Joint Commission, 2016b). Since nurses are the staff most involved in responding to alarms, nurses should assume leadership in meeting this requirement and improving effective responses.

In a systematic review of 24 studies on alarm characteristics, 8 studies focused on evaluating alarm fatigue interventions and noted that most of the time the alarm does not mean there is a problem; it is a false alarm. The review recommends additional strategies to address this problem: widening alarm parameters that set off the alarm, using alarm delays, and frequently changing telemetry electrodes and wires (Paine et al., 2016). As this research and others demonstrate, HCOs are making efforts to understand alarm fatigue and resolve this problem.

In a study on drug allergy alerts integrated into EMR/EHRs, it was noted that overall there was an increase in alert overrides by providers, from 83.3% (2004) to 87.6% (2013) (Topaz et al., 2015). These overrides are dangerous and are not an effective response to increased alarms/alerts. The Joint Commission recommends that the culture of safety increase a shared sense of responsibility among all staff. HCOs are reluctant to remove alarms due to legal concerns, and alert override and removal of alarms compromise effective response for patients who require surveillance and effective, rapid response for their care needs. The following are examples of effective strategies that might be used to reduce problems with alarm fatigue (The Joint Commission, 2013):

- Tailor alerts to patient characteristics and critical integrated clusters of physiologic indicators.
- Tier alerts according to severity. Warnings could be presented in different ways in order for key clinicians to be alerted to more clinically consequential events.
- Make only high-level (severe) alerts interruptive.
- Apply human factor principles when designing alerts (e.g., format, content, legibility, color of alerts).

Workarounds

A **workaround** occurs when a staff member avoids a problem without eliminating it (Lalley & Malloch, 2010). Workarounds are used in many different situations. Medication administration is one of them. In a study that examined 986 medication errors that were either reported through a trigger system or that staff voluntarily reported, approximately half of the errors were not prevented by information technology system such as CPOE and/or bar codes (Stultz & Nahata, 2015). Staff used workarounds to avoid using the informatics systems that were established to avoid errors, and in doing so, errors occurred.

Workarounds can result in positive or negative outcomes. Errors can result, which could be due to a lack of awareness of a risk of error and what should be done to prevent an error. Sometimes the use of workarounds may provide opportunities for creative change or improvement and may identify areas that need to be improved. The AHRQ offers the following insights regarding the place of workarounds in care delivery:

What does matter is that the motivation for a workaround lies in getting work done, not laziness or whim. Thus, the appropriate response by managers to the existence of a workaround should not consist of reflexively reminding staff about the policy and restating the importance of following it. Rather, workarounds should trigger assessment of workflow and the various competing demands for the time of frontline personnel. In busy clinical areas where efficiency is paramount, managers can expect workarounds to arise whenever policies create added tasks for frontline personnel, especially when the extra work is out of proportion to the perceived importance of the safety goal. (HHS, AHRQ, PSNet, 2016)

Health Informatics

More information about HIT is provided in other chapters. It is, however, important to note in this chapter that HIT is an important part of the QI program and plans. The use of HIT can improve care outcomes by providing methods for data collection and analysis and can even provide strategies to prevent and respond to quality care problems. HIT, however, also increases risk of errors and problems with communication and documentation, the focus of this chapter.

Staff Competence

Staff need to be competent in the work they are required to do. When staff are not competent, risk of harm to patients may occur. Competence is the responsibility of individual nurses and employers, including direct supervisors and staff educators. Professional organizations and regulators such as boards of nursing and licensure requirements also have an impact on competence. The critical bottom line is each staff member must feel comfortable admitting they need help; they must be able to ask questions and seek out assistance to take steps to improve their practice. Other chapters discuss competence and staff continuing education required to improve care.

Communication

Communication is mentioned frequently in this text, and it is behind all aspects of health care. Problems with communication are the number one cause of errors and difficulties meeting expected outcomes, increasing risk. The list of situations when communication occurs is unending. Critical examples are patient–staff interactions, reports and rounds, delegation of responsibilities, and performance evaluation. Interprofessional factors are important, such as work difficulties between staff (discussed in other areas relating to teams in this text). During communication, nurses need to be aware of the significance of the facts as they relate to a situation in their practice to reduce errors and improve communication to meet outcomes of care. The process requires that information be updated and evaluated, and this must be an active process, not a passive one, to decrease risk of errors.

Chronic Illness: Complex Patients

Chronic illness has an important impact on CQI and cost of care, with one in four Americans having multiple chronic conditions (MCC). This care consumes two-thirds of the U.S. healthcare costs (HHS, 2015). **A commonly used** chronic care model can be accessed through the Connect to Current Information section at the end of the chapter. Embedded within this model are elements that relate to the five healthcare professions core competencies, and the model also reflects the aims (STEEEP) to improve care. Chronic illness and complex treatment needs increase risk for patients, impacting patient outcomes and possible errors.

In 2010, the U.S. Department of Health and Human Services (HHS) developed a strategic framework to address MCC and risk of quality care problems with this patient population. The framework goals are as follows (HHS, 2010):

- Strengthen the healthcare and public health systems.
- Empower the individual to use self-care management.
- Equip healthcare providers with tools, information, and effective interventions.
- Support targeted research about individuals with MCC and effective interventions.

In support of the framework and the need to improve care, the HHS provides training modules to improve healthcare profession knowledge of MCC. The reason for all of this activity is recognition that the quality of care for these patients has an impact on overall HCO CQI outcomes and cost of care with increased risk for quality care problems.

Pain Management

Pain is a common health problem that is complex (impacted by biological, behavioral, environmental and societal factors), increasing risk of errors, and individuals respond differently to pain. Effectively managing pain is a critical element of patient-centered care. Patients expect that healthcare providers will help them with pain management to maintain or improve their quality of life, including activities of daily living. To meet this expectation, we must have a better understanding of pain and improve how we prevent, assess, and treat pain, as reported in a major report on pain described in **Figure 8-2** (IOM, 2011).

Addiction has increased rapidly in the past few years. It is thought that the increasing use of prescription pain medication has led to people going on to using other types of addictive drugs or these prescriptions providing a source of drugs for others (e.g., family members, friends). This is a major healthcare problem and requires careful assessment. There is also the danger of going too far in limiting pain medication due to concern about addiction and then not assisting patients who need pain management. This undermedicating then impacts their health status. Staff need to be aware of this risk early in the process of pain management. All

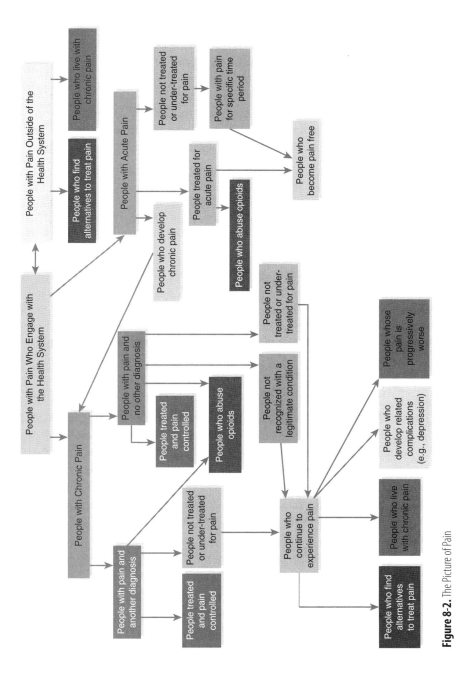

Figure 8-2. The Picture of Pain

Reproduced from Institute of Medicine (IOM). (2011). *Relieving pain in America. A blueprint for transforming prevention, care, education, and research*. Washington, DC: The National Academies Press. Courtesy of the National Academies Press, Washington, DC.

of these factors are directly related to quality care for patients with pain, whether short term or long term.

Some of the barriers to improving pain management are need for more knowledge, staff attitudes toward pain, system issues such as how medication is delivered, use of computerized records, staffing levels to respond to patients when they need help with pain, rehabilitative services, planning and coordination of care, and patient education about pain. Effective pain management requires effective teamwork and may require effective medication administration. The Healthy People 2020 initiative (2016) includes a product safety objective related to pain management: "Increase the safe and effective treatment of pain." Related subobjectives are as follows:

> Reduce the proportion of patients suffering from untreated pain due to lack of access to pain treatment, reduce the number of non-FDA-approved pain medications, reduce serious injuries from the use of pain medicines, and reduce deaths from the use of pain medicines. (Healthy People, 2016)

Nurses are involved directly in pain management in all types of settings. They can influence the quality of care for pain and reduce risk for errors and patient harm. Assessment and interventions, particularly medication administration, are used to ensure effective pain management. Use of pain intensity scales is common now and recommended by experts for assessment and effective treatment decisions.

Responding to High-Risk Situations for Errors and Reduced Quality Care

In 2010, a study was undertaken to expand a 2005 study that was referred to as the Silence Kills study. Findings from more than 6,500 nurses and nurse managers were used to examine other aspects of the problem of communication and errors. The conclusion was that safety tools do not address a second category of communication breakdowns referred to as "undiscussables." Undiscussables, or what we do not like to talk about or are not able to talk about, such as dangerous shortcuts, incompetence, and disrespect, have a direct impact on CQI. Often, they represent risks that are widely known by staff but not discussed. For staff to fully engage in CQI and share concerns, they need active support from other staff and management. As Maxfield, Grenny, Levandero, and Goah (2010) articulate, "Tools don't create safety; people do."

Several examples of high-risk situations when errors may occur and quality of care may be reduced have been identified and described. This list is not complete, but it describes examples to think about and provides a basis for identifying other examples. In summary, nurses need to consider the following general guidelines related to high-risk situations:

- Every staff person has a role in ensuring quality care.
- Understand the many aspects to quality and risk and how they relate to your work daily.

- Understand why it is important for the HCO to commit to QI.
- Commit to participating in the CQI process in your work.
- Recognize higher-risk situations.
- HCOs and individual nurses need to commit to expanding their knowledge and understanding of risk for errors through staff education and continuing education.
- Patients and families need to be engaged in the process.

Stop and Consider #3
Nurses are involved in all of the high-risk situations for errors and reduced quality care.

Examples of Two Major National Initiatives Focused on Potential Risks of Inadequate Quality Care

With the recognition that there are high-risk situations that may have an impact on quality care, more initiatives have been developed and implemented to focus on these concerns to decrease their risk. The initiatives apply the CQI process and planning. Nongovernmental organizations and some governmental organizations at the state and federal levels have developed these initiatives. There are two major national initiatives directed by the HHS that have become very important to HCOs and nursing. These relate to hospital-acquired conditions and 30-day unplanned readmission. Although both of these programs focus on Medicare patients and some Medicaid patients through the CMS, they have an impact on most, if not all, acute care hospitals. Few hospitals do not have Medicare-covered patients, and many have Medicaid-covered patients. In addition, the requirements from these programs have influenced other third-party payer requirements and have a major impact on nursing practice and management.

Hospital-Acquired Conditions

Use of "never events" began in 2001 as part of the efforts to drive greater interest in CQI. The CMS defines **hospital-acquired conditions (HACs)** as "reasonably preventable conditions that were not present at the time of admission to the hospital" (Austin & Pronovost, 2015; HHS, CMS, 2008b). The National Quality Forum identified a list of these events; later The Joint Commission developed its sentinel event list; and then the CMS identified its list of events that would not be covered by CMS payment. Some third-party payers also have similar lists. Data on these events are used for more than determination of payment; for example, some states require that these events be reported, although individual HCOs may have different methods for collecting and reporting the data (Austin & Pronovost, 2015). These conditions are classified by the CMS as follows (HHS, CMS, 2008a):

1. High cost, high volume, or both
2. Identified through the International Classification of Diseases as complicating or major complicating conditions that when present and included in secondary diagnoses may result in a higher-paying diagnosis-related group (DRG), the diagnosis classification system developed by the CMS
3. Conditions that are reasonably preventable through use of evidence-based guidelines

Care for these events are not covered by CMS nor can Medicare and Medicaid patients be personally charged for the additional care needs. This can lead to a significant financial problem for the HCO, and consequently, HCOs are making efforts to reduce HACs. Quality management, including patient safety, teamwork, staffing effectiveness, and patient, staff, and physician satisfaction, has an impact on preventing HACs (Bartlett & Kelly, 2009). Since the HAC program focuses on effectiveness, it is considered to be a type of pay-for-performance program.

Types of HACs

The types of HACs may change over time based on data collected and analysis of the data to determine if there is improvement, although there were no changes in the list for 2014 and 2015. The goal is to identify the most significant potential problems or high-risk events. The HACs for 2015 are listed here, and the most current list can be found on the CMS website (HHS, CMS, 2015b):

- Foreign object retained after surgery
- Air embolism
- Blood incompatibility
- Stage III and IV pressure ulcers
- Falls and trauma: fractures, dislocations, intracranial injuries, crushing injuries, burns, other injuries
- Manifestations of poor glycemic control: diabetic ketoacidosis, nonketotic hyperosmolar coma, hypoglycemic coma, secondary diabetes with ketoacidosis, secondary diabetes with hyperosmolarity
- Catheter-associated urinary tract infection
- Vascular catheter-associated infection
- Surgical site infection, mediastinitis, following coronary artery bypass graft
- Surgical site infection following bariatric surgery for obesity: laparoscopic gastric bypass, gastroenterostomy, laparoscopic gastric restrictive surgery
- Surgical site infection following certain orthopedic procedures: spine, neck, shoulder, elbow
- Surgical site infection following cardiac implantable electronic device
- Deep vein thrombosis or pulmonary embolism following certain orthopedic procedures: total knee replacement, hip replacement
- Iatrogenic pneumothorax with venous catheterization

To provide a basis for understanding the relevance of HACs to CQI, the following content discusses two HAC examples—falls and hospital-acquired infections—in greater detail. **Figure 8-3** provides some data from the AHRQ describing overall HACs.

Example: Strategies to Reduce Falls and Trauma

Falls can result in a number of adverse consequences for patients in a variety of HCOs, including reduced quality of life, increased fear of falling and restricted

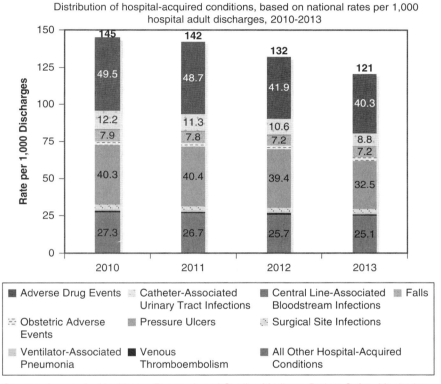

Figure 8-3. Overall Hospital-Acquired Conditions

Reproduced from Agency for Healthcare Research and Quality (AHRQ). (April 2015). 2014 national healthcare quality and disparities report: Chartbook on patient safety. AHRQ Publication No. 15-0007-2. Retrieved from http://www.ahrq.gov/sites/default/files/wysiwyg/research/findings/nhqdr/2014chartbooks/patientsafety/2014nhqdr-ptsafety.pdf

Source: Agency for Healthcare Research and Quality, Medicare Patient Safety Monitoring System, 2010-2013; Centers for Disease Control and Prevention, National Healthcare Safety Network, 2010-2013; and Agency for Healthcare Research and Quality, Healthcare Cost and Utilization Project, Nationwide Inpatient Sample, 2010-2011, and 2012 State Inpatient Databases quality analysis file.

Notes: Data are for patients age 18 years and over. Estimates are rounded to the nearest tenth. All Other HACs includes the following: inadvertent femoral artery puncture for catheter angiographic procedures, adverse event associated with hip joint replacement, adverse event associated with knee joint replacement, contrast nephropathy associated with catheter angiography, hospital-acquired methicillin-resistant *Staphylococcus aureus* (MRSA), hospital-acquired vancomycin-resistant *Enterococcus*(VRE), hospital-acquired antibiotic-associated *C. difficile*, mechanical complications associated with central venous catheters, postoperative cardiac events for cardiac and noncardiacsurgeries, postoperative pneumonia, iatrogenic pneumothorax, postoperative hemorrhage or hematoma, postoperative respiratory failure, and accidental puncture or laceration.

activities, decreased ability to function, serious injuries, and increased risk of death (HHS, AHRQ, 2012). The factors that increase risk of falls are effects of aging on gait, balance, and strength; acute medical conditions and also chronic diseases that weaken the patient or impact function; deconditioning from inactivity; behavioral symptoms and unsafe behaviors; medication side effects; environmental hazards such as poor lighting, improper footwear, and unsafe flooring/carpeting; spills; lack of support such as handrails; clutter and unsafe furniture; and unsafe use of equipment such as walkers, crutches, and wheelchairs (HHS, AHRQ, 2012).

In the past, HCOs that had an increase in patient falls typically made changes in how care was provided; for example, staff might identify some patients at risk and increase paperwork to describe these incidents. Concern about risk of lawsuits also increased, although the HCOs were more concerned about receiving payment for additional care that patients might need due to falls in the HCO. With the establishment of the HAC initiative, HCOs are changing their approaches and monitoring risk and events so that the HCO does not experience loss of CMS payment for care when falls occur. This acts as a very strong incentive to reduce falls.

When a patient is in an HCO, there are many interventions that can be used to prevent falls, including the following (Quigley & White, 2014; Rodak, 2013; Volz & Swaim, 2013):

- Screen for high-risk patients, ensuring that the method used to identify risk is clear but does not embarrass the patient.
- Identify patients with recent fall or fall injury present at time of admission.
- Reassess fall risk as needed or by policy.
- Clarify and communicate patient interventions per patient with the team, noting changes as they occur.
- Assess patients on pain and sleep medications or any medications that may cause drowsiness and/or dizziness.
- Provide safety companions to attend to and assist high-risk patients.
- Consider impact of staff level and mix.
- Educate family and significant others about risks and interventions.
- Use bed and chair alarms, set for time interval so that when the patient gets out of bed, staff can get to the patient in time to prevent a fall.
- Implement safety rounds and hourly rounds to help patients with ambulation and toileting, and clear clutter in the room.
- Provide and encourage use of handrails.
- Keep beds low when there is no need for them to be higher.
- Use restraints per policy and procedure.
- Install bathroom safety features and explain use to patients.
- Keep call lights and personal items within reach of the patient.
- Assist patients with ambulation and when patients are out of bed with intravenous equipment and other equipment that might limit mobility.

- Suggest patient use of nonskid socks or appropriate shoes.
- Provide staff training about falls and prevention.
- Implement a safety culture that supports reporting of near-miss falls and falls.
- Track fall data and use analysis to identify improvement or need for improvement; engage staff in this process.

The Joint Commission considers falls with injuries, most of which occur in acute care hospitals but also occur in other HCOs such as long-term care facilities, as one of the top 10 sentinel events reported (The Joint Commission, 2015). Along with the preceding strategies, The Joint Commission recommends that HCOs use the following overall strategies to reduce falls (The Joint Commission, 2015, p. 2):

- Increase awareness.
- Establish an effective interprofessional falls injury prevention team.
- Implement use of a standardized, validated tool to identify risk.
- Develop individualized care plans based on risk and need.
- Apply standardized interventions such as handoff communication and patient education.
- Conduct post-fall management—post-fall huddle, transparent reporting, analysis and trending of falls to make decisions about care improvement.

A critical strategy to reduce falls is identifying patients at risk for falls. Identifying these patients allows HCOs to plan care for them that incorporates fall prevention. The AHRQ developed a fall self-assessment tool that covers the organization, healthcare providers, and patient concerns (HHS, AHRQ, 2014a). In addition to HAC monitoring by HCOs and the CMS, the National Database of Nursing Quality Indicators, the National Quality Forum, the AHRQ Patient Safety Indicators, and The Joint Commission all measure falls and include measures/indicators associated with the following (Quigley & White, 2014): fall rates, fall injury rates, fall assessment completed, repeat fall rates, injury rates with level of injury, and percentage of patients who fell. Some measures/indicators specify type of injury or trauma, such as hip fracture, dislocations, and intracranial injury, as noted in the list of HACs. The following are two examples of tools used to identify fall risk:

- *Tool 3H: Morse Fall Scale for Identifying Fall Risk Factors.* This tool is used by staff nurses along with regular clinical assessment and review of medications. The tool assists in identifying fall risk factors in hospitalized patients. The tool's total score can predict falls, but the best use of the scale is to integrate identification of risk factors into care planning. The AHRQ provides details about the scale and directions for its use. It is a simple scale that includes six categories of data: history of falling; secondary diagnosis; ambulatory aid such as nurse assist, crutches, cane, walker, furniture; bed rest; gait; and mental status. Patients are ranked from no risk to low, moderate, or high risk (HHS, AHRQ, 2013b).

- *Hendrich II Fall Risk Model.* This model is different from the previous one. Based on the research done using this model, the history of falls is not as critical an assessment factor. This tool is not based on a government model (Upright®, 2013).

The Connect to Current Information section at the end of the chapter provides links to more detailed information about the tools.

Example: Strategies to Reduce Hospital-Acquired Infections

Hospital-acquired infections (HAIs) are of concern in health care, and several infections (UTIs, vascular catheter-associated, and various surgical site infections) are identified in the list of HACs provided in this chapter.

One of the most common HAIs is central line–associated bloodstream infections (CLABSIs). These infections can result in great harm to patients and are costly to treat. Nurses are in the primary position to reduce CLABSIs (Sandoval, 2015). The Centers for Disease Control and Prevention (CDC) notes that there were an estimated 30,100 CLABSI events in hospitals (HHS, CDC, 2015). The CDC provides extensive resources to address this problem. For a CLABSI to be considered an HAI, it must occur after admission; however, whether the patient is admitted with an infection or gets an infection after admission, the risk for patient harm is still high. For the infection to be classified as an HAI, it must also be confirmed by laboratory test and not be due to any infection in other parts of the body.

Surgical site infections (SSIs) are also a serious problem that puts patients at risk postsurgery, increasing costs, length of stay, and also readmission rates (Greene, 2015). The most common type of hospital infection is SSIs associated with pneumonia, representing 21.8% of total infections. Nurses are involved in the care of surgical patients during all phases of the surgical process and can help reduce the risk of SSIs occurring.

Ventilator-assisted pneumonia (VAP) is a pneumonia that develops within 48 hours of endotracheal intubation. The incidence of VAP is decreasing; however, it continues to exhibit a high incidence, 4.4 cases per 1,000 patients (Shay, 2015). Prevention strategies should consider three causative mechanisms: bacterial colonization of the respiratory and upper gastrointestinal tracts, aspiration of contaminated secretions, and contaminated respiratory equipment.

Nurses should assume a major role in preventing catheter-associated urinary tract infection (CAUTI) and providing care for harm caused from CAUTIs. Three major strategies to accomplish these goals are to (1) use fewer catheters, (2) adhere to timely removal of catheters, and (3) follow effective procedures for insertion, maintenance, and postremoval care. A flowchart of care decisions is provided in a recent issue of *American Nurse Today* (Trevellini, 2015). Publications like this one demonstrate the critical nature of HAIs and nursing responsibilities (ANA, 2015a). Studies also indicate that education regarding infections is important in reducing HAIs. An AHRQ-funded study found that in a sample of 5 hospitals and 394 nurses, there were problems in nurses' knowledge and application of correct procedures that impact CAUTIs (Jones, Sibai, Battjes, & Fakih, 2015). The results noted that recommended procedures were not followed; for example, over half of the respondents did not think that their peers complied with the procedures. The study also found that nurses were not commonly evaluated on their skills in placing and maintaining urinary catheters. This study demonstrates that there are major problems with nursing care that need to be addressed.

Due to the growing concern about HAIs, the American Nurses Association (ANA) published a special report on HAIs that includes information to help prevent HAIs, focusing on zero tolerance of HAIs and on the use of a CAUTI prevention tool (ANA, 2015b). The report also discusses the need to use other methods to prevent CLABSIs and SSIs. There is also now greater emphasis on applying evidence-based strategies to prevent VAP, which is not included in the 2015 HAC list, but it is an important infection problem (ANA, 2015a). There are more than 700,000 HAIs in hospitals annually, and at least 75,000 people die in hospitals from this cause, with direct costs estimated at $10 billion (Hessels, 2015). This is a major healthcare problem that has an impact on clinical outcomes and financial outcomes. Though infection control has long been emphasized in HCOs, with nurses assuming an active role, HCOs continue to have major problems with HAIs. Understanding the reasons for this outcome is critical to improving and thus reducing HAIs.

Nursing and HACs

HACs are related to nursing care, and some of the burden for preventing and responding to HACs is a nursing responsibility (Kurtzman & Buerhaus, 2008). HACs require that more effort be spent on system improvements, and nursing services are often tasked with "fixing this." When HACs occur, nursing management and other staff examine the types of HACs, review data about incidence related to the measures/indicators, analyze possible causes, identify interventions, implement the interventions, monitor results, and make adjustments as needed. This is an ongoing process and is part of CQI. Should nursing alone be responsible for improving problems with HACs? If one accepts that there are more system issues related to CQI than were recognized in the past and there is greater need to consider interprofessional teams and practice, then nursing should not be solely responsible for HACs. If an HCO is committed to a culture of safety rather than blame, then this requires a more comprehensive response. Policies, procedures, processes, communication, documentation, staff competencies, and so on are part of this culture. Achieving this comprehensive approach requires strong nursing leadership that will stand up and agree that many, if not all, the HACs relate directly to nursing care, but this is not enough for improvement. Engaging all critical healthcare professionals makes a difference in an effective response. Tools discussed in this text provide methods for staff to examine and respond to problems with HACs. The pressure of no payment is strong, but it should not drive the HCO to take limited steps in responding, such as just focusing on nurses and nursing care.

Impact of the Centers for Medicare and Medicaid Services HAC Initiative

Hospital patient safety substantially improved from 2010 to 2013, with a 17% decline in HACs (HHS, AHRQ, 2016). This represents 1.3 million fewer incidents of patient harm, approximately 50,000 fewer patient deaths in hospitals, and $12 billion less spent on health care. From 2010 to 2014, the data indicated even more improvement, with approximately 2.1 million harmful events avoided, 87,000 fewer deaths, and $20 billion less spent on health care, but disparities in health care for blacks and Asians continued. The HACs included in the data are ADEs, CAUTIs, CLABSIs, pressure ulcers, SSIs, and several other types of adverse events. Several initiatives targeted these problems and had a strong influence on this improvement. However, as promising as these statistics are, other recent studies indicate that if errors were identified as a disease, they would represent the third leading cause of death in the United States (Makary, 2016).

In 2016, the CMS further reduced its payments by 1% to 758 hospitals due to their HAC levels. These hospitals had unacceptable levels of potentially avoidable infections and other complications (blood clots, pressure ulcers, and falls) (Rau, 2015c). This response impacts HCO finances, and maybe this will then motivate these HCOs to focus on improving care and reducing these patient problems. The CMS also notes that for 3 years hospital injury rates decreased, but at the end of 2015, they plateaued (Rau, 2015a). It is thought that HCOs most likely resolved the problems or areas of risk that were easier to identify and resolve; however, the more difficult and higher-risk aspects of care remain. The improvements are also important; for example, from 2010 to 2014, an estimated 87,000 fewer patients died from HACs. Hospitals are safer than they were in 2010 due to efforts made to improve care, but more improvement is still needed (Brady, 2015).

HAC data and analysis of the data are now an important part of CQI and are used in a variety of ways. For example, a study examined the relationship of receiving HAC penalties to factors such as HCO accreditation status and teaching hospitals, which typically have more complex patients. Safety-net hospitals also have similar types of patients. Compared to non-safety-net and non-teaching hospitals, these hospitals received more HAC penalties. One of the results of this study identifies concerns that some experts predicted would be problems with pay-for-performance approaches. HCOs that are not teaching hospitals or safety-net hospitals tend to attract and seek patients that are healthier with less complex health needs and socioeconomic problems. This then leads to controlling greater health disparities and selective treatment and is known as "cherry-picking" of healthier patients (Rajaram et al., 2015).

Thirty-Day Unplanned Readmission

Discharge from hospital care usually does not mean the patient is fully recovered, and this recovery may take a short time or a long time, or may never be complete. As such, there is risk for problems following discharge that may lead to readmission. The AHRQ notes that some of the concerns or problems that occur are ADEs, the most common problem; infections; complications from procedures; and pending test results or testing scheduled postdischarge that may then require a change in treatment (HHS, AHRQ, 2014b). After examination of the problem of readmissions, the CMS decided to initiate a change to reduce 30-day unplanned readmissions. According to the CMS, **30-day unplanned readmission** "measures are estimates of unplanned readmission for any cause to an acute care hospital within 30 days of discharge" (HHS, CMS, 2016). Because readmissions over longer periods may be influenced by factors outside the hospital's control (e.g., other illnesses, the patient's behavior or lack of follow-up on treatment, or care provided to the patient after discharge), the CMS decided it was best to measure unplanned readmission within 30 days instead of over longer periods.

The AHRQ identifies some of the common HCO barriers that may limit success in reducing readmissions (HHS, AHRQ, 2014b, p. 32):

- "We're still studying the root causes of readmissions."
- "The senior leadership doesn't care about Medicaid readmissions because we don't get penalized by Medicaid."
- "We don't have the money to hire any FTEs [staff]."
- "We're waiting for the new electronic medical record system to be implemented."
- "We have really limited access to primary care."
- "There's no peer-reviewed literature to support this readmission reduction strategy."
- "Our community has very limited resources."

The problem of readmissions does not apply only to Medicare patients; for example, adult Medicaid patients have a higher rate of 30-day discharge readmissions than do Medicare patients, and other patient populations also have risk of readmission (HHS, AHRQ, 2014b).

Examples of Strategies Used to Reduce Unplanned Readmission

Discharge is a major example of transition of care and handoffs. It is at this time that the patient has the highest risk of disconnection from healthcare providers. For example, there may be system problems such as ineffective communication between provider and patient, between a new provider and past provider, between the hospital pharmacist and the patient's community-based pharmacist, and so on.

Obtaining medications needed after discharge may be a problem; for example, the patient may be unable to get a prescription filled due to economic reasons, lack of transportation, or lack of support to get the medication from the pharmacy. Admission, discharge, and readmission data should be shared with unit staff, and these data should provide a foundation for an open discussion of problems and sharing of ideas to solve the problems.

Due to these potential events, the AHRQ recommends the following general strategies to prevent 30-day unplanned readmission (HHS, PSNet, August 2014; IHI, March/April 2011):

- Use structured discharge communication that includes information about medications, pending tests, and follow-up, shared with the patient and with providers the patient will see postdischarge.
- Use medication reconciliation, checking all medications to ensure there are no conflicts and safety concerns with prescriptions given to the patient.
- Educate the patient (and when patient agrees, the family) so that there is understanding of diagnosis, follow-up, and whom to contact with questions or problems after discharge. Specific contact information in written form should be provided with directions for follow-up care.
- Focus on the patient, not the patient's diagnosis, to better understand needs such as patient education, transportation needs, nutrition, needs in the home (e.g., equipment, bed, ambulatory assistive devices), and emotional support.
- Set outcomes for evaluation of discharges and readmission.
- Evaluate and improve the discharge process.
- Use interprofessional teams.
- Consider how to improve and develop new transitional interventions.
- Determine how to engage and listen to patients and families.
- Use readmission prevention programs to try to reduce this risk.
- Assess patients, focusing on the whole patient, not just the diagnosis; for example, consider psychological needs, home status, transportation to get prescriptions and to medical appointments, support after discharge, ability to function, and so on.
- Ask patients, and when the patient agrees, the family, what they need postdischarge.
- Ensure that the patient participates in discharge planning and agrees to the plan.
- Track data over time to understand types of patients who get readmitted and reasons, and then use this information to make changes.
- Establish a consistent policy and procedure for preparing patients for discharge.
- Provide greater support for high-risk patients.
- Ensure that the patient has medications (prescriptions), supplies, and equipment that may be needed immediately after discharge to allow time for the patient to get what is needed long term.
- Use follow-up telephone calls to check how the patient is doing.

The AHRQ published a guide to assist hospitals in reducing readmissions in adult, non-obstetric Medicaid beneficiaries and describes strategies to reduce Medicaid readmissions, as shown in **Figure 8-4**.

HCOs should develop specific readmission reduction programs. Staff should then apply these programs to meet individual patient needs. An effective readmission reduction program includes the following practices (HHS, AHRQ, 2014b, p. 5):

- *Analyze the root causes of readmissions.* Understand patterns and trends for the HCO and the local community for comparison; understand the patient's perspective (e.g., effectiveness of communication and coordination). Data should be tracked routinely.
- *Inventory and align the current readmission reduction efforts to meet the needs of the HCO's targeted patients.* This should be an in-depth inventory; the AHRQ guide provides several tools (e.g., Hospital Inventory, Cross-Continuum Team Inventory, and Conditions of Participation Checklist) so that the HCO can understand what they currently do to prevent and/or respond to the problem to better plan changes.
- *Examine the extent to which the current readmission reduction efforts meet the needs of the HCO's targeted patients.* Combine previous information.
- *Improve hospital-based processes to better target and serve targeted patients' needs.* Using the preceding information, set aims and objectives, and then identify strategies that will be part of the program. Examples of strategies are using checklists, arranging for postdischarge follow-up, flagging in the chart patients who have experienced readmission more than 30 days postdischarge, developing transitional plans, engaging the patient and, if the patient consents, the family, and identifying high-risk patients based on HCO criteria.

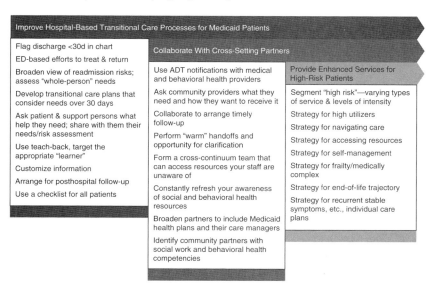

Figure 8-4. Portfolio of Strategies to Reduce Medicaid Readmissions
Reproduced from Agency for Healthcare Research and Quality (AHRQ). (August 2014). Hospital guide to reducing Medicaid readmissions. AHRQ Publication No. 14-0050-EF. Retrieved from http://www.ahrq.gov/professionals/systems/hospital/Medicaidreadmitguide/index.html

Key: ED = emergency department; ADT = admission, discharge, transfer.

- *Expand and strengthen cross-setting partnerships.* Implement strategies to increase collaboration with cross-setting partners.
- *Provide enhanced services to patients at high risk of readmission.* Implement strategies for high-risk patients.

One example of a specific program addressing readmission is Better Outcomes for Older Adults Through Safe Transitions (BOOST), which is supported by the Society of Hospital Medicine in collaboration with the AHRQ (SHM, 2015). This program's toolkit has been implemented by at least 180 hospitals. Some of the results indicate that prior to implementation of BOOST, six of the hospitals experienced a 14.7% 30-day readmission rate compared to a rate of 12.7% after implementation, with a 13.6% reduction in all-cause readmission rates (HHS, NQMC, 2012). More data that provide a long-term perspective are needed to understand the long-term perspective of outcomes.

An example of an initiative that recognizes the need to improve health literacy to reduce readmission is a new tool provided by the AHRQ. This tool is the Re-Engineered Discharge (RED) Toolkit (HHS, AHRQ, 2013a).

The Affordable Care Act includes a provision to establish the Community-Based Care Transitions Program (CCTP), which is focused on improving care transitions and handoffs, particularly to reduce readmission for high-risk Medicare beneficiaries (HHS, CMS, 2015a). CCTP is part of the Partnership for Patients, which is a national public–private partnership that works to reduce errors in hospitals by 40% and to reduce hospital readmissions by 20%. As of September 2015, there were 72 participating CCTP sites. Approximately 2.6 million senior adults experience readmission within 30 days of discharge, costing $26 billion annually. Discharge planning is not new; however, it is clear that this planning has not been adequate in reducing readmissions. CCTP is a 5-year program that began in February 2012 to determine if this type of program can decrease the rate. As part of CCTP, the government funds Community-Based Organizations (CBOs) to provide care transition services to assist Medicare patients and improve care. Acute care hospitals can partner with CBOs to provide transition services. The CMS requires that CBOs meet at least one of the following criteria (HHS, CMS, 2015a):

- Care transition services that begin no later than 24 hours prior to discharge
- Timely and culturally and linguistically competent postdischarge education to patients so patients understand potential additional health problems or a deteriorating condition
- Timely interactions between patients and postacute and outpatient providers
- Patient-centered self-management support and information specific to the beneficiary's condition
- A comprehensive medication review and management, including, if appropriate, counseling and self-management support

To apply for CBO funding, CBO proposals must describe the applicant's community-specific root causes of readmissions, target population, strategies to identify high-risk patients, interventions and services, communication with providers, culturally appropriate strategies, set outcomes, budget, and prior experience with transition care.

Readmission: Impact on Nursing

Process mapping is used to understand all steps that lead to discharge (Endo, 2015). The following questions might be included when applying this method to readmissions (SHM, 2015):

- What standardized processes already exist for care transitions?
- How often are steps in these processes actually followed?
- What other elements of the discharge process can/should we standardize?
- What elements of the discharge process need to be more customized to a specific patient population?
- What checks exist to ensure critical processes occur?
- Who owns each process?

By using this information, the HCO and its nurses can better develop strategies/interventions for the patient and family/caregiver to help them prepare for discharge, identify medication safety needs at the time of discharge, and plan follow-up care after discharge. Having greater understanding of discharge needs and how these needs might impact readmission risk provides information that should then be applied to staff education to ensure that staff are prepared to assess patients carefully, implement the interventions, and improve care transitions.

Inpatient nurses need to be aware of community resources for patients and maintain relationships with home health agencies and other service providers. Many HCOs have specific staff assigned to discharge planning; however, this does not mean that nurses working directly with patients are exempt from active participation in preparing patients for discharge. Leaving discharge preparations solely to designated staff relates back to our earlier discussion of "working in silos." If key staff do not lend input when patients are being prepared to leave the hospital, important information, needs, and problems may be missed. An effective discharge planning process includes all relevant members of the care team, the patient, and the family, when appropriate. Discharge is a critical handoff, and it is a time of risk for near misses, errors, and ineffective care.

Readmission data can be used to assist HCOs and nurses to be more alert and plan strategies to reduce these unplanned readmissions. Important data to consider are the common types of diagnoses that result in readmission within 30 days postdischarge. Individual HCOs should track the data, but there is also national data from the Healthcare Cost and Utilization Project (HCUP). Data published in 2015 identify the five most common diagnoses experiencing readmission, in the following order: (1) septicemia, (2) congestive heart failure, nonhypertensive, (3) pneumonia, (4) mood disorders, and (5) chronic obstructive pulmonary disease and bronchiectasis (HHS, HCUP, 2015). Data change over time and thus common diagnoses may change, but it is important to be alert and use the most current information to improve care. The HCUP website provides a new Nationwide Readmission Database (NRD), which offers a valuable source of data and trends, representing all types of insurers (Medicare, Medicaid, commercial payers) and the uninsured.

Impact of the Centers for Medicare and Medicaid Services Readmission Initiative

There are now financial penalties for hospitals with above-average readmission rates within 30 days of discharge for target diagnoses. According to the AHRQ, as of 2014,

> more than 2200 hospitals had up to two percent of their annual Medicare reimbursements withheld due to excess readmissions. Hospitals also receive "bundled" payments for target illnesses that cover all costs associated with patient care for a 30-day period providing a financial incentive to ensure continuity of care. (HHS, AHRQ, 2014b)

Expected costs are used to determine the retrospective payment amount per patient. In this model, if a patient was admitted for treatment of a myocardial infarction, then the HCO would be paid a specific bundled amount for that diagnosis that would include all expected services, such as laboratory tests, medications, hospital room and food, nursing services, and so on. If the patient receives more care than was considered in the bundled payment established by the payer with the HCO, such as more medication or more laboratory tests, then there would be no additional payment for these services. Readmissions have decreased since the CMS initiative began, but the majority of hospitals are still penalized, as there is much more that needs to be done to reduce these unplanned readmissions (Rau, 2015b).

Some factors that may have an impact on outcomes, although more research is needed, are factors such as weekend discharge and discharges during July when there are changes in some medical staff. Same-hospital readmission or patient discharged and readmitted to the same hospital is the most common readmission scenario, but this varies from state to state and per condition. According to data reported in 2015, readmission occurred at the original place of treatment in three-quarters of the discharges. Typical age ranges for the highest rate of readmission was 65 to 84, and women had a higher rate than men across all conditions. The diagnosis with the highest rate was heart failure, and the lowest rate was hip and knee arthroplasty (Henke et al., 2015).

Medicare state-based Quality Improvement Organizations (QIOs) are groups of QI experts, healthcare providers, and consumers who have organized to assist Medicare patients and improve care. QIOs have made a difference in reducing hospital readmissions within 30 or fewer days after discharge. The results of a 2013 study indicated that in 14 sites, QIOs assisted the 14 communities in reducing readmissions.

It is recognized that this is a complex process, involving patients who often have complex needs, and requires multiple strategies (Brock et al., 2013).

Stop and Consider #4

HCOs are now penalized financially if they do not meet certain care outcomes.

Conclusions

Health care continues to be fragmented, with great variation due to patient characteristics and problems, differences in individual healthcare providers and HCOs, and differences from state to state, with a healthcare system struggling with improving care. This chapter sets the stage for greater examination of how CQI works—what is done to better understand CQI and then how best to improve. HCOs need to plan an effective QI program, and other sections of this text offer greater detail on methods used to monitor and measure quality. This chapter focuses on high-risk events. Using this information helps HCOs and staff take steps to prevent these problems when possible and also be prepared to respond if problems occur. The federal government has assumed more responsibility in trying to direct CQI efforts that identify high-risk events on a national basis. Two initiatives are part of these efforts; they relate to HACs and 30-day unplanned readmission.

Apply CQI

Chapter Highlights

- Three major concerns in healthcare delivery are important in CQI. These are point of care, fragmentation of care, and variation of care. All impact risk of errors and occurrence of quality problems.
- Surveillance should be used throughout the care process in order to assess the patient and situations and allow for appropriate response—for example, to prevent failure to rescue. Surveillance also provides critical information for CQI and allows nurses providing direct care to initiate interventions to prevent or respond to CQI problems and errors.
- HCOs and healthcare providers experience many high-risk error situations and reduced quality of care during care, and they need to be alert to these situations. This chapter highlights some of the high-risk situations: working in silos, application of the annual Joint Commission National Patient Safety Goals, care during transitions/handoffs, failure to rescue, diagnosis and errors, medication administration, alarm/alert fatigue, workarounds, health informatics, staff competence, communication, chronic illness, and pain management.

- Two national initiatives address two major types of high-risk events that apply to most hospitals: hospital-acquired conditions and 30-day unplanned readmission.

Critical Thinking and Clinical Reasoning and Judgment: Discussion Questions and Learning Activities

1. How do you use surveillance in your practice to assist patients and support CQI? Provide specific examples.
2. Select one of the high-risk situations for errors and reduced quality care discussed in this chapter. Provide a brief summary based on content and research of other information via the Internet and literature. Provide two examples that demonstrate why your selection is a high-risk area and two strategies/interventions you might use to improve care and prevent problems with the two high-risk examples.
3. Discuss how HACs might impact your practice. Provide two specific examples.
4. Why are nurses involved in strategies to reduce 30-day unplanned readmissions?

Connect to Current Information

- Institute for Safe Medication Practices
  http://ismp.org/default.asp
- National Coordinating Council for Medication Error Reporting and Prevention
  http://www.nccmerp.org/report-medication-errors
- FDA: MedWatch Reporting Program
  http://www.fda.gov/Safety/MedWatch/default.htm
- The Joint Commission: National Patient Safety Goals
  http://www.jointcommission.org/standards_information/npsgs.aspx
- The Joint Commission: Patient Flow Resources
  http://www.jointcommission.org/accreditation/patient_flow_resources_.aspx
- AHRQ: Falls Management Program Self-Assessment Tool
  http://www.ahrq.gov/professionals/systems/long-term-care/resources
      /injuries/fallspx/fallspxmanapb1.html
- AHRQ: Tool 3H: Morse Fall Scale for Identifying Fall Risk Factors
  http://www.ahrq.gov/professionals/systems/hospital/fallpxtoolkit/fallpxtk-
      tool3h.html
- CMS: Hospital-Acquired Conditions
  https://www.cms.gov/Medicare/Medicare-Fee-for-Service-Payment/
      HospitalAcqCond/index.html?redirect=/HospitalACqCond06_Hospital-
      Acquired_Conditions.asp
- CMS: Thirty-Day Unplanned Readmission
  https://www.medicare.gov/hospitalcompare/Data/30-day-measures.html

- The Chronic Care Model
  http://www.improvingchroniccare.org/index.php?p=The_Chronic_
  CareModel&s=2

EBP, EBM, and Quality Improvement: Exemplar

Durham, M., Suhayda, R., Normand, P., Jankiewicz, A., & Fogg, L. (2016). Reducing medication administration errors in acute and critical care: Multifaceted pilot program targeting RN awareness and behaviors. *Journal of Nursing Administration,* 46(2), 75–81.

    This study describes a medication safety pilot program focused on RN sensitivity and impact on errors.

Questions to Consider:

1. What is the design used for this study, including research question(s), sample, interventions, data collection, and analysis?
2. What are the results of the study?
3. How might you apply these results in a clinical setting to improve care?

Evolving Case Study

As nurse manager for an intensive care unit, you have been sent data about HACs in your unit. You are particularly concerned with the following data about the CLABSI rate: 7 per 1,000 central line days over the last year resulting in one death and extended length of stay by 3 days. This represented a 10% increase in CLABSIs over the last year. You know you need more information, and then you have to figure out what to do to improve. You know that sources such as the CDC and the AHRQ offer important information and resources.

Case Questions A:

You begin your process by gathering information about CLABSIs and your own situation regarding CLABSIs.

1. What other data might you want from the QI program to better understand your problem and how it has changed?
2. What method(s) might you use to describe the data? Provide an example of its use.

Case Questions B:

You are now ready to address next steps using the information you have.

1. Develop a plan with strategies/interventions to address this problem.
2. How will you engage your staff in the planning and implementing the plan? Be specific.

References

American Nurses Association (ANA). (2015a). Special report: Infection prevention. Retrieved from http://www.americannursetoday.com/resources/special-report-infection-prevention/

American Nurses Association (ANA). (2015b). Catheter-associated urinary tract infection prevention. *American Nurse Today, 10*(9), 3–4.

Anathhanam, S., Powis, R., Cracknell, A., & Robson, J. (2012). Impact of prescribed medications on patient safety in older people. *Therapeutic Advances in Drug Safety, 3*(4), 165–174.

Anderson, P., & Townsend, T. (2010). Medication errors: Don't let them happen to you. *American Nurse Today, 5*(3), 23–27.

Austin, J., & Pronovost, P. (2015). "Never events" and the quest to reduce preventable harm. *Joint Commission Journal of Quality Patient Safety, 41*, 279–288.

Barach, P., & Johnson, K. (2013). Assessing risk and harm in clinical microsystems. In W. Sollecito & J. Johnson (Eds.), *McLaughlin and Kaluzny's continuous quality improvement in health care* (4th ed., pp. 249–274). Burlington, MA: Jones & Bartlett Learning.

Barlett, M., & Kelly, K. (2009). Hospital-acquired conditions: A leadership challenge for nursing quality management and performance improvement. *Nurse Leader, 7*(6), 26–28.

Brady, J. (2015, December 3). Sustained efforts continue drop in national rate of hospital-acquired conditions. Retrieved from http://www.ahrq.gov/news/blog/ahrqviews/120315.html

Brock, J., Mitchell, J., Irby, K., Stevens, B., Archibald, T., Goroski, A.,... Care Transitions Project Team. (2013). Associations between quality improvement for care transitions in communities and rehospitalizations among Medicare beneficiaries. *JAMA, 309*(4), 381–391.

Cipriano, P. (2011). When medication regulations collide with common sense. *American Nurse Today, 6*(2). Retrieved from http://www.americannursetoday.com/when-medication-regulations-collide-with-common-sense/

Clark, A., & Flanders, S. (2012). Interruptions and medication errors. Part II. *Clinical Nurse Specialist, 26*(5), 239–243.

Cole, G., Stefanus, D., Gardner, H., Levy, M., & Klein, E. (2015, August 20). The impact of interruptions on the duration of nursing interventions: A direct observation study in an academic emergency department. *BMJ Quality Safety*. Published first online at http://qualitysafety .bmj.com/content/early/2015/08/20/bmjqs-2014-003683.abstract?sid=161de7be-65a9-40a5 -b337-74433203c93f

Cooper, E. (2014). Nursing student medication errors: A snapshot view from a school of nursing's quality and safety officer. *Journal of Nursing Education, 53*(3S), S51–54.

Dickson, G., & Flynn, I. (2012). Nurses' clinical reasoning: Processes and practice in medication safety. *Quality Health Research, 22*(1), 3–16.

Disch, J., & Barnsteiner, J. (2014). Developing a reporting and tracking tool for nursing student errors and near miss. *Journal of Nursing Regulation, 5*(1), 5–7.

Ehlert, D., & Rough, S. (2013). Improving the safety of the medication use process. In B. Youngberg (Ed.), *Patient safety handbook* (2nd ed., pp. 461–493). Burlington, MA: Jones & Bartlett Learning.

Endo, J. (2015, October 1). Five steps for creating value through process mapping and observation. Retrieved from http://www.ihi.org/communities/blogs/_layouts/ihi/community/blog/itemview .aspx?list=7d1126ec-8f63-4a3b-9926-c44ea3036813&id=166

Finkelman, A., & Kenner, C. (2012). *Implementing IOM. Implications of the Institute of Medicine reports for nursing education* (3rd ed.). Silver Spring, MD: American Nurses Association.

Finkelman, A., & Kenner, C. (2016). *Professional Concepts. Competency for quality leadership*. (3rd ed.). Burlington, MA: Jones & Bartlett Learning.

Gleason, K., McDaniel, M., Feinglass, J., Baker, D., Lindquist, L., Liss, D., & Noskin, G. (2010). Results of the medications at transitions and clinical handoffs (MATCH) study: An analysis of medication reconciliation errors and risk factors at hospital admission. *Journal of General Internal Medicine, 25*(5), 441–447.

Graber, M. (2014). Minimizing diagnostic error: 10 things you could do tomorrow. Lists for physicians, healthcare organizations, and patients. *Inside medical liability* (first quarter), 22–26.

Grayson, D., Boxerman, S., Potter, P., Wolf, L., Dunagan, C., Sorock, G., & Evanoff, B. (2014, October). Do transient working conditions trigger medical errors? Patient safety executive walkarounds. *Advances in patient safety*, 53–64.

Greene, L. (2015). Preventing surgical site infections. *American Nurse Today, 10*(9), 10–11.

Hagman, J., Oman, K., Kleiner, C., Johnson, E., & Nordhagen, J. (2013). Lessons learned from the implementation of a bedside handoff model. *JONA, 43*(6), 315–317.

Healthy People. (2016). Medical product safety. Retrieved from http://www.healthypeople.gov/2020 /topics-objectives/topic/medical-product-safety/objectives

Henke, R., Karaca, Z., Hollis, L., Wier, L., Marder, W., & Wong, H. (2015). Patient factors contributing to variation in same-hospital readmission rate. *Medical Care Research Review, 72*(3), 338–358.

Henneman, E., Gawlinski, A., Blank, F., Henneman, P., Jordan, D., & McKenzie, J. (2010). Strategies used by critical care nurses to identify, interrupt, and correct medical errors. *American Journal of Critical care, 19*(6), 500–509.

Hessels, A. (2015). Moving toward zero hospital-acquired infections. *American Nurse Today, 10*(9), 2.

Institute for Healthcare Improvement (IHI). (2011, March/April). Reduced readmissions: Reform's low-hanging fruit. Retrieved from http://www.ihi.org/resources/Pages/Publications/Reduced ReadmissionsReformsLowHangingFruit.aspx

Institute for Safe Medication Practices (ISMP). (2010). CMS 30-minute rule for drug administration needs revision. Retrieved from https://www.ismp.org/newsletters/acutecare/articles/20100909.asp

Institute for Safe Medication Practices (ISMP). (2015). Frequently asked questions. Retrieved from http://ismp.org/faq.asp

Institute of Medicine (IOM). (1999). *To err is human: Building a safer health system.* Washington, DC: The National Academies Press.

Institute of Medicine (IOM). (2001). *Crossing the quality chasm.* Washington, DC: The National Academies Press.

Institute of Medicine (IOM). (2004). *Keeping patients safe.* Washington, DC: The National Academies Press.

Institute of Medicine (IOM). (2011). *Relieving pain in America: A blueprint for transforming prevention, care, education, and research.* Washington, DC: The National Academies Press.

Jones, D., DeVita, M., & Bellomo, R. (2011). Rapid response teams. *New England Journal of Medicine, 365*, 139–146.

Jones, K., Sibai, J., Battjes, R., & Fakih, M. (2015). How and when nurses collect urine cultures on catheterized patients: A survey of 5 hospitals. *American Journal of Infection Control, 44*(2), 173–176.

Kaplan, M. (2016, January 25). Diagnosis is a process: Experts offer advice on diagnostic error and delays in patient safety. Institute for Healthcare Improvement. Improvement blog. Retrieved from http://www.ihi.org/communities/blogs/_layouts/ihi/community/blog/itemview .aspx?List=7d1126ec-8f63-4a3b-9926-c44ea3036813&ID=186

Keroack, M., & Rhinehart, E. (2013). The investigation and analysis of clinical incidents. In B. Youngberg (Ed.), *Patient safety handbook* (2nd ed., pp. 125–142). Burlington, MA: Jones & Bartlett Learning.

Kripalani, S., LeFevre, F., Phillips, C., Williams, M., Basaviah, P., & Baker, D. (2007). Deficits in communication and information transfer between hospital-based and primary care physicians. *JAMA, 297*(8), 831–841.

Kronick, R. (2013, September). New report outlines goals and recommendations to reduce diagnostic errors. Blog Agency for Healthcare Research and Quality. Retrieved from http://www .ahrq.gov/news/blog/ahrqviews/092315.html

Kurtzman, E., & Buerhaus, P. (2008). New Medicare payment rules: Danger or opportunity for nursing? *AJN, 108*(6), 30–35.

Lalley, C., & Malloch, K. (2010). Workarounds: The hidden pathway to excellence. *Nurse Leader, 8*(4), 29–32.

LeBlanc, R., & Choi, J. (2015). Optimizing medication safety in the home. *Home Healthcare Nurse, 33*(6), 313–310.

Makary, M. (2016, May 3). Medical error—the third leading cause of death in the U.S. *BMJ.* Retrieved from http://www.bmj.com/content/353/bmj.i2139

Manojlovich, M., & Talsma, A. (2007). Identifying nursing processes to reduce failure to rescue. *Journal of Nursing Administration, 37*(11), 504–509.

Maxfield, D., Grenny, J., Levandero, R., & Goah, L. (2010). The silent treatment. American Association of Critical Care Nurses, AORN, VitalSmart. Retrieved from http://www.silenttreatmentstudy .com/Silent%20Treatment%20Executive%20Summary.pdf

Mayor, E., Bangerter, A., & Aribot, M. (2012). Task uncertainty and communication during nursing shift handovers. *Journal of Advanced Nursing, 68*(9), 1956–1966.

Nanji, K., Patel, A., Shaikh, S., Seger, D., & Bates, D. (2016). Evaluation of perioperative medication errors and adverse drug events. *Anesthesiology, 124*(1), 25–34.

National Academies of Sciences, Engineering, and Medicine (NAS), Health and Medicine Division (HMD). (2015). *Improving diagnosis in health care.* Washington, DC: The National Academies Press.

National Coordinating Council for Medication Error Reporting and Prevention (NCCMERP). (2001). NCCMERP index for categorizing medication errors algorithm. Retrieved from http:// www.nccmerp.org/sites/default/files/algorBW2001-06-12.pdf

National Coordinating Council for Medication Error Reporting and Prevention (NCCMERP). (2008). Statement of medication error rates. Retrieved from http://www.nccmerp.org /statement-medication-error-rates

National Coordinating Council for Medication Error Reporting and Prevention (NCCMERP). (2015). Types of medication errors. Retrieved from http://www.nccmerp.org/types-medication-errors

Onder, G., Petrovic, M., Tangiisuran, B., Meinardi, M., Markito-Notenboom, W., Somers, A., ... van der Cammen, T. (2010). Development and validation of a score to assess risk of adverse drug reactions among in-hospital patients 65 years or older: The GerontoNet ADR Risk Score. *Archives of Internal Medicine, 170*, 1142–1148.

Paine, C., Goel, V., Ely, E., Stave, C., Stemler, S., Zander, M., & Bonafide, C. (2016). Systematic review of physiological monitor alarm characteristics and pragmatic interventions to reduce alarm frequency. *Journal of Hospital Medicine, 11*(2), 136–144.

Patterson, E., Roth, E., Woods, D., Chow, R., & Gomes, J. (2004). Handoff strategies in settings with high consequences for failure: Lessons for healthcare operations. *International Journal of Quality Health care, 16*(2), 125–132.

Perry, S., Wears, R., & Patterson, E. (2008). High-hanging fruit: Improving transitions in health care. In K. Henriksen, J. Battles, E. Marks, & D. Lewin (Eds.), *Advances in Patient Safety: From Research to Implementation* (Vol. 2., pp. 159–267). Research Findings. AHRQ Publication No. 05-0021-1. Rockville, MD: AHRQ.

Quigley, P., & White, S. (2014). Hospital-based fall program measurement and improvement in high reliability organizations. *OJIN, 18*(2). Retrieved from http://nursingworld.org /ainMenuCategories/ANAMarketplace/ANAPeriodicals/OJIN/TableofContents/Vol-18-2013 /No2-May-2013/Fall-Program-Measurement.html

Rajaram, R., Chung, J., Kinnier, C., Barnard, C., Mohanty, S., Pavey, E.,... Bilimoria, K. (2015). Hospital characteristics associated with penalties in the Centers for Medicare and Medicaid hospital-acquired condition reduction program. *JAMA, 314*, 375–383.

Rau, J. (2015a, December 1). After 3 years of decline, hospital injury rates plateau, report finds. Kaiser Health News. Retrieved from http://khn.org/news/after-3-years-of-decline-hospital-injury-rates-plateau-report-finds/

Rau, J. (2015b, August 13). Half of the nation's hospitals fail again to escape Medicare's readmission penalties. Kaiser Health News. Retrieved from http://khn.org/news/half-of-nations-hospitals-fail-again-to-escape-medicares-readmission-penalties/

Rau, J. (2015c, December 10). 758 hospitals penalized for patient safety in 2016: data table. Kaiser Health News. Retrieved from http://khn.org/news/758-hospitals-penalized-for-patient-safety-in-2016-data-table/

Risenberg, L., Leitzsch, J., & Cunningham, J. (2010). Nursing handoffs: A systematic review of literature. *AJN, 110*(4), 24–34.

Robert Wood Johnson Foundation (RWJF), Interdisciplinary Nursing Quality Research Initiative (INQRI) (2012). Impact of medical surgical acute care microsystem characteristics and practices on patient outcomes. Robert Wood Johnson Foundation. Nursing Research Network. Interdisciplinary research that demonstrates the role of nurses in improving the quality of patient care, p. 6. Retrieved from http://www.inqri.org/sites/default/files/INQRI%20Booklet%20web%205-9-12.pdfl

Rodak, S. (2013). Prevent patient falls now: Five strategies. *Becker's Infection Control & Clinical Quality.* Retrieved from http://www.beckersasc.com/asc-quality-infection-control/prevent-patient-falls-now-5-strategies.html

Sandoval, C. (2015). Preventing central line-associated bloodstream infections. *American Nurse Today, 10*(9), 8–9.

Schnock, K., Dykes, P., Albert, J., Ariosto, D., Call, R., Cameron, C.,... Bates, D. (2016). The frequency of intravenous medication administration errors related to smart infusion pumps: A multihospital observational study. *BMJ Quality Safety*, February 26. doi:10.1136/bmjqs-2015-004465

Sehgal, N. (2014). Annual perspective 2014: Handoffs and transitions. AHRQ Patient Safety Network. Retrieved from http://psnet.ahrq.gov/perspective.aspx?perspectiveID=170

Shay, A. (2015). Evidence-based strategies to prevent ventilator-assisted pneumonia. *American Nurse Today, 10*(9), 12–13.

Singh, H. (2014). Editorial: Helping healthcare organizations to define diagnostic errors as missed opportunities in diagnosis. *Joint Commission Journal Quality Patient Safety, 40*(3), 99–101.

Singh, H. (2015, November 23). Measurement of diagnostic errors is a key first step to their reduction. Retrieved from https://www.qualitymeasures.ahrq.gov/expert/expert-commentary/49659/measurement-of-diagnostic-errors-is-a-key-first-step-to-their-reduction

Society of Hospital Medicine (SHM). (2015). Overview project BOOST® implementation toolkit. Retrieved from http://www.hospitalmedicine.org/Web/Quality_Innovation/Implementation_Toolkits/Project_BOOST/Web/Quality___Innovation/Implementation_Toolkit/Boost/Overview.aspx

Society to Improve Diagnosis in Medicine. (2016). Clinical reasoning toolkit. Retrieved from http://www.improvediagnosis.org/?Remedies

Stultz, J., & & Nahata, M. (2015). Preventability of voluntarily reported or trigger tool-identified medication errors in pediatric institution by information technology: A retrospective study. *Drug safety, 38*(7), 661–670.

The Joint Commission. (2013). Sentinel event alert. Medical device alarm safety in hospitals. Retrieved from http://www.jointcommission.org/sea_issue_50

The Joint Commission. (2015, September). Sentinel alert: Preventing falls and fall-related injuries in health care facilities. Retrieved from http://www.jointcommission.org/new_sentinel_event_alert_focuses_on_preventing_patient_falls/

The Joint Commission. (2016a). 2016 National patient safety goals. Retrieved from http://www.jointcommission.org/standards_information/npsgs.aspx

The Joint Commission. (2016b). Hospital national patient safety goals. Retrieved from http://www.jointcommission.org/assets/1/6/2016_NPSG_HAP_ER.pdf

Topaz, M., Seger, D., Slight, S., Goss, F., Lai, K., Wickner, P.,... Zhou, L. (2015). Rising drug allergy alert overrides in electronic health records: An observational retrospective study of a decade of experience. *Journal American Medical Informatics Association.* Retrieved from http://jamia.oxfordjournals.org/content/early/2015/11/17/jamia.ocv143

Trevellini, C. (2015). Operationalizing the ANA CAUTI tool in Acute-care settings. *American Nurse Today, 10*(9), 5–7.

Upright®. (2013). Hendrick II Fall Risk Model. Retrieved from http://uprightfallprevention.com/hendrich-ii-fall-risk-model/

U.S. Department of Health and Human Services (HHS). (2010). Multiple chronic conditions: A strategic framework. Retrieved from http://www.hhs.gov/ash/initiatives/mcc/mcc_framework.pdf

U.S. Department of Health and Human Services (HHS). (2015). HHS initiative on multiple chronic conditions. Retrieved from http://www.hhs.gov/ash/initiatives/mcc

U.S. Department of Health and Human Services (HHS), Agency for Healthcare Research and Quality (AHRQ). (2012). Chapter 1. Introduction and program overview. Retrieved from http://www.ahrq.gov/professionals/systems/long-term-care/resources/injuries/fallspx/fallspxman1.html

U.S. Department of Health and Human Services (HHS), Agency for Healthcare Research and Quality (AHRQ). (2013a, March). Tool 1: Overview. Retrieved from http://www.ahrq.gov/professionals/systems/hospital/red/toolkit/redtool1.html

U.S. Department of Health and Human Services (HHS), Agency for Healthcare Research and Quality (AHRQ). (2013b, January). Tool 3H: Morse fall scale for identifying fall risk factors. Retrieved from http://www.ahrq.gov/professionals/systems/hospital/fallpxtoolkit/fallpxtk-tool3h.html

U.S. Department of Health and Human Services (HHS), Agency for Healthcare Research and Quality (AHRQ). (2014a) Appendix B1: The Falls Management Program Self-Assessment Tool. Retrieved from http://www.ahrq.gov/professionals/systems/long-term-care/resources/injuries/fallspx/fallspxmanapb1.html

U.S. Department of Health and Human Services (HHS), Agency for Healthcare Research and Quality (AHRQ). (2014b, August). Hospital guide to reducing Medicaid readmissions. Publication No. 14-0050-EF. Retrieved from http://www.ahrq.gov/professionals/systems/hospital/medicaidreadmitguide/index.html

U.S. Department of Health and Human Services (HHS), Agency for Healthcare Research and Quality (AHRQ). (2014c). Improving patient flow and reducing emergency department crowding: A guide for hospitals. Retrieved from http://www.ahrq.gov/research/findings/final-reports/ptflow/index.html

U.S. Department of Health and Human Services (HHS), Agency for Healthcare Research and Quality (AHRQ). (2016, March). Chartbook on patient safety AHRQ Publication No. 16-0006-EF. Retrieved from http://www.ahrq.gov/sites/default/files/wysiwyg/research/findings/nhqrdr/chartbooks/patientsafety/qdr2015-ptschartbook.pdf

U.S. Department of Health and Human Services (HHS), Agency for Healthcare Research and Quality (AHRQ), Patient Safety Network (PSNet). (2014a, August). Adverse events after discharge. Retrieved from http://psnet.ahrq.gov/primer.aspx?primerID=11

U.S. Department of Health and Human Services (HHS), Agency for Healthcare Research and Quality (AHRQ), Patient Safety Network (PSNet). (2014b, November). Handoffs and signouts. Retrieved from http://psnet.ahrq.gov/primer.aspx?primerID=9

U.S. Department of Health and Human Services (HHS), Agency for Healthcare Research and Quality (AHRQ), Patient Safety Network (PSNet). (May 2015). Alert fatigue. Retrieved from https://psnet.ahrq.gov/primers/primer/28

U.S. Department of Health and Human Services (HHS), Agency for Healthcare Research and Quality (AHRQ), Patient Safety Network (PSNet). (2016). Glossary: Workaround. Retrieved from https://psnet.ahrq.gov/glossary/workaround

U.S. Department of Health and Human Services (HHS), Centers for Disease Control and Prevention (CDC). (2015, January). Bloodstream infection event (central line-associated bloodstream infection and non-central line bloodstream infection. Retrieved from http://www.cdc.gov/nhsn/PDFs/pscManual/4PSC_CLABScurrent.pdf

U.S. Department of Health and Human Services (HHS), Centers for Medicare and Medicaid Services (CMS). (2008a). Hospital-acquired conditions. Retrieved from http://www.cms.gov/HospitalACqCond06_Hospital-Acquired_Conditions.asp

U.S. Department of Health and Human Services (HHS), Centers for Medicare and Medicaid Services (CMS). (2008b, July 31). Never events. Retrieved from https://downloads.cms.gov/cmsgov/archived-downloads/SMDL/downloads/smd073108.pdf

U.S. Department of Health and Human Services (HHS), Centers for Medicare and Medicaid Services (CMS). (2011, November 18). Memo: Updated guidance on medication administration, hospital appendix A of the state operations manual. Retrieved from https://www.cms.gov/Medicare/Provider-Enrollment-and-Certification/SurveyCertificationGenInfo/downloads/SCLetter12_05.pdf

U.S. Department of Health and Human Services (HHS), Centers for Medicare and Medicaid Services (CMS). (2015a, September). Community-Based Care Transitions Program (CCTP). Retrieved from http://innovation.cms.gov/initiatives/CCTP/index.html

U.S. Department of Health and Human Services (HHS), Centers for Medicare and Medicaid Services (CMS). (2015b). Hospital-acquired conditions. Retrieved from https://www.cms.gov/Medicare/Medicare-Fee-for-Service-Payment/HospitalAcqCond/Hospital-Acquired_Conditions.html

U.S. Department of Health and Human Services (HHS), Centers for Medicare and Medicaid Services (CMS). (2016). Thirty-day unplanned readmission. Retrieved fromhttps://www.medicare.gov/hospitalcompare/Data/30-day-measures.html

U.S. Department of Health and Human Services (HHS), Food and Drug Administration (FDA). (2015). Medication errors. Retrieved from http://www.fda.gov/Drugs/DrugSafety/edicationErrors/default.htm

U.S. Department of Health and Human Services (HHS), Healthcare Cost and Utilization Project (HCUP). (2015, Winter). eNews, HCUP nationwide readmissions database, Issue #45. Retrieved from https://www.hcup-us.ahrq.gov/news/newsletters/newsltrQ4_2015.html

U.S. Department of Health and Human Services (HHS), National Quality Measures Clearinghouse (NQMC). (2012, June 25). Eliminating hospital readmissions: "No hospital left behind"? Retrieved from http://www.qualitymeasures.ahrq.gov/expert/expert-commentary.aspx?id=37562&search=boost

Volz, T., & Swaim, T. (2013). Partnering to prevent falls. *JONA, 43*(6), 336–441.

Wachter, R. (2008). *Understanding patient safety.* New York, NY: McGraw-Hill.

Walton, B. (2014). Are you prepared to prevent medication errors? *Ohio Nurse,* March, 10–15.

Welsh, C., Flanagan, M., & Ebright, P. (2010). Barriers and facilitators to nursing handoffs: Recommendations for redesign. *Nursing Outlook, 58*(3), 148–115.

CHAPTER 9

The Quality Improvement Plan

CHAPTER OBJECTIVES

At the conclusion of this chapter, the learner will be able to:

- Examine the relevance of quality improvement (QI) programs and planning.
- Discuss the purpose of continuous quality improvement (CQI) planning.
- Examine the structure and functions of a QI program.
- Critique the process of developing CQI plans: strategic, operational, and project.

OUTLINE

Introduction

Previous content laid the groundwork for understanding continuous quality improvement (CQI) in healthcare organizations (HCOs) and within states and nationally. This information is critical background information that is related to quality improvement (QI) program planning and measurement. Developing, implementing, and maintaining an effective QI program require planning—strategic, operational, and project. Other chapters discuss the change process and planning for change, and this content applies to CQI planning. Following the development of plans, the QI program must then focus on measurement based on the plans. Measurement is discussed in other chapters.

Quality Improvement Program: Structure to Support CQI

Each HCO typically has some type of structure within its organization that guides its CQI activities. The structure may have many different titles, but for this discussion QI program will be used. Integrated into the QI program is planning, a key function, to meet the CQI needs of the HCO.

The HCO needs to carefully consider who will be on the QI program team and how leadership will be provided. Engagement at all levels of the organization is important, and this then impacts representation in the CQI process. Since the QI program is complex and ongoing, who participates, how, and when may vary, but this all must be carefully considered. The HCO board of directors must have an understanding of CQI and participate in the discussion to identify overarching goals. Senior management is responsible for providing information and open discussion with the board so that it has an understanding of the importance of CQI. The board has ultimate responsibility for HCO actions and outcomes of the organization. The board also approves the budget, which impacts care delivery in many ways, including through the allocation of funds for initiatives such as the QI program. Not only does the HCO board need initial information and education about CQI, but board members also need ongoing reports of progress prepared by senior management.

Many HCOs have designated QI staff—for example, a QI program director (although the title may vary)—and other formal staff positions. Once the QI program is implemented, there is much work to be done, and relying only on committees/teams will not be effective. The organization structure needs to be described for the QI program staff. For example, staff need to know to whom they report and their responsibilities. Ideally, the staff should have CQI experience. They are often also part of the organizational structure that is responsible for accreditation and regulatory issues and also risk management and utilization review/management. All of these activities relate to the same overarching goals.

CQI activities need to be integrated throughout the HCO, and it is the QI program that guides the activities. However, all senior management, such as the chief executive officer, chief nursing executive, chief operating officer, and chief financial officer (titles vary from one HCO to the other) must be committed and participate in key decisions regarding CQI, including development of plans, receive and respond to CQI information, and share updated information on progress with staff, the board, and other relevant stakeholders external to the HCO.

CQI communication must move both ways in the organization: down from the board and management and up from the staff. CQI that is solely directed and managed by management will not be effective; teams are a critical aspect of the process. Various teams work on different parts of the planning and implementation. A core team develops the overall QI program plan (strategic plan) and the operational plan. However, this team and all teams that get involved in CQI need to reach out to others for input and expertise, which later helps to engage other staff when their help may be needed. Teams are discussed in several chapters, and the content in this chapter applies to other discussions about teams. Team membership includes representatives from management and administration services such as finance, data management and information technology, and medical records; clinical support services such as pharmacy and laboratories; and medical and nursing representation. The consumer (patient) should be represented at some point during planning, as should community representatives. Membership and responsibilities need to be clearly defined. Support staff to assist the QI program staff and CQI teams are also important; for example, they help maintain documentation of meetings and CQI activities, track data, and so on. CQI work takes time, and staff members who participate need time to complete required work, which may require adjustment in position responsibilities.

Stop and Consider #1

The QI program requires a structure to support its functions.

Purpose of the Quality Improvement Program and Planning

QI program staff develop a comprehensive quality improvement plan that relates to current standards and benchmarks, performance appraisal, interprofessional assessment and improvement, and specific HCO CQI needs. Developing such a plan requires understanding of and effective application of the change process (Fuji et al., 2011). The **quality improvement (QI) plan**, or the strategic plan, is a detailed, organizational plan describing an HCO's CQI goals and proposed activities. The purpose of the HCO's QI plan is "to provide a formal ongoing process by which the organization and stakeholders utilize objective measures to monitor and evaluate the quality of services, both clinical and operational, provided to the patients" (HHS, AHRQ, 2014). The QI plan serves as a road map for all QI program activities and includes the following (HHS, AHRQ, 2014):

- A systematic process with identified leadership, accountability, and dedicated resources
- Use of data and measurable outcomes to determine progress toward relevant, evidence-based benchmarks
- Focus on linkages, efficiencies, and provider and patient expectations in addressing outcome improvement
- Continuous process that is adaptive to change and fits within the framework of other programmatic quality and CQI activities (e.g., The Joint Commission, Centers for Medicare and Medicaid Services [CMS], accreditation)
- Assurance that goals are accomplished and are concurrent with improved outcomes based on data collected

These plans should address performance measures, performance measurement, and performance management, focusing on core areas of clinical care, operations, and finance (HHS, HRSA, 2011b).

- **Performance measures** are designed to measure systems of care and are derived from clinical or practice guidelines. Data that are sorted into specific measurable elements provide an HCO with a meter to measure the quality of its care.
- **Performance measurement** is a process by which an HCO monitors important aspects of its programs, systems, and processes. In this context, performance measurement includes the operational processes used to collect data necessary to assess performance measures.
- **Performance management** is a forward-looking process used to set goals and regularly check progress toward achieving those goals. In practice, an HCO sets goals and evaluates its success in achieving those goals by reviewing the actual data of its performance.

Nurses should be involved in all of these focus areas as direct care providers and managers/leaders.

Stop and Consider #2
The purpose of a QI program plan is similar to that of a nursing care plan.

Planning and Implementation

Each HCO should develop and implement a QI plan and then evaluate and revise it on a scheduled basis. Change is a major concern throughout the process. Effective change requires leadership and also staff engagement. A QI plan that is dictated from management will not be effective. Effective QI planning results from proactive leadership with staff (Finkelman, 2016). Planning requires input from all levels of the staff. When the CQI plan recognizes and integrates nurses into the plan, there is greater chance that their involvement will be expected in all steps of the CQI process. Planning is a key competency for nurse leaders, who need to assume more active responsibility in QI planning. It is important for the HCO to have a structured process for approval of the plan and for plan modification. This ensures that planning changes are considered carefully and that goals and commitment to CQI are maintained.

A QI program uses three types of planning: (1) strategic, (2) operational, and (3) project. The **strategic plan** is the overall plan; it considers long-term goals and outcomes, noting the gaps or what needs to be improved over time. The **operational plan** describes detailed steps needed to ensure outcomes are met, describes roles and responsibilities, identifies timelines, plans evaluation, and describes the revision process. As the CQI strategic and operational plans are implemented, the QI program will need **project plans** focused on specific needs, such as implementing use of structured communication methods in the HCO or a change in the medication administration procedure for the emergency department. There are many smaller initiatives or projects that are undertaken to reach overall CQI goals.

An initial step is to clearly identify the HCO's overarching CQI goals or aims, which must connect with the HCO's vision, mission, and goals. Today, many HCOs apply the aims identified in the *Quality Chasm* reports discussed in this text to the HCO's overarching goals or aims (IOM, 2001)—safe, timely, effective, efficient, equitable, and patient-centered (STEEEP)—and integrate the triple aim (better care, healthy people/healthy communities, affordable care). The HCO may also choose to apply one of the QI theories or models discussed in other chapters to its QI program.

Planning is never static and requires ongoing review and revision as situations change, problems are resolved, and new problems are identified. QI plans are used to implement systematic CQI activities that incorporate processes, structure, outcomes, patients, teams and teamwork, and measurement.

Assessment to Prepare for CQI Planning

In order to develop an effective QI program and plans, the HCO needs to complete a careful self-assessment. Clear goals and timelines require understanding of the current status of the organization. The QI team also needs to consider factors such as internal policies and procedures, healthcare trends, healthcare policies and legislation at the state and national levels, professional standards and other types of standards, state requirements, accreditation, national quality measurement and reporting systems, and third-party payer requirements such as those of the CMS relating to hospital-acquired conditions and 30-day unplanned readmissions. With the increasing importance of information management and technology in all phases of CQI, the QI program needs to consider the functioning of the HCO's health informatics technology. Can it provide effective support for CQI activities, including data collection, measurement, and analysis? During self-assessment, the HCO may identify weaknesses in its system that may impact the QI plans, such as ineffective data management requiring a change in software.

As HCOs prepare to develop or expand and improve their QI programs, it is important to determine **organizational readiness**. As is discussed in content relating to change, knowing when staff and the organization are better able to handle change is important to success. To determine HCO readiness for CQI, the HCO should undertake a "systematic analysis of an organization's ability to undertake a transformational process or change" (HHS, HRSA, 2011c). What does the HCO gain from this analysis? It should have a better understanding of its processes, structures, and outcomes; its culture and environment; barriers; and gaps—what needs to be improved or better analyzed. There are two levels of readiness assessment—organizational QI program readiness and QI project readiness (HHS, HRSA, 2011c). The first level considers the overall organization and its readiness for CQI planning, implementation, and evaluation. The second is much more specific, and it is ongoing as new CQI projects are undertaken. HCO self-assessment should consider the following areas (HHS, HRSA, April 2011b, pp. 2–3):

- *Organizational readiness.* Readiness is marked by high levels of executive commitment to the QI initiative from key decision makers; an understanding of the financial investment and time commitment that QI requires; consensus throughout the organization that the QI initiative is aligned with organizational goals, physicians and clinicians who support the initiative and understand its value, and clinicians who enjoy a collaborative working environment.
- *Staff characteristics.* A critical staff characteristic is the provider's adoption of the CQI initiative. The provider may be considered supportive of adoption if the provider believes that it is relatively easy to care for patients at the facility, and the improvement strategy will improve this experience; the relationship between the provider and the organization's administration and other clinicians is open and collaborative; the provider actively participates in initiatives that promote evidence-based practice (EBP) and leading clinical practices; and the provider is willing to assume a leadership role while implementing an integrated care system by taking responsibility for key objectives and helping to promote the system to other providers within the organization.
- *Resource readiness.* The organization's ability to support the CQI initiative requires assessment to determine if healthcare decision makers are knowledgeable about the type and availability of organizational resources required for initial implementation of a CQI initiative/project and for

ongoing support of CQI. Resource readiness encompasses a wide range of assets, such as, money, space, technology, training availability, supervisors, and sometimes consultation services.

There are many approaches that could be taken to planning, but this text focuses on the Agency for Healthcare Research and Quality (AHRQ) recommendations for CQI planning. Its QI resources for HCOs use an EBP approach and include input from multiple stakeholders. The AHRQ developed and offers assessment tools or surveys for HCOs to use as they assess their CQI readiness and CQI activities. There are tools for hospitals, nursing homes, ambulatory outpatient medical offices, community pharmacies, and ambulatory surgery services. Using these surveys also provides opportunities for HCOs to compare their results with those of similar HCOs. The AHRQ surveys are designed to meet the following goals for the HCO culture of safety (HHS, AHRQ, 2016):

- Raise staff awareness about patient safety.
- Diagnose and assess the current status of patient safety culture.
- Identify strengths and areas for patient safety culture improvement.
- Examine trends in patient safety culture change over time.
- Evaluate the cultural impact of patient safety initiatives and interventions.
- Conduct internal and external comparisons.

Strategic and Operational Plans

HCO self-assessment provides information needed to develop effective CQI strategic and operational plans that meet the current needs of the HCO. Typically, these plans include the following information, with the operational plans providing more details and covering a shorter period of time:

- Goals and objectives
- Establishment of a culture of safety, including consideration of how to accomplish and maintain it
- Description of QI program structure and functions, including roles and responsibilities
- Identification of budgetary requirements
- Clarification of communication and engagement at all levels in the HCO structure—for example, executive, departmental, and unit meetings, and meetings with clinical and nonclinical staff
- Reporting methods to ensure that all are informed of CQI status
- Description of required planning for projects, including consideration of what needs to be included and who determines when a project should be initiated
- Current analysis of quality status, including identification of best practices and problems (gaps) with prioritization of problems and actions to take

- Description of the process to be used to identify and develop measures/indicators with thresholds
- Description of measurement process and methods, including data required and data availability or need for new data collection methods
- Identification and prioritization of QI project plans, including consideration of the focus, teams, and timeline
- Description of staff education needs regarding CQI and a plan to meet these needs in orientation and other staff education activities
- Required evaluation of the QI program and project plans

Engaging staff in the QI program should be part of planning, implementation, and evaluation of plans. The following are examples of methods that an HCO might use to increase staff engagement (Fallon, Begun, & Riley, 2013, p. 199):

- Screen new hires for attitudes toward practice, management, and CQI.
- Take advantage of management levers to enhance motivation—recognize, reward, and reinforce high motivation.
- Invest in employee learning.
- Experiment with creative forms of recognition.
- Search for and recognize positives in employee performance.
- Demonstrate the impact of the employee's work on patients and consumers.

Impact of Analysis on CQI Planning

During data collection and analysis, an HCO examines its performance and often compares its performance to that of other HCOs. During this phase, the HCO analyzes data to determine if HCO performance meets the desired quality level based on the measures/indicators identified in the CQI plan. As the HHS, AHRQ, 2014 states, "Interpreting data is the process of assigning meaning or determining the significance, implications, and conclusions of data collected; it is used to evaluate and improve activities, identify gaps, and plan for improvement." Based on analysis, a decision is made regarding the next step: (1) Continue the process as is, with the same measures/indicators and data monitoring, (2) continue the process with modifications (i.e., implement additional interventions/strategies), (3) add new measures/indicators, or (4) stop monitoring. There may need to be changes in measure/indicator thresholds, or the decision may be to maintain current targets. Adjustments to the plan are made as needed. This process is applied to clinical and administrative/management measures/indicators and should be ongoing.

Project Plans

Project plans are a critical element, as this is where the HCO focuses on improving care for specific concerns or gaps in care quality. Plan-do-study-act (PDSA), discussed in other sections of this text, is one method that is commonly used. **Figure 9-1** reviews the key PDSA elements. This approach identifies the problem based on analysis of data. Then the project team plans and implements a strategy/intervention to improve. After implementation, results are measured and analyzed to evaluate whether outcomes were met. If so, then the strategy/intervention may be standardized in the HCO. An HCO may be implementing several CQI projects at the same time—for example, use of a new checklist to improve emergency department admissions, patient education on discharge needs for a postsurgical patient, ongoing evaluation of bar coding for medication administration, and use of hand washing in the clinic. The identification and prioritization of these projects depend on data and data analysis. Since data and outcomes change, these projects are revised, or new projects are begun. Key project plan questions include the following (Sollecito & Johnson, 2013, pp. 38–39):

1. What are we trying to accomplish?
2. What changes can we predict will be an improvement?
3. How will we know when the change (strategy/intervention) is an improvement?
4. What do we expect to learn from the test run (pilot)?
5. As the data come in, what have we learned?
6. If we get positive results, how do we hold on to the gains?
7. If we get negative results, what needs to be done next?
8. When we review the experience, what can we learn about doing a better job in the future to improve our CQI processes?

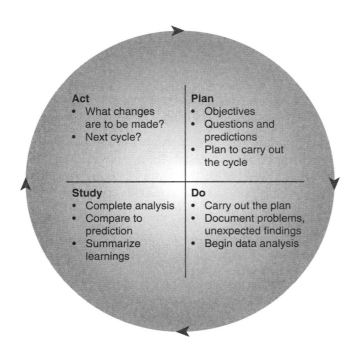

Figure 9-1. PDSA Cycle

Reproduced from U.S. Department of Health and Human Services & Health Resources and Services Administration. (April 2011). Testing for improvement. Methods for testing changes. Retrieved from http://www.hrsa .gov/quality/toolbox/methodology /testingforimprovement/index .html.

A CQI project plan typically includes the following elements (HHS, AHRQ, 2014; HHS, HRSA 2011a):

1. Problem(s) identified through a variety of sources (e.g., patient and other stakeholder complaints, providers, over- or underutilization, clinical quality or safety gaps and errors, administrative problems, changes in third-party payer requirements such as monitoring of 30-day discharge readmissions, changes in standards and regulations, accreditation concerns)
2. Identification of issues with the greatest impact on the selected population based on demographics, utilization and cost of care, and so on (use of prioritization)
3. Development or selection of measures/indicators related to the problem(s) (e.g., what will be measured), including thresholds
4. Description of data needed and data source(s) per measures/indicators
5. Detailed data collection plan, including identification of data collection methods and who will collect data, training for data collectors, data recording methods, methods to describe data, timelines
6. Identification of data collection barriers and if possible resolution before data collection
7. Description of data analysis methods
8. Ongoing evaluation of plan implementation to ensure work is done and the plan is effective in collecting and analyzing data

After an appropriate time, new data may be gathered to assess the success of the plan and may be collected at regular intervals on an ongoing basis for continuous assessment of performance.

Patient-Centered Care and CQI Planning

Patient-centered care is the core of healthcare delivery today and thus needs to be the core element in the QI program. The patient's needs and expectations are part of CQI, and services that are typically used to meet patient needs should be considered in planning. Examples include the following (HHS, HRSA, April 2011a):

- Systems that affect patient access
- Care provision that is evidence-based
- Patient safety
- Support of patient engagement
- Coordination of care with other parts of the larger healthcare system
- Cultural competence, including assessing health literacy of patients, patient-centered communication, and linguistically appropriate care

Evaluation of Planning and Plans

The QI program and its plans should be reviewed according to a schedule, which should be identified in the plans. Evaluating its own processes and plans is often a weak part of the QI program. Objective feedback should be obtained, such as data and feedback from all levels of staff. Evaluation of whether the HCO met its goals is typically done annually; however, throughout the implementation of the QI program, leaders need to be attuned to ongoing evaluation to ensure the program is functioning effectively. An ineffective CQI process should not be allowed to continue. This will lead to flawed data and analysis, which then impact decision-making, often leading to incorrect decisions. As noted elsewhere in this text, change is difficult enough, but if not done well, then it will be a barrier to future effective change. Effective QI programs should also look ahead. QI programs are often able to predict trends and problems. In doing so, they can be proactive in their responses to problems.

In summary, it is important to note that the AHRQ, under its mandate to focus on healthcare quality for the nation, provides many resources for HCOs to use in QI planning, including implementation and evaluation. It recommends steps that should be taken. The AHRQ tools may be used to help HCOs develop action plans based on the analysis of an HCO's self-assessment and assessment of its culture of safety (HHS, AHRQ, 2016). One of the AHRQ tools is a template focused on the critical elements that should be considered: goals, planned initiatives, needed resources, process and outcome measures, and timelines. The AHRQ identifies the following questions as a guide for HCOs to use as they develop their plans (HHS, AHRQ, 2014):

1. *Understand your AHRQ survey results.* It is very important for HCOs to recognize that collecting data about CQI status and analyzing data are not endpoints but rather critical first steps in planning effective CQI. The following are important questions for staff to initially consider:
   - Which areas were most and least positive?
   - How do your HCO results compare with the results from the database hospitals?

   Next, consider examining your AHRQ survey data broken down by work area/unit or staff position. (The AHRQ provides surveys for specific types of HCOs.) Questions to consider include the following:
   - Are there different areas for improvement for different HCO units (e.g., departments, services, clinical units)?
   - Are there different areas for improvement for different HCO staff?
   - Do any patterns emerge?
   - How do your HCO results for these breakouts compare with the AHRQ hospital database (or other survey setting you have selected)?

If your HCO administered the survey more than once, compare your most recent results with your previous results to examine change over time. Consider the following:

- Did your HCO have an increase in its scores on any of the survey composites or items?
- Did your HCO have a decrease in its scores?
- When you consider the types of patient safety actions that your hospital implemented between each survey administration, do you notice improvements in those areas?

Then review your results and select two or three areas for improvement. Focusing on too many at one time is not effective.

2. *Communicate and discuss survey results.* To engage staff at all levels, it is important to share results from the survey and also identify decisions made based on the results and analysis and input on planning.

3. *Develop focused action plans.* These plans should be SMART: specific, measurable, achievable, relevant, and time bound. A typical major barrier is lack of resources, including expertise and staff (e.g., number, levels, mix).

4. *Communicate action plans and deliverables.* All aspects of the plans need to be shared with staff who need to know and may be directly involved. Leaders/managers need to assume responsibility for ensuring that this communication occurs. Roles and responsibilities need to be clear to all who are involved in implementing the plan.

5. *Implement action plans.* This is the most difficult step. Many methods are used during this step, as discussed in other chapters on measurement.

6. *Track progress and evaluate impact.* Measures/indicators are used to review progress and evaluate the change. If this review indicates that outcomes are not being met, then adaptations in the plan need to be made. Assessing HCO culture can be overdone, as change takes time. If HCOs assess outcomes too soon, they may not be able to clearly identify the outcome results. If an HCO is using one of the AHRQ assessment surveys and different staff complete the survey from an earlier use of the survey, it will be difficult to compare the survey with earlier survey results.

7. *Share what works.* Once a strategy/intervention works and outcomes are met, typically the strategy/intervention is spread to other areas of the HCO, if this applies to the specific strategy/intervention or change. Throughout the process, results need to be shared with staff and other stakeholders.[1]

---

[1] Modified from Agency for Healthcare Research and Quality. (March 2014). 2014 User Comparative Database report: Chapter 8. What's next? Action planning for improvement. Retrieved from http://www.ahrq.gov/professionals/quality-patient-safety/patientsafetyculture/hospital/2014/hosp14ch8.html

---

Stop and Consider #3

An emphasis on patient-centered care should be integrated into all CQI planning.

Conclusions

This chapter provides critical information about CQI planning that a QI program might use to develop its strategic, operational, and project plans. Nurses should be involved in all of the planning and assume active roles in implementing and evaluating the CQI plans. The CQI plans provide the framework for CQI measurement, discussed in other chapters.

Apply CQI

Chapter Highlights

- QI programs need to develop strategic, operational, and project plans to provide guidance for the CQI work that needs to be done. Nurses need to be involved in all phases of planning.
- The plans need to be detailed plans to meet outcomes.
- Preparing for planning requires an understanding of the organization and its readiness to develop, implement, and evaluate plans.
- Planning and implementing the plan need to be done carefully. The AHRQ provides resources to assist HCOs.

Critical Thinking and Clinical Reasoning and Judgment: Discussion Questions and Learning Activities

1. Compare and contrast the three types of QI planning, and identify when they are used.
2. Why is organizational readiness important in planning CQI?
3. Apply the CQI planning process to a clinical problem you select.
   - Review the AHRQ: Creating Quality Improvement Teams and QI Plans
4. Make a list of information that would be useful to your understanding of QI planning. Compare with the Institute for Healthcare Improvement: Project Planning Form

Connect to Current Information

- AHRQ: QI™ Toolkit Roadmap
  http://www.ahrq.gov/professionals/systems/hospital/qitoolkit/index.html

- Health Resources and Services Administration: Developing and Implementing a QI Plan
  http://www.hrsa.gov/quality/toolbox/methodology/developingandimplementingaqiplan/
- AHRQ: Creating Quality Improvement Teams and QI Plans
  http://www.ahrq.gov/professionals/prevention-chronic-care/improve/system/pfhandbook/mod14.html
- Institute for Healthcare Improvement: Project Planning Form
  http://www.ihi.org/resources/Pages/Tools/ProjectPlanningForm.aspx

EBP, EBM, and Quality Improvement: Exemplar

U.S. Department of Health and Human Services (HHS), Agency for Healthcare Research and Quality (AHRQ). (2014, October). QI™ toolkit roadmap. Retrieved from http://www.ahrq.gov/professionals/systems/hospital/qitoolkit/qiroadmap.html

This website provides several toolkits that can be used to develop effective plans.

Questions to Consider:

Select one of the toolkits. Summarize why it may be useful to an HCO. Develop a rationale for using the toolkit. This may be done in a PowerPoint slide presentation or using a visual method (e.g., figure, poster).

Evolving Case Study

As a nurse manager for a medical unit, you have been asked to serve on a CQI project committee to develop a plan to address an increase in the number of patient falls in the five medical units in the hospital. The committee includes you, representing the nurse managers, a staff nurse and a physician from the medical units, a QI program staff member, a staff educator, and an administrator.

Case Questions:

1. Before you begin planning, what other plans should you review? Why is this important?
2. What data should you review as part of your planning?
3. What should be in the project plan? Provide an outline.
4. Describe how you will engage staff (clinical and nonclinical) in this CQI project.

References

Fallon, L., Begun, J., & Riley, W. (2013). *Managing health organizations for quality performance.* Burlington, MA: Jones & Bartlett Learning.

Finkelman, A. (2016). *Leadership and management for nurses* (3rd ed.). Upper Saddle River, NJ: Pearson Education.

Fuji, K., Hoidal, P., Galt, K., Drincic, A., & Abbott, A. (2011). Safe patient care systems. In K. Galt & K. Pascal (Eds.), *Foundations in patient safety for health professionals* (pp. 161–180). Burlington, MA: Jones & Bartlett Learning.

Institute of Medicine (IOM). (2001). *Crossing the quality chasm.* Washington, DC: The National Academies Press.

Sollecito, K., & Johnson, J. (2013). The global evolution of continuous quality improvement: From Japanese manufacturing to global health services. In W. Sollecito & J. Johnson (Eds.), *McLaughlin and Kaluzny's continuous quality improvement in health care* (4th ed., pp. 3–47). Burlington, MA: Jones & Bartlett Learning.

U.S. Department of Health and Human Services (HHS), Agency for Healthcare Research and Quality (AHRQ). (2014, October). QI™ toolkit roadmap. Retrieved from http://www.ahrq.gov/professionals/systems/hospital/qitoolkit/index.html

U.S. Department of Health and Human Services (HHS), Agency for Healthcare Research and Quality (AHRQ). (2016, February). Surveys on patient safety culture. Retrieved from http://www.ahrq.gov/professionals/quality-patient-safety/patientsafetyculture/index.html

U.S. Department of Health and Human Services (HHS), Health Resources and Services Administration (HRSA). (2011a, April). Developing and implementing a QI plan. Retrieved from http://www.hrsa.gov/quality/toolbox/methodology/developingandimplementingaqiplan/

U.S. Department of Health and Human Services (HHS), Health Resources and Services Administration (HRSA). (2011b, April). Performance management and measurement. Retrieved from http://www.hrsa.gov/quality/toolbox/508pdfs/performancemanagementandmeasurement.pdf

U.S. Department Health and Human Services (HHS), Health Resources and Services Administration (HRSA). (2011c, April). Readiness assessment and developing project aims. Retrieved from http://www.hrsa.gov/quality/toolbox/methodology/readinessassessment/

CHAPTER 10

A Toolbox to Monitor, Measure, and Analyze Care Quality

CHAPTER OBJECTIVES

At the conclusion of this chapter, the learner will be able to:

- Examine the use of measurement in continuous quality improvement (CQI).
- Critique methods used to monitor care and collect data for CQI.
- Critique methods used to analyze care quality.
- Compare and contrast examples of national healthcare measurement programs.
- Appraise roles of nurses in CQI measurement, including monitoring, collecting data, and analyzing care quality.

OUTLINE

KEY TERMS

Baseline data	Flowchart	Prevalence
Benchmarking	Gap analysis	Primary CQI data
Check sheet	Generic measure/indicator	Process measure/indicator
Common format	Global trigger	Qualitative data
Core measure set	Healthcare delivery measures	Quantitative data
Dashboard	Incidence	Report card
Data	Incident report	Risk management
Database	Indicator	Root cause analysis (RCA)
Deep dive	Measure	Run chart
Define and measure-analyze-design-verify (DMADV)	Metric	Secondary CQI data
	Morbidity	Sentinel measure
Disease-specific measure/indicator	Mortality	Structure measure/indicator
Enterprise data warehouse	Outcome measure/indicator	Tally sheet
Failure mode and effects analysis (FMEA)	Pareto chart	Utilization review/management
	Performance measure	Validity
Fishbone analysis	Population health measure	Value stream mapping

Introduction

Continuous quality improvement (CQI) has expanded with greater emphasis on measuring, monitoring, and analyzing care quality. Each healthcare organization (HCO) selects the methods it will use and identifies them in its quality improvement (QI) program planning, as discussed in other sections of this text. This chapter discusses measurement, providing nurses with a toolbox to understand the methods and their application. If nurses are to be actively engaged in CQI, they must have this information and know how to use the methods effectively. Nurses may not actually use all the methods, but they need to understand the methods and their application in order to participate in analyzing results and making changes necessary to respond to problems and improve care.

Measurement

With the increasing emphasis on CQI since the *Quality Chasm* reports were first published in 1999, there has been expansion in the development of measures; however, many of them are duplicative or similar. This expansion can get out of control and make the situation even more complicated. The report *Vital Signs: Core Measures for Health and Health Care Progress* describes a set of core measures to support measurement efficiency and effectiveness, as described in **Figure 10-1** (NAS/HMD, 2015). Collecting, analyzing, tracking, and storing data for multiple measure options is a time-consuming and costly endeavor that has an impact on understanding performance.

Description and Purpose

Why measure healthcare quality? Measures/indicators drive improvement by providing performance data to better understand actual practice, identify problems, and assist in best practice changes to improve. The Health Resources and Services Administration (HRSA) of the U.S. Department of Health and Human Services (HHS) describes the importance of measuring healthcare quality as follows:

> Measuring a health system's inputs, processes, and outcomes is a proactive, systematic approach to practice-level decisions for patient care and the delivery systems that support it. Data management also includes ongoing measurement and monitoring. It enables an organization's CQI team to identify and implement opportunities for improvements of its current care delivery systems and to monitor progress as changes are applied. Managing data also helps a CQI team to understand how outcomes are achieved, such as, improved patient satisfaction with care, staff satisfaction with working in the organization, or an organization's costs and revenues associated with patient care. (HHS, HRSA, 2011a, p. 1).

1. Life expectancy
Infant mortality
Maternal mortality
Violence and injury
    mortality

 2. well-being
Multiple chronic conditions
Depression

 3. Overweight and obesity
Activity levels
Healthy eating patterns

 4. Addictive behavior
Tobacco use
Drug dependence/illicit use
Alcohol dependence/
    misuse

 5. Unintended pregnancy
Contraceptive use

6. Healthy communities
Childhood poverty rate
Childhood asthma
Air quality index
Drinking water quality index

 7. Preventive services
Influenza immunization
Colorectal cancer screening
Breast cancer screening

 8. Care access
Usual source of care
Delay of needed care

9. Patient safety
Wrong-site surgery
Pressure ulcers
Medication reconciliation

 10. Evidence-based care
Cardiovascular risk
    reduction
Hypertension control
Diabetes control composite
Heart attack therapy
    protocol
Stroke therapy protocol
Unnecessary care
    composite

 11. Care match with patient goals
Patient experience
Shared decision-making
End-of-life/advanced care
    planning

 12. Personal spending burden
Health care–related
    bankruptcies

 13. Population spending burden
Total cost of care
Healthcare spending
    growth

14. Individual engagement
Involvement in health
    initiatives

15. Community engagement
Availability of healthy food
Walkability
Community health benefit
    agenda

Figure 10-1. Core Measure Set with Related Priority Measures
Reproduced from Institute of Medicine. (2015). *Vital signs: Core metrics for health and health care progress.* Washington, DC: The National Academies Press. Courtesy of the National Academies Press, Washington, DC.

The expansion of CQI measurement led to positive and negative results for the HHS. The negative results are concerned with the following (HHS, National Quality Strategy [NQS], 2014):

- There has been an increase in the number of measures used by HHS agencies.
- There are redundancies and overlaps in the measures that lead to increased work, conflicting results, inefficient use of resources, and missed opportunities to improve.
- There is no formal systematic mechanism to align, coordinate, and approve development, maintenance, implementation, and retirement of measures across the HHS department.

These results are important, as they indicate areas that need to be addressed if the processes for measuring care are effective in providing reliable and valid data to best describe quality status and then to use for decision-making to improve.

It is critical that an HCO's QI program and plans identify clear steps to be taken to ensure that the CQI activities have direction. This direction is provided by over-all goals, which typically are fairly universal and often focus on the six aims—safe, timely, effective, efficient, equitable, and patient-centered (STEEEP); however, more specific direction is required. Measures/indicators provide this direction to assist in reaching the overarching goals. They identify the topics that will be monitored to determine performance and expected outcomes. Data are used to identify potential quality concerns and areas that require more examination and to track changes over time (HHS, AHRQ, 2004). The function of these data is expressed by the Agency for Healthcare Research and Quality (AHRQ): "We cannot really measure 'quality care,' per se, so we use measures as an 'indicator' of quality—although they are not a direct measure of quality care" (HHS, AHRQ, 2004).

Measures and Indicators

A **measure** is a "standard used as a basis for comparison, a reference point against which other things can be evaluated" (HHS, AHRQ, 2014). **Indicators** are aggregate measures for a specific operation. **Metrics** allow HCOs to quantify some aspect of care by comparing it to a specified criterion in categories; for example, **Figure 10-2** shows a hierarchical view of quality measures, indicators, and metrics related to the major aims, STEEEP (HHS, HRSA, 2015; Sadeghi, Barzi, Mikhail, & Shabot, 2013). Using the measure or indicator helps to determine whether a lower or higher score for a measure or indicator means care is better or not (HHS, AHRQ, NQMC, 2015b).

A measure/indicator provides a quantitative method for assessing care and has several parts (HHS, AHRQ, 2014). They are expressed as "proportions or rates, ratios, or mean values for a sample population" (Mainz, 2003, p. 524). The first part

Figure 10-2. A Hierarchical View of Quality Measures, Indicators, and Metrics

Reproduced from Sadeghi, S., Barzi, A., Mikhail, O., & Shabot, M. (2013). Integrating quality and strategy in healthcare organizations. Burlington, MA: Jones & Bartlett Learning.

of the measure/indicator is the focus of the measurement, what will be measured; for example, it might measure performance of a procedure or a diagnosis outcome and may include specific identifier information such as age, sex, diagnosis code, admission date, and provider. The numerator includes the number related to what is measured; for example, it may be number of admissions of patients diagnosed with pulmonary edema who experience need for rapid response team, number of patient falls getting out of bed, or number of medication errors at time of discharge. The denominator is the population at risk; for example, it might be patients with pulmonary edema, number of patient falls regardless of cause or situation, or number of discharges. Observed rate is the numerator over denominator. A measure or indicator should identify a threshold/criterion, the preestablished level that should be achieved; for example, 100% of medical records should include information about allergies. If the result is less than the identified threshold level, then a problem is indicated.

Measures/indicators serve many purposes, one of which is to inform patients and others, such as policy makers and insurers, about quality care status. Publicly reported measures/indicators are now more accessible via the Internet. Measurement influences payment, and both public and private payers may use measures/indicators to determine payment. The overall result should be a better picture of the status of healthcare quality. Increased experience with measurement has influenced the development of government CQI initiatives such as the hospital-acquired conditions (HACs) and 30-day unplanned readmission initiatives discussed in other chapters. As defined by the HHS, HRSA (2011c), "**performance measures** are designed to measure systems of care. . . . Data that is defined into specific measurable elements provides an organization with a meter to measure the quality of its care."

Who determines what will be measured? Within HCOs, leadership and CQI staff or teams make this decision based on data and needs of the HCO, its patients, and staff. HCOs should also use healthcare literature (evidence-based practice and evidence-based management), healthcare professional organization standards, accreditation requirements, and government resources (local, state, and federal). As the National Academy of Medicine (NAS/HMD) describes, however, current health measurement practices have room for improvement:

> A case can be made that, while the health measurement landscape today consists of a great many high-quality measures, meaningful at some level for their intended purpose, the effectiveness of the health measurement enterprise as a whole is limited by a lack of organizing focus, interrelationship, and parsimony in the service of truly meaningful accountability and assessment for the health system. (NAS/HMD, 2015, p. S-5)

Selecting what should be measured is a critical measurement step in the CQI process. Data should not be collected just to demonstrate that data are collected. There are general guides for what should be measured, and then each HCO needs to customize its QI program to meet its own CQI needs. Some of the guides include HAC incidence, 30-day unplanned readmission rate, STEEEP or the six major CQI aims, Centers for Medicare and Medicaid Services (CMS) requirements and measures/indicators, and the National Quality Strategy (NQS). Quality measures/indicators relate to concerns about accessibility, appropriateness, continuity, effectiveness, efficacy, efficiency, timeliness, patient perspectives, and safety. HCOs monitor clinical outcomes such as mortality rates, complications, adverse events, patient/family satisfaction, and outcomes that relate to the organization structure and functions, such as staffing levels, staff retention, reasons for staff turnover, budget goals, and staff satisfaction (Gottlieb, 2006).

Should HCOs continue focusing on broad-stroke measurement—blunt measures such as measuring adverse events (Shojania, 2015)? After an HCO identifies its specific problems, it should focus more on them. To determine long-term effectiveness, the HCO should apply follow-up measurement to changes that have been made. For example, if the HCO changes its bar-coding procedure, then evaluating the new procedure should be the focus, not overall medication adverse events. This is a more efficient and effective approach for a QI program. As HCOs make plans for measuring CQI and identify or develop their measures/indicators, they should consider questions such as the following (Casey, 2006, p. 94):

1. What are the goals in attempting to measure outcomes? In other words, why bother?
2. What sort of outcomes management (OM) expertise is available to assist with the measurement of outcomes? OM is not for the amateur and requires specific prerequisite skills, knowledge, and experience.
3. What resources, especially computer software and hardware, are necessary and available to support the process of OM?
4. What are the costs and benefits of measuring outcomes?
5. Can other published or unpublished experiences be identified, consulted, and utilized that will assist in short-cutting the process of developing and measuring outcomes without sacrificing scientific accuracy? This effort includes identifying information that can be used in conjunction with or instead of information that might be generated by an expensive process.
6. What is the process for interpretation and identification of limitations of the OM that are generated?

The Joint Commission accreditation focuses on accountability measures, which are measures of evidence-based care closely linked to positive patient outcomes. The Joint Commission use the following criteria to identify accountability measures (The Joint Commission, 2012, p. 4):

1. *Research.* There should be strong evidence demonstrating that the evidence-based process improves health outcomes.

2. *Proximity.* Performing the process is closely connected to the patient outcomes, with few clinical processes occurring after the one that is measured before improved outcome occurs.

3. *Accuracy.* The measure accurately assesses whether the care process has actually been provided.

4. *No adverse effects.* Implementing the measure has little or no chance of inducing unintended adverse consequences.

The Agency for Healthcare and Research Quality (AHRQ) Quality Indicators Toolkit also describes criteria that HCOs should consider in selecting measures, remembering that not everything can be or should be measured (HHS, AHRQ, 2012):

- Processes, utilization, and outcomes measures
- Importance of the factor being measured—should focus on most important outcomes met for new processes implemented
- Ability to interpret and act on findings
- Feasibility of measurement—most efficient data collection is from existing automated information systems
- Identifiable and measureable denominators

This type of criteria system may be used in conjunction with the criteria used by The Joint Commission mentioned earlier. The critical point is that each QI program should approach selection of measures/indicators in a systematic manner and apply clear criteria.

Ideally, measures/indicators should be based on best evidence, and their validity and reliability are important so that results can be used to effectively improve care. Mainz (2003) describes these concepts as follows:

> **Validity** is the degree to which the measure/indicator measures what it is intended to measure. . . . **Reliability** is the extent to which repeated measurements of a stable phenomenon by different data collectors, judges, or instruments, at different times and places, get similar results. Reliability is important when using a measure/indicator to make comparisons among groups or within groups over time. A valid measure/indicator must be reproducible and consistent.

Table 10-1 describes some attributes used to evaluate measures.

There are several different types of measures/indicators. A common approach is to use the three quality elements described by Donabedian (1980): structure (how work is organized), process (how work is done), and outcomes (results of work). The following are examples of the application of these elements of quality to measures/indicators (Mainz, 2003; NQF, 2010):

- **Structure measures/indicators.** Examples are access to specialists, clinical guidelines based on evidence-based practice, staffing level met as required

TABLE 10-1 Attributes Used to Evaluate Measures	
Attribute	**Definition**
1. Importance of topic area addressed by the measure	
A. High priority for maximizing health of person population	For example, measure focuses on medical condition as defined by high prevalence, incidence, mortality, morbidity, or disability.
B. Financially important	Measure focuses on clinical conditions or area of health care that requires high expenditures on inpatient or outpatient care; a condition is financially important if it has either high per-person costs or if it affects a large number of people.
C. Demonstrated variation in care and/ or potential for improvement	Measure focuses on an aspect of health care for which there is a reasonable expectation of wide variation in care and/or the potential for improvement; if the measure is used for internal QI and professional accountability, then wide variation in care across physicians is not necessary.
2. Usefulness in improving patient outcomes	
A. Based on established clinical recommendation	Evidence indicates that process improves health outcomes; there are processes or actions that providers can take to improve the outcome.
B. Potentially actionable by the user	The measure addresses an area of health care that potentially is under the control of the physician, other healthcare provider, HCO, or healthcare system that is assesses.
C. Meaningful and interpretable to the user	The results of the measure are reportable in a manner that is interpretable and meaningful to the intended use. For example, results need to be of use to improve care, help make administrative decisions, compare health systems, and so on.
3. Measure design	
A. Well-defined specifications	The following need to be well defined: numerator, denominator, sampling methodology, data sources, allowable values, methods of measurement, and method of reporting.
B. Documented reliability	The measure will produce the same results when repeated in the same population and setting; use of test of reliability; inter-rater; and internal consistency.
C. Documented validity	The measure has face validity—i.e., it should appear to a knowledgeable observer to measure what is intended. The measure should also correlate well with other measures or the same measures.

Modified from Casey, D. (2006). Fundamentals of outcomes measurement. In D. Nash & N. Goldfarb (Eds.), *The quality solution* (pp. 93–113). Sudbury, MA: Jones & Bartlett Publishers.

per standard, access to procedure (specify) in timely manner (specify), and amount of admission wait time from emergency department to inpatient.

- **Process measures/indicators**. Examples are proportion of patients with infection that receive appropriate antibiotic, nurse assessment of newly admitted patients within half an hour of admission, rate and type of specific medication errors, and rapid response team called when patient's blood pressure changes per guidelines.
- **Outcomes measures/indicators**. Examples are blood pressure maintained per guidelines, blood sugar maintained per guidelines, mortality, morbidity, quality of life, patient satisfaction, and patient functional status. Multiple factors may impact outcomes, and these need to be considered, particularly when comparing with other HCOs. For example, smoking and weight have an impact on health outcome, so if you are comparing groups of patients where these factors vary, then comparing outcomes is not really possible unless this factor is included in the sample.

Combining these measures/indicators provides a clearer picture of the status of healthcare quality and the organization.

There are other types of measures/indicators commonly used by HCOs. The **sentinel measure/indicator** "identifies individual events or phenomena that are intrinsically undesirable, and always trigger further analysis and investigation" (Mainz, 2003). All sentinel events must be assessed. Examples would be number of patients who die during labor or number of suicides in the hospital. For this type of measure/indicator, the threshold is zero, as no sentinel event is acceptable. **Generic measures/indicators** are relevant to most patients—for example, the proportion of physicians to a population. **Disease-specific measures/indicators** focus on a disease and apply to patients with that disease—for example, the number of patients with lung cancer who have surgery or the number of patients receiving chemotherapy who require support for extreme nausea and loss of weight.

An example of a national program that includes indicators used by many hospitals is the Inpatient Quality Indicators, which includes 28 provider-level indicators established by the AHRQ and applied to hospital inpatient discharge data. These indicators provide aggregate data from multiple acute care hospitals and are grouped into the following four categories (HHS, AHRQ, 2014):

- *Volume indicators* are proxy, or indirect, measures of quality based on counts of admissions during which certain intensive, high-technology, or highly complex procedures were performed. They are based on evidence suggesting that hospitals performing more of these procedures may have better outcomes.
- *Mortality indicators for inpatient procedures* include procedures for which mortality has been shown to vary across institutions and for which there

is evidence that high mortality may be associated with poorer quality of care.

- *Mortality indicators for inpatient conditions* include conditions for which mortality has been shown to vary substantially across institutions and for which evidence suggests that high mortality may be associated with deficiencies in the quality of care.
- *Utilization indicators* examine procedures whose use varies significantly across hospitals and for which questions have been raised about overuse, underuse, or misuse.

CQI needs to focus on the goals of improved health status, care, quality, affordability, and public engagement; however, nationally there are differences in the domains of influence on health and health care, including disparities by race, ethnicity, income, education, gender, geography, and urban or rural populations (NAS/HMD, 2015). There are many individual measures/indicators that HCOs and organizations have developed and use, many of which are very specific to HCO needs and may not provide broader data about CQI. The growth in measures/indicators is positive, but it has negative aspects as it has resulted in "a measurement system that lacks standardization for the assessment and reporting of data on commonly assessed health concepts" (NAS/HMD, 2015, p. S-5).

In 2012, the HHS decided that it was time to address the concern about expanding measurement and need for greater control. To address this concern, it focused on clarifying criteria for measures, determining a strategic implementation plan that provides greater coordination, and developing measurement policy and management. This effort needed to be based on the three aims of better care, healthy people/healthy communities, and affordable care. This was related to the development of the National Quality Strategy, which is discussed in other chapters. Core measure sets have now been developed; however, these measures do not cover all areas of CQI. A **core measure set**, as defined by the NAS/HMD (2015), is a

set of measures that provide a quantitative indication of current status on the most important elements in a given field, and that can be used as a standardized and accurate tool for informing, comparing, focusing, monitoring, and reporting change, reducing reporting burden while improving impacts. (pp. S-8–S-9)

Data

Data are "discrete entities described objectively without interpretation" (Finkelman & Kenner, 2016, p. 421). The purpose of using data is to help identify potential quality concerns and describe problems, gaps, trends, patterns, and so on. **Primary CQI data** are found in original sources—information collected for the purpose of CQI. Examples are using observation to determine if staff respond to patient call lights when needed and collecting information about medication errors. **Secondary CQI data** are found in second-hand sources, and in the case of CQI, these sources are often sources that are primarily used in care delivery such as the electronic medical record/electronic health record (EMR/EHR) or a preoperative checklist. The data are collected routinely for other purposes and then may also be used for CQI data collection, although this was not the original intent of the documentation.

The medical record is a rich source of data for multiple measures/indicators. Many HCOs now use electronic records, making data collection easier and more accurate; quicker; and less costly, as data collection takes less staff time. Electronic records also make the data accessible in real time. Hard copy records are often illegible, incomplete, and less accessible over time. Administrative data are also used, and most administrative records provide some secondary data for CQI purposes. For example, tracking utilization data about admissions and discharges is important for HCO financial and planning purposes, but the data can also be used in conjunction with CQI needs. Pharmacy records also provide valuable CQI data, although most of the data are not collected for the primary purpose of CQI.

Data are classified as quantitative or qualitative: (1) **Quantitative data** focus on numbers and frequencies so that measurable data can be obtained and statistics used to analyze the data—for example, calculating the average of a specific laboratory value, frequencies of readmissions, and percentages of patients who meet standards for health screening. (2) **Qualitative data** provide information about descriptive characteristics, used to make inferences based observable data, not measurable data. **Baseline data** are collected prior to a change or an improvement. The data are then used to compare against after the change is implemented to determine if outcomes were met (HHS, HRSA, 2010, pp. 4–5). HCOs and CQI initiatives use the three types of data in their data collection efforts.

With any data collection, one needs to be concerned about the quality of the data. Is it accurate, clear, and concise? Is there missing information? Is the information accessible? Can it be accessed in a timely manner? As mentioned earlier in this chapter, validity and reliability are important in evaluating the quality of CQI data and results.

Databases

A **database** is a method used to organize data so information is easy to store, manage, and access. Given the large amount of data used in QI programs, databases are critical, storing large amounts of data, typically computerized, and providing easier access to the data for analysis and for CQI decision-making. The federal government has a number of healthcare databases used by the government, HCOs, healthcare providers, healthcare professional organizations, insurers, and accreditors. An example is the Healthcare Cost and Utilization Project (HCUP). There are also databases provided by nongovernment sources, such as the National Database of Nursing Quality

Indicators (NDNQI) (HHS, AHRQ, HCUP, 2015b; Press Ganey, 2015). An **Enterprise data warehouse** provides a collection of databases that can then be accessed and analyzed. This makes it easier to search for different data from multiple databases to gain access to more data and to use data more effectively (HHS, AHRQ, PSNet, 2015). HCOs and healthcare professionals are inundated with data today. Methods that help to organize the data are critical to effective use of data in a QI program. The Connect to Current Information section at the end of the chapter provides links to sites with examples of healthcare databases.

Along with the development of the Network of Patient Safety Databases (NPSD), the AHRQ has developed **Common Formats**, which constitute a set of definitions and reporting formats that offer HCOs consistency across one another when reporting data external to the HCO, such as to the AHRQ. The NPSD was developed with input from multiple stakeholders, including the National Quality Forum (NQF) and the Food and Drug Administration (FDA). A common concern about reporting CQI data is consistency, particularly using the same terms with the same meanings when data are collected. Using common terms avoids comparing "apples to oranges." For a long time, the United States did not have a national system that provided CQI data and guidance, but now there are major efforts to develop and maintain an effective CQI system that considers the issue of consistency and the CQI reporting process. According to the AHRQ and its CQI initiative, three situations should be reported (HHS, AHRQ, PSO, 2016b):

- *Incidents* are patient safety events that reached the patient, whether there was harm or not.
- *Near misses or close calls* are patient safety events that did not reach the patient; they may be precursors to adverse events.
- *Unsafe conditions* are circumstances that increase the probability of a patient safety event.

The Common Formats "focus on generic common formats or all patient safety events and on event-specific common formats or frequently occurring and/or serious types of patient safety events, and the list expands as needed" (HHS, AHRQ, PSO, 2016a). Currently, the settings for application of the Common Formats are acute care and skilled nursing facilities; however, the plan is to expand into other healthcare settings. Types of information collected are circumstances of the event, patient information, and reporting, reporter, and report information. **Table 10-2** describes information the AHRQ recommends that HCOs report for generic and event-specific events.

Prevalence and Incidence

Prevalence and incidence rates are used in CQI. **Prevalence** is the rate of the number of cases at a given time divided by the number in the at-risk population. This rate provides

Table 10–2 Information Required for Common Formats: Generic and Event-Specific Events
Generic Common Formats
Type of Event
1. Class of patient safety concern being reported
a. Incident
i. Harm
ii. No harm
b. Near miss (close call)
c. Unsafe condition
2. Category of patient safety concern
Circumstances of Event
1. Date and time that the event was discovered
2. Where the event occurred or unsafe condition exists
3. Factors contributing to the event, known at the time of the initial report
4. Association of the event with a handover (handoff)
5. Preventability of the event, as noted at the time of the initial report
6. Reason the near miss did not reach the patient
7. Narrative descriptions (for facility and PSO use)
a. Narrative by the initial reporter
b. Summary comments by the patient safety manager
Patient Information
1. Identifying information about the patient affected
2. Degree of harm—AHRQ's Harm Scale—including when the harm was assessed
3. Rescue—interventions made within 24 hours after discovery of an incident to reduce or halt the progression of harm to the patient
4. Increased length of stay attributed to an adverse outcome (hospital setting only)
5. Notification of the patient, patient's family, or guardian
Reporting, Reporter, and Report Information
1. Unique identifier assigned to the event/condition
2. Report date
3. Reporter information
Event-Specific Common Formats
Definition of the Event
1. Brief narration of the name of the event category, with specifications of the event.
2. Processes of care—delineation of process error(s) that caused/are the (defined) event; these can include near misses.
3. Patient outcomes—delineation of outcomes that are associated with/are the (defined) event; includes no-harm events; by definition, unsafe conditions do not result in patient outcomes.

(*Continued*)

Table 10-2 Information Required for Common Formats: Generic and Event-Specific Events (*Continued*)

Event-Specific Common Formats (Continued)

Scope of Reporting

Separate Common Formats are developed for each overall type of setting, such as a hospital or skilled nursing facility. Furthermore, scope delineates the applicability of specific event descriptions to incidents, near misses, and unsafe conditions. For example, the description for *fall events* pertains to incidents only (not near misses or unsafe conditions), whereas the description for *medication and other substance events* pertains to incidents, near misses, and unsafe conditions.

Risk Assessments and Preventive Actions

Event-specific Common Formats list assessments, preventive actions, or other measures that should have been performed or established prior to the event to prevent or mitigate its occurrence. This includes the precise circumstances in which such actions should have been taken. The Event-specific Common Formats do not include routine protocols that apply to all patients, such as the universal protocol (used in the operating room).

Note: If precise specification is not possible, such actions cannot be delineated in an event-specific Common Format; this type of information/opinion can be entered into a narrative field to assist in the analysis of any individual event.

Circumstances of the Event

1. Identifying or descriptive information pertaining to the category of patient safety concern (e.g., product name, drug name, ICD-9/ICD-10)
2. Risk factors specific to the event. Risk factors increase the probability of an event and are known in advance of its occurrence.
3. Contributing factors specific to the event. Contributing factors are determined only retrospectively, after the event has occurred. These factors are different from those that could apply to any event and that are found in the generic event descriptions.

To access the most current versions of the Common Formats, go to Connect to Current Information section at the end of the chapter. There, you will find the full list of event-specific formats for both acute care hospital settings and skilled nursing facility settings. Future versions of the Common Formats will be developed for ambulatory settings to include ambulatory surgery centers and physicians' and practitioners' offices.

Common Formats for Surveillance—Hospital

Most recently, AHRQ and the interagency Federal Patient Safety Workgroup released *Common Formats for Surveillance—Hospital.* Until now, Common Formats have been designed to support only traditional event reporting. *Common Formats for Surveillance—Hospital* are designed to provide, through retrospective review of medical records, information that is complementary to that derived from event reporting systems. These formats will facilitate improved detection of events and calculation of adverse event rates in populations reviewed. To view the Federal Register notice announcing *Common Formats for Surveillance—Hospital*, go to http://www.gpo.gov/fdsys/pkg/FR-2014-02-18/html/2014-03492.htm.

a close-up of a particular concern. For CQI purposes, the goal is to understand how common something is, and then if an improvement intervention is implemented, it is possible to determine if there was a change in prevalence. **Incidence** is an estimate of how frequently new events, cases, etc., develop (Storme, 2013, p. 13). These methods help HCOs identify occurrence patterns. To ensure arriving at an incident rate that provides a clear picture, the population at risk should be described as concisely as possible. This can be useful in CQI, but it should not be the only approach taken. There are many CQI reports, both from individual HCOs and from state and national sources. What is critical is not how data are presented in the reports, but whether the report is useful, accurate, timely, relevant to the question(s) asked, directed toward the best stakeholders, analyzed appropriately based on types of data and questions, and visualized in a way that is helpful (Keroack & Rhinehart, 2013).

Stop and Consider #1
CQI measurement needs to be individualized for each HCO.

Monitoring Care Quality

There is a lot of information and discussion about errors, mostly with the focus on what happens after they occur or retrospective review; however, there needs to be more done to prospectively identify safety hazards (HHS, AHRQ, 2015a). There are methods to detect these hazards, but more are needed.

Transparency, public reporting, and benchmarking are now important aspects of healthcare delivery. There is need for measurement systems that are effective and meet the multiple needs of individual departments, HCOs, agencies, and programs; individual healthcare professions; accreditors; insurers; and government regulations and standards.

Data Collection to Improve Care

In an HCO's QI program and its plans, a critical part of the work is to clearly identify measures/indicators, but the QI program needs to identify the data that are needed to assess the measures/indicators in a clear data collection plan. This task requires careful consideration of the data that are available, such as from secondary sources, or the need to develop new effective data collection methods. The CQI team and staff should avoid repetitive work, such as collecting data that are already available, and also should avoid collecting data that are not needed. An effective data collection plan must do the following for each measure/indicator (HHS, HRSA, 2011b, 2011c):

- Identify the measure/indicator.
- Describe the denominator in detail with inclusions and exclusions; this needs to clarify whom or what will be included in the sample/population.

- Identify the data source for the denominator and include any specific queries to be run or report parameters that must be entered in the digital system.
- Describe the numerator in detail with inclusions and exclusions (e.g., "Documentation in the medical record must note the date on which the laboratory test was performed and the results, or the record notates the date and results of a test ordered by another provider.").
- Use randomized sampling when possible. Randomized sampling is the most recommended method for performance improvement because it ensures every patient or selected event has an equal chance of inclusion in the sample without bias.
- Identify data sources for the numerator and include specific computer queries to be run, manual steps, or specific sampling parameters.
- Identify who collects each data element and calculates the measure.
- Describe the calendar for measure-performance reporting.
- Describe data collection procedures, timelines, and any required data collection training.

An important attribute of the AHRQ Quality Indicators Toolkit is that there is more than one way to develop a system of monitoring sustainability of performance. There are, however, some critical elements of effective monitoring that HCOs need to consider in their CQI planning. According to the HHS, AHRQ (2012), the HCO should choose a limited set of effective measures, establish a schedule for regular reporting, develop report formats for acting on problems identified, and assess sustainability on a periodic basis.

Human factors, as noted in other parts of this text, impact our understanding of risks and harms in healthcare delivery. In cultures of safety where the staff are recognized for their contributions, they can add important information to this understanding of care processes and the use of policies and procedures, thereby expanding the CQI prospective. This contribution, however, requires that management listen to staff and that staff feel they can make comments without retribution. An effective CQI environment is one in which staff do not feel they must wait to be asked for feedback.

Data collection is typically retrospective, prospective, or a combination. There are no universal effective prospective and retrospective methods for detecting errors and safety hazards. Retrospective, the most common approach, reviews safety hazards typically focused on two types of methods (HHS, AHRQ, PSNet, 2015):

- Screening large datasets for preventable adverse event evidence for further examination
- Screening and analyzing adverse events or strongly suspected adverse events, including use of trigger tools; screening administrative data sets; and using more in-depth methods such as root cause analysis and mortality reviews

There are many methods used for screening these datasets for evidence of adverse events. One of these methods is the AHRQ Patient Safety Indicators (PSIs). These screening measures/indicators identify potential problems within an HCO that require more analysis and should not be used to compare data from one HCO to another; nor are they useful in estimating overall incidence of adverse events. For example, if a hospital notes an increased incidence of postoperative sepsis PSI, then the specific HCO may have a systematic problem with failure to rescue in postoperative patients with problems, but making a definitive determination requires more examination (HHS, AHRQ, PSNet, 2015).

When one considers national CQI data and data collection methods, the first source for the data is often the medical record. This source does offer considerable data, but there are also barriers to obtaining accurate and relevant data from this source (Rosen, 2010). Collecting data is costly and labor-intensive. Before the development of the EMR/EHR, it was even more difficult to get data from hard copies of records, although both types of documentation have potential problems. It is not legitimate to say that electronic methods are perfect; they are not. They present numerous problems, including variation, inaccuracies, and missing information. Electronic methods and use of technology are discussed further in other chapters.

This text discusses transfers or handoffs, situations that add to the difficulty of keeping and sharing data. When patients move within a system or between systems, we do not always get the information we need in documentation that is then retrievable for CQI purposes. Once the data are collected, they must be put into some type of database so that they can be analyzed.

Methods Used in Data Collection

HCOs and other organizations involved in CQI use a number of methods to collect data. Staff may be involved in data collection, but even if not directly involved, they need to understand these methods in order to provide feedback and consider how the results impact their work.

Check/Tally Sheets

Check sheets or **tally sheets** are a simple way to collect data and document data. It is not difficult to develop a data collection check/tally sheet focused on a particular event. An example might be a check/tally sheet used to document data on observations of hand washing. Check/tally sheets should be clear and easy to use. After data are collected, another method needs to be used to aggregate the data. The Connect to Current Information section at the end of the chapter provides a link to a site with examples of check/tally sheets.

Questionnaires/Surveys

Questionnaires/surveys are used by HCOs to collect data, although this is not a common method. It takes time and requires cooperation from staff to complete the surveys. It also takes time to develop effective surveys and then to analyze the data, although electronic methods have made this method easier to use. One needs to keep in mind data analysis. The HCO also needs to identify who should respond to the questionnaire and how this will be communicated. For example, if the problem is the need to improve documentation in the intensive care unit, then data given by staff who work in dietary services may not be relevant, but data given by the nutritionist who works with these patients would be important to include. Also, questionnaires/surveys are often used with patients, such as patient satisfaction surveys. These methods are discussed in greater detail elsewhere in this text. In this chapter, it is important to recognize that this method may be used to collect data.

Interviews

Interviews may be used to learn more about care and how to improve care. Interviews may focus on individuals or may be done in a group, such as a focus group. Questions may be highly structured, using specific questions and no variation; structured questions may be used, with additional questions based on the responses; or questions may be open-ended, with the interviewer introducing the topic and then asking group members to share their thoughts. The interviewer needs to use a clear method for recording the responses so that data can then be used; for example, the interviewer can use a form listing the questions, then record the responses on the form. When using this method, it can be time consuming to collect, aggregate, and analyze the data.

Observation

Observation is used for collecting data, although it is a time-consuming method and thus can be costly. Observer subjectivity may be a potential barrier to obtaining objective data, although observer training and using consistent data collection documentation methods reduces subjectivtity. Management uses observation routinely to determine performance and identify situations that require immediate response as well as long-term concerns. When changes are made to improve care, observation might be used. For example, are staff using hand washing when required? Is the new staff call system effective? Is a change in a treatment or procedure improving outcomes?

Examples of Methods Used to Describe Data

Before data collection is begun, it is important to determine how the data will be described. What format or method will best provide a visual of the data so that they can be understood, analyzed, and applied? Understanding the purpose for the data collection is important and allows you to apply the best method. Describing data is important and serves a variety of purposes. Methods commonly used include the following (Kelly, Johnson, Sollecito, 2013, p. 93):

- *Flowcharts* enable reviewing or updating of information and help keep it current.

- *Cause and effect diagrams* stratify and examine causes.
- *Pareto diagrams/charts* stratify causes and demonstrate change.
- *Histograms (frequency distribution)* are used in presentations to provide a visual of data, assess patterns, and enable monitoring.
- *Run charts* relate data to changes and examine the relationship of improvement to change(s).
- *Control charts* relate data to changes and help determine if a process is or remains under control.
- *Regression analysis* helps assess strength of association and test hypotheses.

The Connect to Current Information section at the end of the chapter provides links to sites that provide visuals of some of the methods. Looking at these examples will help to better understand the methods and how they might be applied in a QI program.

Run Charts

Run charts display data to illustrate or plot change and patterns over time. They assist in identifying problems and when they occurred. Other terms used for these charts are line graphs, trend charts, and time-series charts.

Pareto Charts

Pareto charts are vertical bar graphs with bars ordered from the longest to the shortest. They are based on the Pareto principle that 80% of the output in a situation is due to 20% of the input. The chart prioritizes frequency of causes related to one another (Kelly et al., 2013).

Flowcharts

Flowcharts are useful tools to gain a better understanding of a process and variations in the process. Flowcharts may be used to display information prospectively, for example to describe an approach to a process such as a description of a unit's admission process. During the root cause analysis process, flowcharts may be used retrospectively to visualize steps that were taken in a specific process such as a procedure for a specific patient; identify possible and potential causes of problems; examine handoffs; identify staff, teams, and departments that were involved in the process; and provide a view of current practice and consideration for improvement (HHS, AHRQ, HIT, 2013a). Staff who understand the process are more effective in developing a flowchart, and typically, this means an interprofessional team. The following questions might be considered when developing a flowchart (Kelly et al., 2013, p. 97):

1. How effective is the process in meeting customer (patient) requirements?
2. Are there performance gaps or perceived opportunities for improvement?

3. Have the relevant stages of the process been represented? If not, what needs to be done to gather feedback and ideas?

4. What inputs are required for the process, and where do they come from? Are the inputs constraining the process or not? Which ones?

5. Are there equipment or regulatory constraints forcing this approach?

6. Is this the right problem process to be working on? To continue working on?

Dashboards

Dashboards provide a clear visualization of data in one view, a compilation of run charts or a summary. Managers need quick information on CQI status, and using dashboards to communicate this status can be effective, sharing results with staff and offering a view of performance of each measure over time.

Examples of Monitoring Methods

In developing its QI plans, an HCO needs to decide not only what, specifically, it will monitor, but also how it will consistently monitor performance in general to identify gaps or problems and key measures/indicators. Some monitoring methods may be determined by external sources such as accreditors, third-party payers, and government agencies, both state and federal (e.g., the CMS). There are many potential methods that could be used, including the examples found in **Table 10-3** and in the following description.

Benchmarking and Report Cards

Benchmarking refers to comparison. For example, consumers might compare hospital ratings, or an HCO may collect data prior to instituting an improvement change and then compare results after the change, with the initial data serving as the benchmark (NAS/HMD, 2015). Using benchmarking to compare data may act as an incentive to stimulate HCOs and individual healthcare providers to improve and also provides positive feedback and recognition of improvement. The process also helps to identify variations and gaps in care. In addition, measurement is a method used to determine if HCOs and individual healthcare providers are compliant with standards and regulations (NAS/HMD, 2015, pp. 2–12). It is important to evaluate the CQI process, and part of this is comparing performance with other similar providers. **Report cards** are summary reports of status, and in the case of CQI, it would be status of the quality of care. Individual HCOs also need to monitor their own CQI and may use a report card format for this purpose. Common data found in these reports are data about admissions and discharges, diagnoses, procedures/treatment, patient satisfaction, staffing, patient outcomes, and other data. Report cards are often published, for example, on the Internet, so that consumers and others can compare HCOs.

Do these rating systems offer clear, accurate, and helpful information? In a study that compared four major rating systems, it was found that none of the rated

Table 10-3 Strategies for Measuring Patient Safety		
Measurement Strategies	**Advantages**	**Disadvantages**
Retrospective chart review	Considered the "gold standard," contains rich detailed clinical information	Costly, labor-intensive, data quality variable due to incomplete clinical information, retrospective review only
Incident reporting systems	Useful for internal QI and case finding, highlights adverse events that providers perceive as important	Capture small fraction of adverse events that occur, retrospective review only based on provider self-reports, no standardization or uniformity of adverse events reported
Automated surveillance	Can be used retrospectively or prospectively, helpful in screening patients who may be at high risk for adverse events using standardized protocols	Need electronic data to run automated surveillance, high proportion of "triggered" cases are false positives
Administrative/ claims data	Low cost, readily available data, useful for tracking events over time across large populations, can identify "potential" adverse events	Lack detailed clinical data, concerns over variability and inaccuracy of ICD-9-CM* codes/ICD-10 codes across and within systems, may detect high proportion of false positives

*International Classification of Diseases, Ninth Revision, Clinical Modification

Reproduced with permission from AHRQ Patient Safety Network, & Rosen, A.K. (November 2010). Are we getting better at measuring patient safety? Retrieved from https://psnet.ahrq.gov/perspectives/perspective/94

hospitals were rated as high performers by all four rating systems. Only 10% of the 844 hospitals rated as a high performer by one system was rated the same by one of the other three systems (Austin et al., 2015). This result is most likely due to differences in HCO methods, focus, measures of performance, and differences in measuring systems. For the consumer, this means there might not be clear and accurate views of an HCO for comparison, and when consumers search for this information, typically online, most consumers do not realize the ratings may not be all that valid and reliable. To decrease these problems, there is need for more consistency in the rating scales that are used, such as using the same definitions for patient safety. The goal should be greater transparency with effective information so that consumers can make more informed choices.

Some noted QI experts have questioned the direction CQI measurement is taking (Wachter, 2016). Dr. Wachter published his concerns in the *New York Times*, noting that there is now an overemphasis on targets, yardsticks, metrics, and outcomes. Such measures seek to determine whether something was or was not done, but often to the exclusion of salient CQI insights. There are many report cards for rating hospitals, and over 1,600 hospitals claim to be in the "top 100." This has led to questions about the value of HCO ratings and measurements. The EMR/EHR has had both a positive and a negative impact. For example, in tracking physician computer use, physicians clicked the mouse 4,000 times in a 10-hour shift (Wachter, 2016). While all this clicking shows their engagement in documentation and technology interfacing, it says very little about the quality of care they are providing. Understanding the sometimes arbitrary or misleading nature of poorly selected or applied CQI measurement methods, The Joint Commission is not reporting hospital ratings any longer, and the CMS is reducing some of its measurement and reporting initiatives related to the EMR/EHR (CMS Blog, 2016; Wachter, 2016). Wachter (2016) expresses his concern for the state of CQI measurement as follows:

> Measurement cannot go away, but it needs to be scaled back and allowed to mature. We need more targeted measures, ones that have been vetted to ensure that they really matter. In medicine, for example, measuring the rates of certain hospital-acquired infections has led to a greater emphasis on prevention and has most likely saved lives. On the other hand, measuring whether doctors documented that they provided discharge instructions to heart failure or asthma patients at the end of their hospital stay sounds good, but turns out to be an exercise in futile box-checking, and should be jettisoned.

We moved into measurement and did not recognize that it may have both positive and negative impacts on healthcare providers. Throughout the discussion on CQI in this text, it is important not to make the CQI process the sole focus or goal. The goal is always focus on the patient, high-quality patient care, and effective performance that make a difference in outcomes.

Mandatory Versus Voluntary Reporting

The *Quality Chasm* reports recommend mandatory reporting, but what is the view of major healthcare delivery organizations, organizations that focus on healthcare delivery, healthcare profession organizations, and government agencies? The American Hospital Association (AHA) is a major organization for hospitals. It is very involved in supporting CQI and reducing errors. It collaborates with the Institute for Safe Medication Practices (ISMP) to identify needs and develop solutions that will help HCOs reduce errors. The recommendation to provide legal protections for those who report errors is supported by the AHA; however, it is not in full agreement with some of the recommendations for reporting. The AHA supports voluntary rather than required reporting of errors, believing this approach best supports staff reporting (Regenstein, 2013). The AHA does not believe that the AHRQ should be the reporting agency, but rather recommends that medication errors be reported to the ISMP, and errors related to devices be reported to the FDA. This demonstrates how complex CQI is, involving multiple stakeholders who do not always agree. **Figure 10-3** describes the National Coordinating Council for Medication Error Reporting and Prevention Index for categorizing medication errors. This categorization of errors, which is important in reporting errors, represents a coordinated effort between nongovernment and government organizations.

The Joint Commission is very involved in CQI due to its focus on accreditation (Regenstein, 2013). It has not made a clear statement for or against mandatory or voluntary reporting of errors, though it does support the need for legal protections for those who report errors. As noted in this text, The Joint Commission has a major impact on HCOs, not only due to its role in accreditation but also due to its annual patient safety goals and reporting requirements for its accredited HCOs.

As Kizer and Stegun (2014) state, "HCOs and healthcare providers through their mission and ethical principles that support public accountability should provide information and transparency to consumers when there is concern about problems and actions taken" (p. 341). Disclosure to patients about errors has been discussed

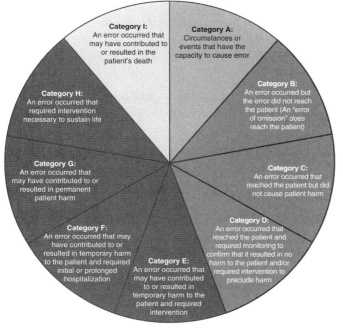

Definitions

Harm
Impairment of the physical, emotional, or psychological function or structure of the body and/or pain resulting therefrom.

Monitoring
To observe or record relevant physiological or psychological signs.

Intervention
May include change in therapy or active medical/surgical treatment.

Intervention Necessary to Sustain life
Includes cardiovascular and respiratory support (e.g., CPR, defibrillation, intubation, etc.)

Figure 10-3. National Coordinating Council for Medication Error Reporting and Prevention Index for Categorizing Medication Errors in this text, and there are conflicting views about its use. HCOs are also obligated to provide information about their performance to external agencies (e.g., state and federal) and accreditors. The question that has become more important today is, how much of this performance information should then be shared with the general public, and should it be mandatory? The HHS, Office of the Inspector General (OIG) (2010) summarizes this issue as follows:

> Public disclosure of adverse event information offers potential benefits, yet may also lead to unintended negative consequences. For example, publicly disclosing adverse event information can educate healthcare providers about the causes of events potentially leading to improvements in patient safety, and assist patients making decisions about their care. However, there is concern that disclosure of event information could undermine patient privacy and that naming the hospital where an event occurred, or the individual providers involved, could discourage reporting of events. (p. 6)

With multiple viewpoints about a universal decision on mandatory reporting, this concern has not yet been resolved.

Two issues that are important to consider are the complexity of reporting and reporting data to multiple entities, such as accreditors, insurers, state agencies, and federal government agencies. Accountability means that all should be focused on improving patient care. Systematic reporting using standard definitions is critical if one is to compare data across HCOs and other entities to which reports are given, but at this time we do not have systematic reporting that meets the needs of multiple organizations and the government (state and federal).

Incident Reports

Incident reports have long been used by HCOs, particularly hospitals, to report and track quality care issues. The AHRQ's Patient Safety Network describes an incident report as follows:

> An incident reporting is general term for all voluntary patient safety event reporting systems, which rely on those involved in events to provide detailed information" (HHS, AHRQ, PSNet, 2014a)

Although this reporting has been used a long time, incident reporting has not done enough to improve care.

HCOs should have a policy that describes when the incident report should be completed and a procedure defining how it should be completed. Typically, HCOs use incident reports to track infections, pharmacy and medication errors, treatment procedure errors, patient complaints, falls, sentinel events, security issues, harm to staff, and regulatory compliance (Levinson, 2012). **Table 10-4** describes an example of a list of serious reportable events.

Table 10–4 List of National Quality Forum Serious Reportable Events	
Event	**Additional specifications**
1. Surgical Events	
A. Surgery performed on the wrong body part	Defined as any surgery performed on a body part that is not consistent with the documented informed consent for that patient. Excludes emergent situations that occur in the course of surgery and/or whose exigency precludes obtaining informed consent.
B. Surgery performed on the wrong patient	Defined as any surgery on a patient that is not consistent with the documented informed consent for that patient
C. Wrong surgical procedure performed on a patient	Defined as any procedure performed on a patient that is not consistent with the documented informed consent for that patient. Excludes emergent situations that occur in the course of surgery and/or whose exigency precludes obtaining informed consent. Surgery includes endoscopies and other invasive procedures.
D. Retention of a foreign object in a patient after surgery or other procedure	Excludes objects intentionally implanted as part of a planned intervention and objects present prior to surgery that were intentionally retained_
E. Intraoperative or immediately post-operative death in an ASA Class I patient	Includes all ASA Class I patient deaths in situations when anesthesia was administered; the planned surgical procedure may or may not have been carried out. Immediately post-operative means within 24 hours after induction of anesthesia (if surgery not completed), surgery, or other invasive procedure was completed

(Continued)

Table 10–4 List of National Quality Forum Serious Reportable Events (*Continued*)

Event	Additional specifications
2. Product or device events	
A. Patient death or serious disability associated with the use of contaminated drugs, devices, or biologics provided by the health care facility	Includes generally detectable contaminants in drugs, devices, or biologics regardless of the source of contamination and/or product
B. Patient death or serious disability associated with the use or function of a device in patient care, in which the device is used for functions other than as intended	Includes, but is not limited to, catheters, drains and other specialized tubes, infusion pumps, and ventilators_
C. Patient death or serious disability associated with intravascular air embolism that occurs while being cared for in a health care facility	Excludes deaths associated with neurosurgical procedures known to be a high risk of intravascular air embolism_
3. Patient protection events	
A. Infant discharged to the wrong person	
B. Patient death or serious disability associated with patient elopement (disappearance) for more than four hours	Excludes events involving competent adults.
C. Patient suicide, or attempted suicide resulting in serious disability, while being cared for in a health care facility	Defined as events that result from patient actions after admission to a health care facility. Excludes deaths resulting from self-inflicted injuries that were the reason for admission to the health care facility.
4. Care management events	
A. Patient death or serious disability associated with a medication error (e.g., errors involving the wrong drug, wrong dose, wrong patient, wrong time, wrong rate, wrong preparation, or wrong route of administration)	Excludes reasonable differences in clinical judgment on drug selection and dose.

Event	Additional specifications
B. Patient death or serious disability associated with a hemolytic reaction due to the administration of ABO-incompatible blood or blood products	
C. Maternal death or serious disability associated with labor or delivery in a low-risk pregnancy while being cared for in a health care facility	Includes events that occur within 42 days post-delivery. Excludes deaths from pulmonary or amniotic fluid embolism, acute fatty liver of pregnancy or cardiomyopathy.
D. Patient death or serious disability associated with hypoglycemia, the onset of which occurs while the patient is being cared for in a health care facility	
E. Death or serious disability (kernicterus) associated with failure to identify and treat hyperbilirubinirnia in neonates	Hyperbilirubinimia is defined as bilirubin levels > 30 mg/dl. Neonates refers to the first 28 days of fife.
F. Stage 3 or 4 pressure ulcers acquired after admission to a health care facility	Excludes progression from Stage 2 to Stage 3 if Stage 2 was recognized upon admission.
G. Patient death or serious disability due to spinal manipulative therapy	
5. Environmental Events	
A. Patient death or serious disability associated with an electric shock while being cared for in a health care facility	Excludes events involving planned treatments such as electric countershock.
B. Any incident in which a line designated for oxygen or other gas to be delivered to a patient contains the wrong gas or is contaminated by toxic substances	
C. Patient death or serious disability associated with a burn incurred from any source while being cared for in a health care facility	

(Continued)

Table 10-4 List of National Quality Forum Serious Reportable Events (Continued)	
Event	**Additional specifications**
D. Patient death associated with a fall while being cared for in a health care facility	
E. Patient death or serious disability associated with the use of restraints or bedrails while being cared for in a health care facility	
6. Criminal events	
A. Any instance of care ordered by or provided by someone impersonating a physician, nurse, pharmacist, or other licensed health care provider	
B. Abduction of a patient of any age	
C. Sexual assault on a patient within or on the grounds of the health care facility	
D. Death or significant injury of a patient or staff member resulting from a physical assault (i.e., battery) that occurs within or on the grounds of the health care facility	

Reproduced from Kizer, K & Stegun, M. (October 2014). Serious reportable adverse events in health care. In Agency for Healthcare Research and Quality (AHRQ). *Advances in patient safety.* Retrieved from http://www.ahrq. gov/professionals /quality-patient-safety/patient-safety-resources/resources/advances-in-patient-safety/index.html

It is not simple to develop and implement effective error reporting systems, and the process requires ongoing attention. Dashboards may be used to routinely share incident report information with staff without inclusion of specific staff information and other identifiers.

Staff members at the point of care, rather than managers, usually identify error or near-miss information, although managers are also involved in some of these errors and near misses. Incident reporting is a passive form of surveillance as compared to active forms such as record reviews, observation of care delivery, and use of trigger tools (HHS, AHRQ, PSNet, 2014a). For the reporting system to be effective, the HCO should have a culture of safety that protects privacy when staff report events, and the HCO should expect any staff involved in an event to use the required incident reporting procedure. The HCO should use structured methods to analyze the data, including root cause analysis, benchmarking, and development of action plans to respond when needed. Today, many HCOs have changed to electronic reporting methods.

The reports and the data should be reviewed by CQI staff and management, and also by risk management for possible malpractice risk. This information is then used to develop needed changes to improve care. However, as commented earlier, this process may not be effective. The incident reporting process has had a major impact on the development of the blame culture, with staff viewing the reports as a way for the HCO administration to identify the staff member who made an error and possibly "punish" that person. It is, however, necessary to have a documentation process for monitoring and examining errors. Attitudes toward monitoring should be positive, focused on identifying opportunities for improvement, not blame or punishment. Although an individual staff member typically completes the incident report, it is critical to move away from just focusing on individuals to a system approach. The documentation then provides information to track errors and identify errors that require examination and use of root cause analysis.

Management and staff attitudes toward incident reporting must be carefully monitored and evaluated long-term. A negative attitude toward incident reporting is difficult to change to a positive experience. HCOs must consider whether the use of incident reports limits reporting. For example, in one review of incident reports, the following was noted, "hospital staff did not report 86 percent of events to incident reporting systems, partly because of staff misperceptions about what constitutes patient harm" (Levinson, 2012, p. i). Incident reporting identified only an estimated 14% of the patient harm events experienced by Medicare beneficiaries (HHS, OIG, 2012). When these events were identified, the HCOs investigated events that were considered to most likely lead to CQI problems. The review noted that few policy or practice changes resulted from data about incidents. As the Office of the Inspector General (2012) reports, "Hospital administrators classified the remaining events (86 percent) as either events that staff did not perceive as reportable (61 percent) or as events that staff commonly report but did not report in this case (25 percent)." Medicare patients represent a large number of hospital admissions, so these comments are disturbing and impact a lot of patients. Even though this review did not include non-Medicare patients, it is easy to wonder about the level of reporting incidents that involve other patients. **Table 10-5** describes the Common Format data elements that were included in the HHS review of incident reports.

There are many common barriers to staff voluntarily reporting events in their HCO system, including the following (Evans et al., 2006): no feedback on incident follow-up, form too long or confusing, lack of time, incident seemed unimportant, unit was busy, forgot to report, and not sure who is responsible for the report. Using this type of information about barriers should help to develop strategies/interventions such as changes to processes and policies, and procedures to prevent barriers so that staff are more engaged in the incident reporting system. Staff orientation and

Table 10–5 Common Format Data Elements Present on the Complete Incident Reports (*n* = 19)	
Element Description	**Number of Reports With Element**
Basic Event Information	
Date the event was discovered	19
Location of the event	19
Whether the event was an adverse event, near miss, or unsafe condition	17
Narrative description of the event	16
Patient Impact Information	
Time between event and assessment of harm	16
Whether rescue steps were taken	16
Level of harm caused by event	14
Whether event prolonged patient's length of stay	2
Contributing Factor Information	
Whether and which factors contributed to event	10
Patient safety staff's summary of event and follow-up	6
Preventability of event	6
Whether event was a National Quality Forum Serious Reportable Event	0
Whether a patient handoff was associated with event	3

Reproduced from U.S. Department of Health and Human Services (HHS) & Office of the Inspector General. (January 2012). Hospital incident reporting systems do not capture most patient harm. OEI-06-09-009. Retrieved from http://oig.hhs.gov/oei/reports/oei-06-09-00091.asp

education should provide information so that staff understand why and how it is done. Reporting results to staff also helps staff better understand incident reporting and why it is important. Staff have limited time and energy to devote to "administrative" tasks, so they need to appreciate the value of these tasks. Lastly, and this is not unimportant, staff need to be recognized for their contributions to CQI—emphasizing their roles and responsibilities in CQI in all aspects of the HCO's QI program. For example, for staff to effectively report incidents such as medication errors they must know an error has occurred, be willing to report it, know the policy and procedure for reporting, and have the time to complete the incident report procedure. Further, it is important that staff do not fear blame and punishment and that they view this activity as part of their commitment to CQI in their daily practice.

It is not enough to rely solely on incident reporting as the major monitoring method in a CQI program. HCOs and healthcare professions have focused a lot of attention on CQI, but there is an aspect of CQI getting less attention that also has an impact on CQI. This issue is staff responses when they are involved in an error. Namely, how do they cope? There is recognition now that many adverse events are system related; however, this does not mean that staff may not have negative personal reactions and responses to situations that lead to adverse events and difficulties reporting them. Staff may respond with anger if they think they are being "accused" of something. Staff may experience depression with lowered self-esteem due to their view of professional status or anxiety about their work. They may become overly careful, checking and rechecking their work process. They may feel embarrassed with their colleagues and supervisors. If an adverse event is not reported and patient harm occurred, staff may find that keeping this event a secret has a negative impact on them personally and professionally. Staff may find that their personal lives are also affected. HCOs need to recognize these human responses pose a potential problem and provide support to staff as needed when errors occur.

Global Triggers

A **global trigger** is a signal or a clue that may be used to identify a potential adverse event, not the event itself. Triggers are used for screening and alerting staff to monitor for a particular situation, for example, by reviewing the medical record or a physician order (Adler et al., 2008).

The Institute for Healthcare Improvement (IHI) provides trigger tools for measuring general adverse events and events that might occur in specific care situations, such as for intensive care, perioperative, and mental health services. Only 10% to 20% of errors are reported; however, of the errors reported, 90% to 95% do not cause any harm. This means that we need more effective methods to identify those events that have greater risk of causing harm, and triggers can help to do this (IHI, 2015a). There is danger in focusing on counting errors rather than examining errors that cause harm to patients (IHI, 2015b). The general tool monitors adverse events per 1,000 patient-days per 100 admissions and percentage of admissions with an adverse event (IHI, 2016a, 2016b). Dr. Shojania, editor in chief of *BMJ Quality and Safety*, offers the following insights about alert systems:

> As with any alert system, the threshold for generating triggers needs to balance true and false positives. The system will lose its value if too many triggers prove to be false alarms. This concern is less relevant when triggers are used as chart review tools, since the "cost" of a false positive is relatively low—mostly sufficient resources for medical record review. (HHS, AHRQ, PSNet, 2015)

Morbidity and Mortality Monitoring

Morbidity (incidence of disease state or condition) and **mortality** (incidence of death) are important outcomes requiring monitoring. Morbidity is determined by scores based on tested systems such as scales rating coma level and pain and special rating scales, such as APACHE II (intensive care unit patient rating mortality risk and rate of disease) and SAPS II (acute care patient rating of mortality risk and rate of disease). The mortality rate is typically described as number of deaths per 1,000 individuals in a year and includes crude death rates; perinatal, maternal, or infant rates; and rates figured by age, gender, diagnosis, and other characteristics.

Acute care HCOs typically have routine meetings in which mortality and morbidity are discussed per specific patients and events. Staff explore system factors that contribute to adverse events and adverse patient outcomes. These meetings are also used for teaching medical staff, residents, and healthcare profession students. How are morbidity and mortality measured? The discussions focus on more than just data; they include details about practice and related problems and solutions. These meetings should be interprofessional and should not be focused on placing blame, but rather on providing opportunities for staff learning, consideration of needs for changes in practice to improve outcomes, and identification of care that is effective.

Utilization Review/Management and Risk Management

Utilization review/management is used by HCOs to routinely collect data about use of services. The data describe the number of admissions, transfers, discharges, procedures, and other pertinent details, and provide other types of data such as patient diagnosis, gender and age, length of treatment, and types of treatment. This information is also used in CQI and HCO marketing to assist in understanding HCO services, finance, and other operations.

Risk management focuses on HCO risk for malpractice claims and thus risk for financial loss. Risk management requires that HCOs do the following (Barach & Johnson, 2013): (1) Identify risk so that the HCO knows what is going wrong, (2) analyze the risk by collecting and understanding data, and (3) control the risk by developing strategies/interventions that will help identify, manage, and prevent problems.

Attorneys are involved in assisting the HCO in this monitoring. The incident reporting system is a critical source of information for CQI but also for risk management. HCO structure often combines utilization review with risk management so that staff work together or are the same staff that provide this monitoring and may also be part of the QI program. Risk managers recognize that there is always risk, and some risk can be identified and prevented or actions may be taken to reduce the risk level. Example methods used to collect risk management data are observation and rounds, medical record reviews, and informal feedback from staff.

Malpractice lawsuits that focus on nurses do occur. A study of closed claims reviewed 516 claims (2006–2010) and identified that the average total incurred payment per nursing claim was $204,594 (Benton, Arm, & Flynn, 2013). Out of 11 nursing specialty areas, the areas with the highest percentage of claims were adult medical/surgical (40.1%), gerontology in an aging services facility (18.0%), and obstetrics (10.3%). The study reviewed the following malpractice categories of problems noted in claims: scope of practice (1.7%); assessment (12.6%); monitoring (6.8%); treatment/care (58.6%); medication administration (14.7%); patients' rights, patient abuse, and professional conduct (5.4%); and documentation (0.2%). The licensure types included in the claims were 84.5% registered nurses and 15.5% licensed practical or vocational nurses. Acute care had the most claims (57.3%). The review of these claims indicates that some of the situations could have been prevented. Nurses need to document according to standards, clearly, and in a timely manner; follow policies and procedures; understand and follow their scope of practice; improve written and oral communication; implement effective handoff methods; and maintain clinical competence through self-assessment, staff education, and continuing education. Each nurse must feel comfortable reporting concerns to supervisors without fear of reprimand.

Stop and Consider #2
Monitoring care quality is a never-ending endeavor.

Analysis of Care Quality

Analysis of CQI data is usually done quantitatively and statistically, but for healthcare multiple variables make this a complicated process. The HHS, HRSA (2011c) describes the key concepts of this process as follows:

> *Analyzing* data is the *review* of performance data to determine if it meets the desired quality level; it is used to define a performance plan. *Interpreting* data is the process of *assigning* meaning or determining the significance, implications, and conclusions of data collected; it is used to evaluate and improve activities, identify gaps, and plan for improvement.

The drivers of CQI are people, information management, infrastructure, processes, and culture, all of which impact desired outcomes (Ettinger, 2006). People are an important component of CQI. They are needed to develop and implement CQI initiatives and then to develop and implement necessary changes. How people work together can make a difference. Even the staffing level has an impact. For example, if staffing is short and staff members are overworked, CQI efforts may be negatively impacted; namely, the HCO may see increased errors, and aspects of the QI program, such as reporting, documenting, collecting, and analyzing data, may be limited, thus harming development of improvement strategies.

Just collecting data is not enough. Analysis and interpretation of data are critical, and mistakes can be made in interpretation (Ettinger, 2006). When focusing too much on mean or average and ignoring variation, data may be misinterpreted; that is, the mean can be improved and yet the variation is still unacceptable. If the analysis focuses just on percentages and not absolute numbers, this too might not provide a clear view of a problem. For example, the HCO might identify that 95% of medication orders were administered according to procedure, but the numerical description is that there were 5,000 errors a year or 15 per day. The latter description clearly indicates an unacceptable result.

Infrastructure is the driver that focuses on physical aspects of the HCO, such as space, lighting, noise, equipment availability, function, and software and hardware. Processes represent another driver and are integral in all HCO functioning and have an impact on CQI (Ettinger, 2006). HCOs use different methods to understand their processes and their impact on quality. Examples of these methods are process mapping and define and measure-analyze-improve-control (discussed later in this chapter). Organizational culture is also a driver and has been discussed in other sections of this text. We pay more attention to organizational culture today in health care. A high-performing culture has "optimistic staff and leaders, [is] open to change and innovation, [has] leaders focused on both customers (e.g., patients and others) and staff, [is] process oriented, [is] committed to excellence, and measures and shares information" (Ettinger, 2006, p. 125). Organizational culture is connected to development of a culture of safety within HCOs.

The data analysis process requires that the CQI team and staff review current performance and then ideally compare performance with baseline data that were collected earlier (benchmarking)—for example, data from the previous year or month. Measures/indicators guide this process to determine if there is any change and, if so, describe the change. To determine if this is acceptable, the "interpretation process provides knowledge of the changes applied to the systems, special events with a potential impact, and lessons learned from the prior month's work that forms the next steps" (HHS, HRSA, April 2011c). The team may use the plan-do-study-act cycle, discussed elsewhere in this text and summarized in **Figure 10-4**, to guide action and make changes to improve. If the QI team decides that progress toward improvement has not occurred, and this includes progress in all the CQI steps, it might then review any of the following (HHS, HRSA, 2011b, 2011c):

- *Ensure data systems are reliable.* Secondary sources are at risk as data are collected for reasons other than CQI and may not meet CQI requirements.
- *Reevaluate potential causes of underlying system problems.* Methods used to identify the causes, effectiveness of the methods, and analysis of results all could have led to errors in identifying causes.
- *Reevaluate changes made for improvement.* A common cause of a change failing to result in improvement is that the change was implemented inconsistently or was unexpectedly discontinued; possible reasons are communication issues, insufficient training, or resistance to change and are the typical challenges that may contribute to an unsuccessful change.
- *Increase number of changes per week/month, etc.* When a team has insufficient resources or time, it may implement changes slowly, which

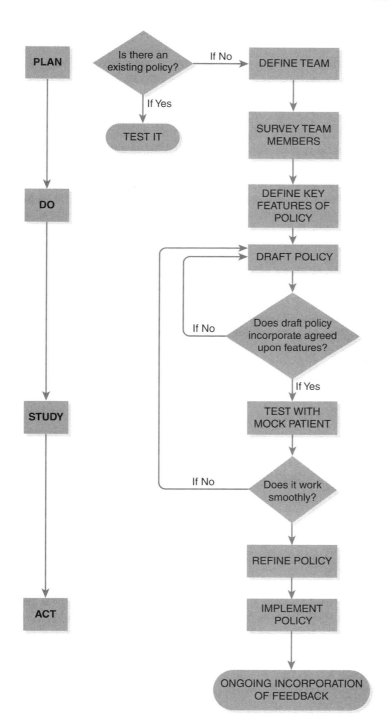

Figure 10-4. Plan-Do-Study-Act Cycle of Policy Development
Reproduced from Bonner, L., Felker, B., Chaney, E., Vollen, K., Berry, K., Revay, B., ... Sherman, S. (February 2005). Suicide risk response: Enhancing patient safety through development of effective institutional policies. In Agency for Healthcare Research and Quality (AHRQ), *Advances in patient safety (Vol. 3: Implementation issues)*. AHRQ publication No. 05-0021-3. Retrieved from http://www.ahrq.gov /professionals/quality-patient-safety/patient-safety-resources /resources/advances-in-patient-safety/index.html

slows the rate of performance improvement. A recommendation for this scenario is to include other staff members to assist with incremental tasks, such as testing the changes so the CQI team can work on multiple factors simultaneously to improve systems.

It is important to not focus just on problems but to also recognize success. What does the HCO do when a CQI project is successful and helpful, meaning care has improved and there is greater understanding of positive staff engagement? HCO and team celebration is just as important as the other steps. Teams need to remember that healthcare delivery is complex, and there is no single magic answer to CQI challenges. For many problems, it takes multiple changes, but celebrating along the way is critical in engaging staff, developing a culture of safety, and improving quality care. The CQI team needs to evaluate the process and consider the HHS, HRSA's (2011b) advice: "Continue on the same path, work on a different part of the system, test changes in more situations, and spread the improvement" (pp. 20–21).

As Kelly and colleagues (2013) state, "Variation is the extent to which a process differs from the norm" (p. 79). Understanding variation within an HCO helps to understand connections with variation within the HCO, its processes, resources used, adverse events, and patient outcomes. HCO management has to determine if the amount of variation is acceptable performance. Understanding a process needs to include consideration of the people involved and technical concerns. Processes have requirements, which are also the criteria that are used to evaluate a process, and impact the inputs needed to design the process and also the outputs of the process. Elements that are important are inclusion of customers such as patients and other stakeholders and listening to their feedback. For example, what do stakeholders expect? How are services selected, designed, and improved? And how are outcomes measured?

Analysis of data requires thoughtful planning and choice of methods. Some of the common methods are described below, although root cause analysis is the most common method used in HCOs. The Connect to Current Information section at the end of the chapter provides links to sites that describe some of the following methods.

Root Cause Analysis

Root cause analysis (RCA) is a method used by many HCOs today to analyze errors, supporting the recognition that most errors are caused by system issues and not necessarily individual staff issues. The HHS, AHRQ's Health Information Technology (2013b) branch explains that RCA is a process that "allows the analyst or analyzing team to identify the exact issue, identify the reason for the problems occurrence, and develop means to prevent the issue from recurring or reduce the probability that it will happen again."

The reasoning behind RCA may seem to imply there is only one cause for an error. Using the Swiss cheese model of errors, discussed elsewhere in this text, the focus is on multiple errors and system flaws that often intersect for a critical incident to reach the patient. Labeling one or even several of these factors as "causes" may overemphasize specific "holes in the cheese" and obscure others, decreasing understanding of the overall relationships between different layers and other aspects of system design (HHS, AHRQ, PSNet, 2014b; NPSF, 2015). The RCA process includes the following steps (HHS, AHRQ, HIT, 2013b):

1. Select the team to complete the RCA. The team should include experts related to the event. For example, if the error occurred in the intensive care unit for postcardiac surgical patients, team members should include representatives from the intensive care unit, operating room, and anesthesiology staffs, as well as other relevant healthcare professionals such as cardiac surgeons and nurses, laboratory technicians, radiologist, infusion team, pharmacy, and infection control. Management should also be represented, and staff educators may participate.
2. Create a flowchart, as described earlier in this chapter.
3. Examine the flowchart for areas of failure.
4. Use team methods to assist the team in discussing and identifying underlying causes.
5. Use CQI tools to relate data collected to possible root causes.
6. Redesign the process for improvement (if required) based on the analysis results.
7. Implement the changes first through a pilot, and then spread to other areas as appropriate for the improvement strategy/intervention.

This analysis is in depth, follows specific steps, and should focus on the system, not individual staff. Its major purpose is to identify causes and then consider changes that might be required to reduce risk of reoccurrence.

The team analyzing the problem or error usually uses brainstorming, flowcharts, and cause–effect diagrams. The goal is to clearly describe the problem and all factors related to it. Typical contributing factors are categorized as follows:

- *Environmental factors* (e.g., work environment, staff safety, safety culture type, ethical/legal concerns)
- *Organizational factors* (e.g., staffing levels/mix, staff availability and roles, support staff, clear policies, administrative support, effective leadership, access to equipment and supplies, documentation, use of rounds and other communication methods, attitudes toward patients and families, patient-centered care)
- *Staff/team* (e.g., supervision of staff, communication, team membership, quality of teamwork, team leadership and functioning, availability of expertise)
- *Individual staff factors* (e.g., level of knowledge, competence, and experience; fatigue; stress; expectations; position description; staff safety)

- *Task factors* (e.g., clear protocols and/or guidelines, use of checklists, lab tests and other procedures, description of tasks, policies)
- *Patient factors* (e.g., stress, communication, accessible patient information, diversity factors, comorbidities, status on admission, past history, 30-day unplanned readmission, discharge plans)

Key questions that are asked during RCA include the following:

- What happened?
- Who was involved?
- When did it happen?
- Where did it happen?
- What is the severity of the actual or potential harm?
- What is the likelihood of reoccurrence?
- What are the consequences?

There are multiple methods used during RCA, but one common method focuses on the "five whys" to "figure out something that went wrong and ask why; then in answer to that reason ask why again and so on" (HHS, HRSA, 2011c). In addition to the preceding questions, the team may ask the following (HHS, HRSA, April 2011a):

- What proof do I have that this cause exists? (Is it concrete? Is it measurable?)
- What proof do I have that this cause could lead to the stated effect? (Am I merely asserting causation?)
- What proof do I have that this cause actually contributed to the problem I'm looking at? (Even given that the cause exists and could lead to this problem, how do I know it wasn't actually something else?)
- Is anything else needed, along with this cause, for the stated effect to occur? (Is it self-sufficient? Is something needed to help it along?)
- Can anything else, besides this cause, lead to the stated effect? (Are there alternative explanations that fit better? What other risks are there?)

RCA results should provide a clearer picture of the problem and options for preventing additional errors or problems. Then choices can be made as to the best approach to take; however, whenever possible, evidence or best practice should also be used to support decisions. The process should include an interprofessional team of staff who are knowledgeable about the issue or problem, thereby increasing the chance that the analysis will be complete and decisions effective (HHS, AHRQ, PSNet, 2014b).

Health care has borrowed and adapted models and methods from a variety of industries; for example, some of the leadership theories and models that are often applied to healthcare delivery originated in other industries. RCA is one of the methods that was adopted. Despite the common use of RCA, there actually are limited data supporting its effectiveness. There are problems with how RCA results are interpreted, and there is no consensus as to how an HCO should analyze data for RCA or follow-up. Another issue is that few formal mechanisms exist for analysis of multiple RCAs across institutions. Each time the RCA process is used, it might be considered to be a case study focused on a specific event in a specific HCO. In addition, there should be an analysis of multiple RCAs from multiple HCOs to identify trends and patterns (macro and aggregate data), and then this information is used to recommend changes in health care that would apply across HCOs. The Joint Commission expects its accredited HCOs to use RCA, and some states require use of RCA as part of their state HCO regulations. Outcomes may then be reported to The Joint Commission or to the state regulators. So despite the need for greater supporting evidence to determine the value of using RCA, it continues to be an important analysis method.

The National Patient Safety Foundation (NPSF) issued a report in 2015 renaming RCA, RCA squared (RCA^2). The reason for this change is to emphasize the need to use RCA to identify adverse events, hazards, and HCOs vulnerable for future events. In doing this, the HCO needs to identify and take steps to prevent a repetition of these events, which is the most important step in the RCA, or RCA^2, process. To improve RCA and establish the RCA^2 approach, the report makes the following recommendations:

- Leadership (e.g., CEO, board of directors) should be actively involved in the RCA and action process, supporting the process. This involvement includes approving and periodically reviewing the status of actions, understanding what a thorough RCA^2 report should include, and taking actions when reviews do not meet minimum requirements.
- Leadership should review the RCA^2 process at least annually for effectiveness.
- Blameworthy events that are not appropriate for RCA^2 review should be defined.
- HCOs should use a transparent, formal, and explicit risk-based prioritization system to identify adverse events, close calls, and system vulnerabilities requiring RCA^2 review.
- An RCA^2 review should be started within 72 hours of recognizing that a review is needed.
- RCA^2 teams should be composed of four to six people. The team should include process experts as well as other individuals drawn from all levels of the organization, and the team should consider inclusion of a patient representative unrelated to the event. Team membership should *not* include individuals who were involved in the event or close call being reviewed, but those individuals should be interviewed for information. (Some HCOs include staff on the team who were involved.)
- Time should be provided during the normal work shift for staff to serve on an RCA^2 team, including attending meetings, researching, and conducting interviews.

- Common RCA[2] tools (e.g., interviewing techniques, flow diagramming, cause and effect diagramming, five rules of causation, action hierarchy, process/outcome measures) should be used by teams to assist in the investigation process and identification of strong and intermediate-strength corrective actions.
- Feedback should be provided to staff involved in the event as well as to patients and/or family members regarding findings of the RCA[2] process.[1]

Some HCOs are now using a new rapid RCA[2] approach, called "SWARMing" (Li et al., 2015). SWARMs may be part of RCAs and are conducted without delay after a reported event. The first step is a preliminary investigation into what happened and who was involved, followed by an in-person meeting with the interprofessional team and any staff directly involved in the event. Following this, a full RCA is conducted.

Failure Mode and Effects Analysis

Failure mode and effects analysis (FMEA) is one example of a prospective analysis method. This method can also be used as a retrospective method when RCA is used in combination with FMEA. When they are combined, the analysis considers the probability of failure and also consequences of failure (Wachter, 2008). FMEA is focused on known or potential problems and errors, with the goal "to prevent errors by attempting to identify all the ways a process could fail, estimate the probability and consequences of each failure, and then take action to prevent the potential failures from occurring" (Hughes, 2008). FMEA requires identification of all steps in the process and a description of potential problems with each step, probability, and impact. In this analysis of the problem, the team identifies those areas or steps that are at higher risk for problems (HHS, AHRQ, PSNet, 2015). FMEA reliability has been questioned by some experts, as there can be variation in opinions when it is used. This factor needs to be considered when FMEA is used.

Fishbone Analysis

Fishbone analysis is a problem analysis tool. It allows the team to identify causes of a problem. It requires the team to be open and consider all possible causes and then add ideas to the fishbone graphic. Brainstorming is typically used to stimulate the process and idea formulation. The visual can then be used to identify and discuss the possible causes.

Define and Measure-Analyze-Design-Verify

Define and measure-analyze-design-verify (DMADV) is a method used by Six Sigma. Using this method, project goals and outcomes are defined, the process is analyzed, a

---

[1] Reproduced from National Patient Safety Foundation (NPSF). (2015). RCA2 : Improving root cause analyses and actions to prevent harm. Retrieved from http://www.npsf.org/?page=RCA2.

detailed description of the process is developed, and then performance is verified. Another method used by Six Sigma is define and measure-analyze-improve-control (DMAIC), which completes the same activities described for the first two DMADV steps. In the third step, however, the process is improved by removing defects so that future performance is controlled. Six Sigma is an approach to QI that is focused on using data, reducing variation, and eliminating defects or deviations in processes. DMADV is typically used when a new process or product needs to be developed or when there is a process or product that has been changed but more improvement is needed (iSixSigma, 2016a).

Gap Analysis

Gap analysis is a method for examining current status. The analysis focuses on where the organization, department, or unit and the staff want to go. The difference in current status and future vision is referred to as the "gap." The gap may then guide actions to improve. Further detailed analysis and planning are then required.

Value Stream Mapping

Value stream mapping is a method used in Six Sigma. It documents, analyzes, and improves the flow of information or supplies that are needed to complete a process or produce a product (iSixSigma, 2016b). Elements include mapping to identify the process boundaries, the process steps, information flows, process data, the timeline, and stakeholders; interpreting data; and planning next steps.

Brainstorming

Brainstorming is a method used to identify the most ideas possible and can also be used during analysis to determine both prospective and retrospective views. Examples of brainstorming are I PASS the BATON, the Delphi technique, and the nominal group. These methods are discussed elsewhere in this text as methods used in the change process; however, here they may also be used in the analysis of CQI problems.

Deep Dive

Deep dive is an in-depth brainstorming technique that is used ideally by an interprofessional team. All members actively participate in the process—engaging frontline staff in the change process to improve care. Deep dive focuses on ensuring that the critical participants in the workplace are involved. It is a structured approach, with a plan for implementing change, including aspects such as agenda, time spent storytelling and identifying what is disturbing staff and possible resolutions, use of methods to post ideas so that they can be viewed by the team for assessment and discussion, and use of voting or selection methods. Deep dive is a critical method used in Transforming Care at the Bedside, an important nursing initiative to improve care and engage nursing staff in the process, which is described elsewhere in this text (IHI, 2016c).

Stop and Consider #3

CQI analysis requires an in-depth view of a CQI problem.

National Healthcare Measurement Programs

The number of national healthcare measurement programs has increased, particularly since the first *Quality Chasm* reports in 1999. The NQS is very important in stimulating further development in aggregate or macro-initiatives rather than just focusing on an individual HCO's QI program (microlevel). There are, however, now many measures/indicators that have been developed to assist efforts to measure care. The following content provides examples of initiatives that identify multiple measures/indicators, illustrating the complexity and choices for CQI measurement (Chassin, Loeb, Schmaltz, & Wachter, 2010, pp. 1–3; HHS, CMS, 2015; NAS/HMD, 2015):

- The Centers for Medicare and Medicaid Services (CMS) Measures Inventory is used by the Medicare and Medicaid programs to assess their quality; it includes nearly 1,700 measures/indicators.
- The NQF measure database includes 620 measures. The NQF does not develop measures, but rather reviews and endorses measures. Its web-based system, Quality Positioning System, provides access to the endorsed measures.
- The National Committee for Quality Assurance's Healthcare Effectiveness Data and Information Set, used by more than 90% of health insurance plans, includes 81 different measures.
- The Joint Commission requires hospitals to provide data for specified measures.

An important example of the impact of new models of care on measurement is the movement to establish accountable care methods by developing accountable care organizations (ACOs), which is a provision in the Patient Protection and Affordable Care Act of 2010 (ACA). This model focuses on replacing the fragmented and uncoordinated care system described by the *Quality Chasm* reports, recognizing the need for a system that integrates care received by a patient, with payment incentives aimed at individual and population health outcomes (Fisher, Staiger, Bynum, & Gottlieb, 2007). The CMS, the federal agency responsible for implementing the ACO model, has launched several programs to support the ACO model, including the Medicare Shared Savings Program, the Pioneer model, the Advance Payment initiative, and Medicaid ACOs. In addition, private insurers, employers, and others support ACOs, and some have established these programs. By early 2015, estimates indicated that 744 ACOs were established, illustrating growth from 64 in 2011 (Muhlestein, 2015). Monitoring care quality is part of the ACO model. In early 2016, the acting administrator of the CMS reported that the following developments can be expected in the near future:

> There will be over 475 new ACOs with 30,000 physicians participating around the country, including 64 that are 2-sided or full risk, up from 19 just last year, and of course zero before the Affordable Care Act. In total, 8.9 million Medicare FFS beneficiaries, or greater than 1 in 5, in 49 states and the District of Colombia, will now be a part of an ACO, with 1.6 million in better, more advanced models. (CMS Blog, 2016)

Due to the ACA, 30% of Medicare payments are now connected to alternative payment models such as the ACO, with 10 million Medicare patients getting improved care due to more time with their physicians and improved coordinated care (HHS, 2016). **Table 10-6** describes a coordinated care model developed by the AHRQ.

Other care delivery changes such as patient-centered medical homes, clinics devoted to high-risk patients, team-based care models, and retail clinics also indicate the need for monitoring measures that meet the needs of these new models of care. The ACA focuses primarily on changes in healthcare payment with "the emphasis on requiring healthcare insurance and penalties for not carrying such insurance and establishment of the insurance marketplaces to expand individual access to insurance plans if not provided by employer" (KFF, 2014). The law does include some CQI provisions, as noted in Appendix A. Changing reimbursement requirements does, however, in itself influence QI. When people have more access to care, there is greater chance that they will get care when needed and reach care outcomes. In addition, the increase in patients requesting care impacts the risk of complications and errors; there may be greater incidence due to the greater number of potential patients, and some of them may have complex needs. Another problem that is increasing is changes in the insurance marketplaces due to some insurers dropping out of participation. This has an impact on patients receiving care when they need from a consistent provider.

Centers for Medicare and Medicaid Services Quality Core Measures

The CMS bases its QI goals on four principles: (1) Eliminate racial and ethnic disparities, (2) strengthen infrastructure and data systems, (3) enable local innovations, and (4) foster learning organizations (HHS, CMS, 2015, p. 9). The CMS is mandated by the ACA to assess the quality of its services. This effort is also connected with the NQS, which was first described in 2011 and provides the broad aims and priorities that guide the HHS and CMS quality initiatives. The overall vision for the CMS Quality Strategy is to optimize health outcomes by improving quality and transforming the healthcare system (HHS, CMS, 2016). The CMS includes many

Table 10-6 Care Coordination Measures		
Type of Care Coordination	**Description**	**Example**
Coordination within a provider team/site	Coordination between individuals employed by or acting for a healthcare organization (defined by a single administrative management)	A measure assessing adequacy and timeliness of follow-up on ordered tests in the ambulatory care setting
Coordination across provider teams/sites	Coordination between individuals employed by or acting for different healthcare organizations that do not share institutional or administrative management systems	A measure assessing the quality of discharge documentation sent from a hospital to a long-term care facility at the time of hospital discharge
Coordination between providers and patient/caregiver	Coordination between healthcare workers and the patient, family members, or caregivers (often nonprofessionals) with responsibility for providing care to the patient	A measure assessing contacts between the primary care team and patients/caregivers between ambulatory visits
Coordination between providers and community	Coordination between healthcare workers and community-based organizations on behalf of the patient	A measure assessing communication between pediatricians and school staff for pediatric patients with developmental disorders

Reproduced from Agency for Healthcare Research and Quality & National Quality Measures Clearinghouse. (June 18, 2015). Finding care coordination measures. Retrieved from https://www.qualitymeasures.ahrq.gov/tutorial/CareCoordination.aspx

partners to ensure a comprehensive approach. Its measure domains are as follows (HHS, CMS, 2015, p. 2):

- Patient safety
- Patient and family engagement
- Care coordination
- Clinical process/effectiveness
- Population/public health
- Efficient use of healthcare resources

These measures are reviewed and changed as needed over time. **Table 10-7** describes the relationship between the NQS and the CMS Quality Strategy per measure.

The CMS believes its efforts are in the best interest of all patients, stating the following:

> Everyone receiving healthcare in the nation is likely to benefit from CMS programs and initiatives, as healthcare professionals engage in delivery system reform to achieve better care for patients, better health for the U.S. population, and lower costs through quality improvement. (HHS, CMS, 2015, p. 7)

The reason for this optimism is that most hospitals have Medicare patients, and in meeting requirements for these patients, the hospitals will improve care for all patients.

Patient Safety Organizations

The AHRQ is mandated by Congress to support the development of patient safety organizations (PSOs), but the federal government does not fund PSOs. To be certified as a PSO requires that the organization collect and analyze data in a standardized manner, such as applying the Common Formats developed by the AHRQ (HHS, AHRQ, PSO, 2016b). A PSO is an entity or component of another organization that may carry out or provide services on behalf of a PSO or a healthcare provider, including the following services (HHS, AHRQ, PSO, 2016a):

1. Efforts to improve patient safety and quality of healthcare delivery
2. Collection and analysis of patient safety work product (PSWP)
3. Development and dissemination of information regarding patient safety, such as recommendations, protocols, or information regarding best practices
4. Utilization of PSWP for the purposes of encouraging a culture of safety as well as providing feedback and assistance to effectively minimize patient risk
5. Maintenance of procedures to preserve confidentiality with respect to PSWP
6. Provision of appropriate security measures with respect to PSWP
7. Utilization of qualified staff
8. Initiation of activities related to the operation of a patient safety evaluation system and provision of feedback to participants in a patient safety evaluation system

In providing these services, PSOs, acting as independent, external experts, assist HCOs in improving healthcare delivery. Since patient data are part of these services, it is important that this communication be protected. PSOs gather data from multiple HCOs and then are able to analyze aggregate data about patient safety events to better understand these events.

Table 10-7 National Quality Strategy and CMS Quality Strategy

National Quality Strategy Priorities	CMS Quality Strategy Goals and Objectives	Measure Domains (Abbreviated)
1. Making care safer by reducing the harm caused in the delivery of care	Goal 1: Make care safer by reducing harm caused in the delivery of care. ■ Improve support for a culture of safety. ■ Reduce inappropriate and unnecessary care. ■ Prevent or minimize harm in all settings.	Patient Safety (Safety)
2. Ensuring that each person and family are engaged as partners in their care	Goal 2: Strengthen person and family engagement as partners in their care. ■ Ensure all care delivery incorporates patient and caregiver preferences. ■ Improve experience of care for patients, caregivers, and families. ■ Promote patient self-management.	Patient and Family Engagement (Patient Engagement)
3. Promoting effective communication and coordination of care	Goal 3: Promote effective communication and coordination of care. ■ Reduce admissions and readmissions. ■ Embed best practices to manage transitions to all practice settings. ■ Enable effective healthcare system navigation.	Care Coordination (Care Coordination)
4. Promoting the most effective prevention and treatment practices for the leading causes of mortality, starting with cardiovascular disease	Goal 4: Promote effective prevention and treatment of chronic disease. ■ Increase appropriate use of screening and prevention services. ■ Strengthen interventions to prevent heart attacks and strokes. ■ Improve quality of care for patients with multiple chronic conditions. ■ Improve behavioral health access and quality care. ■ Improve perinatal outcomes.	Clinical Process/ Effectiveness (Effective Treatment)

National Quality Strategy Priorities	CMS Quality Strategy Goals and Objectives	Measure Domains (Abbreviated)
5. Working with communities to promote wide use of best practices to enable healthy living	Goal 5: Work with communities to promote best practices of healthy living. ■ Partner with and support federal, state, and local public health improvement efforts. ■ Improve access within communities to best practices of healthy living. ■ Promote evidence-based community interventions to prevent and treat chronic disease. ■ Increase use of community-based social services support.	Population/Public Health (Healthy Communities)
6. Making quality care affordable for individuals, families, employers, and governments by developing and spreading new healthcare delivery models (affordable care)	Goal 6: Make care affordable. ■ Develop and implement payment systems that reward value over volume. ■ Use cost analysis data to inform payment policies.	Efficient Use of Healthcare Resources (Affordable Care)

Reproduced from Centers for Medicare and Medicaid Services (CMS) & Center for Clinical Standards and Quality. (March 2, 2015). 2015 national impact assessment of the Centers for Medicare & Medicaid Services (CMS) quality measures report. Retrieved from https://www.cms.gov/Medicare/Quality-Initiatives-Patient-Assessment-Instruments/QualityMeasures/Downloads/2015-National-Impact-Assessment-Report.pdf

Healthcare Effectiveness Data and Information Systems

Nurses primarily think about CQI in relation to healthcare providers and HCOs that provide care. There is, however, more than CQI focused on clinical practice, as the issue of insurer/third-party payer quality is also important. The Healthcare Effectiveness Data and Information Set (HEDIS®) is a tool that is supported by the National Committee for Quality Assurance. It is used by more than 90% of U.S. health plans to measure their performance, but it also provides performance measurement options for physician provider organizations (PPOs), physicians, and other HCOs.

Its 81 measures cover five domains, providing data for plans to compare themselves (NCQA, 2016). The HEDIS® report card, Quality Compass®, is an interactive web-based comparison tool that assists employers and consumers in choosing the best health insurance plan for them by comparing plans that participate in this report card or performance measurement report. The Connect to Current Information section at the end of the chapter provides a link to the HEDIS® site.

National Healthcare Quality and Disparities Reports

The *National Healthcare Quality and Disparities Report* is discussed elsewhere in this text. In this chapter, it is important to note that this national report provides national data focused on specific indicators related to quality and diversity. This information is useful to HCOs as they plan their QI programs because the reports identify national elements of care delivery that are improving, and those that are not should then be considered when HCOs identify specific areas of concern for their CQI planning (HHS, AHRQ, 2015b).

AHRQ QI™

The AHRQ QI™ is used to "highlight potential quality concerns, identify areas that need further study and investigation, and track changes over time" (HHS, AHRQ, 2015a). As an HHS agency, the AHRQ provides free software to hospitals. This software is used to collect data and submit data to the AHRQ based on indicators identified by the AHRQ. This tool allows hospitals to compare their data to national benchmarks. This is an example of a national effort used to monitor some aspects of care and provide individual hospitals with tools to collect data and guidelines for improving care. Examples of these indicators, which were identified in 2009, include the following (HHS, AHRQ, 2015a):

- *Prevention quality indicators.* These indicators focus on preventing additional hospitalization or are used to indicate need for early intervention to avoid complications and change negative change in disease status. The indicators rely on use of inpatient discharge data and help communities assess needs and patient self-management needs.
- *Inpatient quality indicators.* Using hospital administrative data, these indicators focus on hospital quality care (e.g., mortality rates; utilization and volume of procedures that might be overused, underused, or misused; risk for mortality).
- *Pediatric quality indicators.* These indicators examine care in hospitals for pediatric patients.
- *Home and community-based services.* These indicators focus on Medicaid beneficiaries who are receiving home and community-based services.

- *Patient safety indicators (PSIs).* These hospital indicators examine hospital complications and adverse events, particularly following procedures, surgery, and childbirth; includes 18 provider-level indicators established by the AHRQ to screen for adverse patient events.

Use of PSI provides aggregate data per hospital applied to a number of events that are identified by the PSIs. A study, using a retrospective, multifacility, cross-sectional chart abstraction, addressed the question of whether the AHRQ PSIs could be used to improve nursing care (Zrelack, Utter, Cuny, & Romano, 2012). The researchers identified specific potential nursing opportunities for the following indicators: central line-related bloodstream infection, postoperative deep vein thrombosis or pulmonary embolus, postoperative respiratory failure, and pressure ulcer. The study notes that there were common trends in the data: "lack of documentation of accurate and timely patient assessment, lack of adherence to national standards of care related to prophylaxis or prevention, and delays in recognition and intervention" (Zrelack et al., 2012, pp. 103–104). The researchers commented there was need for greater recognition of the importance of nursing roles to prevent and identify complications before they become worse. Data from the PSI are a good source for nurses to better understand nursing care improvement.

Healthcare Cost and Utilization Project

The Healthcare Cost and Utilization Project (HCUP) is an online resource that includes a number of databases developed and maintained by the AHRQ to provide data about hospital discharges from the majority of the states. Data from state data organizations, hospital associations, private data organizations, and the federal government are updated quarterly and annually. HCUP, with its extensive data collection of longitudinal hospital data, is an important source for providers, policy makers, and others who need this information (HHS, AHRQ, HCUP, 2015a). Currently, the databases focus on national inpatient data, state inpatient data, state ambulatory surgery and services, pediatric services, and emergency departments. Over time, additional data and information may be added to this source.

National Quality Measures Clearinghouse

The National Quality Measures Clearinghouse (NQMC) is a government/public resource that describes evidence-based quality measures and measure sets that may be used by HCOs (HHS, AHRQ, NQMC, 2015b). The AHRQ manages this resource. It is a database of measures that meet specific inclusion criteria. The goal is to provide more consistent measures for CQI and provide a resource that organizes measures so that HCOs and healthcare providers have a more accessible source of multiple measures. The measures found in the NQMC are used to assess the performance of clinicians, clinical delivery teams, delivery organizations, or health insurance plans (HHS, AHRQ, NQMC, 2015a).

This clearinghouse of measures focuses on two major categories of measures. **Healthcare delivery measures** are measures of care delivered to individuals and populations defined by their relationship to clinicians, clinical delivery teams, delivery organizations, or health insurance plans. **Population health measures** are measures that address health issues of individuals or populations defined by residence in a geographic area or a relationship to organizations that are not primarily organized to deliver or pay for healthcare services (such as schools or prisons) (HHS, AHRQ, NQMC, 2015a). **Figure 10-5** describes the NQMC Domain Framework.

Stop and Consider #4
National healthcare measurement programs provide important guidance to HCOs.

Multiple Roles of Nurses in Quality Improvement: Monitoring, Collecting Data, and Analyzing

As discussed in this chapter, there are multiple methods used to identify and track errors or potential errors. However, no matter how much is done to identify and/or track errors, if staff do not report problems or potential problems, and then if little or nothing is done to take action to improve, CQI will not be effective. Use of these tools requires more than just applying the tools. It requires analysis and use of critical thinking. CQI is commonly assumed to be a management function. In the long run, this view removed nurses from CQI or led nurses to believe it was not their responsibility to participate, let alone lead, CQI activities. It is clear that such thinking has not been helpful. Nurses provide much of the direct care and in this role can provide quality care, intervene to prevent problems, and participate in all phases of the CQI process. Nurses should be active in, monitoring, data collection, analysis, and developing strategies/interventions to prevent or respond to CQI problems. Including nurses in all levels of CQI planning helps ensure that nurses are involved and their ideas and experience are added to the QI program.

Each HCO needs to communicate and commit to engaging all staff, not just clinical staff, in CQI. Efforts include improving documentation, providing a cleaner environment, ensuring that equipment is maintained and functioning safely, monitoring drug supplies so they are available when needed, keeping supplies current and accessible, helping to make food nutritious and attractive to patients, answering telephones, and helping to keep computers working effectively. As Harrington (2009) states, "Quality improvement is about ensuring that the organization works

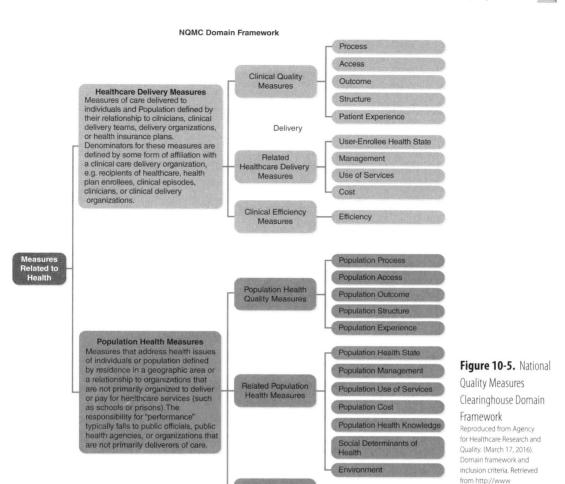

Figure 10-5. National Quality Measures Clearinghouse Domain Framework
Reproduced from Agency for Healthcare Research and Quality. (March 17, 2016). Domain framework and inclusion criteria. Retrieved from http://www .qualitymeasures.ahrq.gov /about/domain-framework.aspx

effectively and efficiently, all aspects of the organization" (p. 44). As such, staff should participate in the following (Harrington, 2009, p. 44):

- Identifying risk situations or situations where work process could be improved
- Communicating concerns in a clear manner to appropriate persons
- Committing to improvement, improving job performance every day
- Participating in organization wide or unit/department focused CQI activities
- Participating in improving knowledge base and competencies
- Caring about the patient, putting the patient in the center of care

Stop and Consider #5

Nurses have often avoided active participation in all phases of CQI measurement.

Conclusions

This chapter provides a toolbox of information about monitoring, measuring, and analyzing care quality. Methods are described to meet the CQI process elements that should be considered when an HCO develops its QI program and associated plans. There are multiple methods that an HCO may choose to use. In addition to the HCO-focused CQI initiatives, there are now more national CQI measurement initiatives that make a difference to healthcare status and influence the HCO's CQI activities. Several examples were discussed, and others are discussed in other sections of this text. As noted in the *Future of Nursing* report (IOM, 2010) and by other experts, the nursing profession needs to assume more responsibilities in CQI activities, as individual nurses providing care, as managers and leaders, and as members of professional organizations, and they must participate in CQI health policy development, implementation, and evaluation. Nurses need to be familiar with the methods used and then participate in their use on a routine basis in the work environment, and they must properly use data to inform decision-making.

APPLY CQI

Chapter Highlights

- Measurement is a complex process that is critical to the success of QI programs.
- There are many methods used to monitor care and collect data for quality improvement (QI). HCOs must choose methods as they plan and implement their QI program.
- Measures/indicators are an important part of an HCO's QI program. They help identify the focus of QI efforts and are used to track progress.
- HCOs use utilization review/management to better understand conditions that impact the quality of care, such as use of nursing services and length of treatment. Risk management is used to identify potential risk, such as financial loss, with the goal of mitigating or eliminating the risk in a timely, effective manner.
- There are many methods used to analyze care quality; however, root cause analysis is the most common method.
- There are a number of national initiatives that address national healthcare measurement, mostly led by the Agency for Healthcare Research and Quality (AHRQ), but also by the Centers for Medicare and Medicaid Services

(CMS). Initiative examples, which are influenced by the National Quality Strategy, are the CMS Quality Core Measures, Healthcare Effectiveness Data and Information Systems, patient safety organizations, Healthcare Effectiveness Data and Information Systems, *National Healthcare Quality and Disparities Report*, and AHRQ QI™, which includes the Healthcare Cost and Utilization Project and the National Quality Measures Clearinghouse.

- Nurses need to be involved in all aspects of QI measurement.

Critical Thinking and Clinical Reasoning and Judgment: Discussion Questions and Learning Activities

1. Develop a comparison chart of the following: dashboard, check sheet, survey, interview, observation, run chart, Pareto chart, flowchart, benchmarking, and report card.
2. What are the advantages and disadvantages of mandatory and voluntary reporting? Do you think nursing students understand this issue and the need for them to report errors as students and then as registered nurses?
3. Compare and contrast the methods used to analyze quality: root cause analysis, fishbone analysis, FMEA, DMADV, gap analysis, brainstorming, and deep dive.
4. What is the nurse's role in CQI measurement?

Connect to Current Information

- CDC: *Morbidity and Mortality Weekly Reports*
  http://www.cdc.gov/mmwr/index.html
- Examples of flowcharts
  https://www.google.com/search?q=flow+charts+templates&client=
    safari&sa=X&rls=en&biw=1324&bih=1019&tbm=isch&tbo=u&
    source=univ&ved=0ahUKEwiM8Pi_253KAhXGyyYKHTXoBDIQsAQINg
- Examples of run charts
  http://www.bing.com/images/search?q=run+chart&qpvt=run+chart&qpvt=
    run+chart&FORM=IGRE
- Examples of fishbone charts
  http://www.bing.com/images/search?q=fishbone+analysis&qpvt=Fish-
    bone+analysis&qpvt=Fishbone+analysis&FORM=IGRE
- Examples of check/tally sheets
  https://www.google.com/search?q=tally+sheets&client=safari&
    rls=en&tbm=isch&tbo=u&source=univ&sa=X&ved=0ahUK
    Ewi-6JuF-p_KAhVHLSYKHT9uAagGsAQIHA&biw=1324&bih=1019
- Examples of dashboards
  Government dashboards
  http://dashboard.healthit.gov/dashboards/dashboards.php

Nongovernment dashboards

https://www.google.com/search?q=health+care+dashboards&client=
    safari&rls=en&tbm=isch&tbo=u&source=univ&sa=X&ved=0ahUKEwiYuurT-5_
    KAhVEPiYKHe9dDTQQsAQITg&biw=1324&bih=1019

- Examples of value stream mapping

https://www.google.com/search?q=value+stream+mapping&client=safari&
    rls=en&tbm=isch&tbo=u&source=univ&sa=X&ved=0ahUKEwitmqHZ16z
    KAhUD4CYKHcC1AM0QsAQIRA&biw=1033&bih=1012

- AHRQ QI™

http://www.qualityindicators.ahrq.gov/

- AHRQ: QI™ Toolkit

http://www.ahrq.gov/professionals/systems/hospital/qitoolkit/index.html

- AHRQ: National Quality Strategy (NQS)

http://www.ahrq.gov/workingforquality/

- AHRQ: Common Formats

http://www.pso.ahrq.gov/common

- NCQA: Healthcare Effectiveness Data and Information Systems (HEDIS®)

http://www.ncqa.org/tabid/59/Default.aspx

- AHRQ: *National Healthcare Quality and Disparities Report* (*QDR*)

http://www.ahrq.gov/research/findings/nhqrdr/index.html

- AHRQ: Patient Safety Indicators (PSI)

http://www.ahrq.gov/health-care-information/topics/topic-patient-safety-
    indicators.html

- AHRQ: Healthcare Cost and Utilization Project (HCUP)

http://www.ahrq.gov/research/data/hcup/index.html

- AHRQ: National Quality Measures Clearinghouse (NQMC)

http://www.qualitymeasures.ahrq.gov/

- National Quality Forum

http://www.qualityforum.org/Field_Guide/List_of_Measures.aspx

- CMS: Quality Measures

https://www.cms.gov/Medicare/Quality-Initiatives-Patient-Assessment-
    Instruments/QualityMeasures/index.html

EBP, EBM, and Quality Improvement: Exemplar

Pham, J., Girard, T., & Pronovost, P. (2013). What to do with healthcare incident reporting systems? *Journal of Public Health, 2*(3). Retrieved from http://www.ncbi.nlm.nih.gov/pmc/articles/PMC4147750/

This article examines incident reporting.

Questions to Consider

1. What is the importance of incident reporting discussed in this article?
2. Is incident reporting always effective, and if not, what are the barriers?
3. What are the challenges in using incident reporting, and how might these challenges apply to nursing?

Evolving Case Study

As nurse manager for the operating room service, you are meeting with the medical director, with whom you have worked for 5 years. You are both overwhelmed with routine work, and now you have to prepare a plan to address CQI in your department. Administration and the QI program recommend that you use the following AHRQ website, which provides a toolkit: http://www.ahrq.gov/professionals/systems/hospital/qitoolkit/index.html.

Case Questions

After reviewing the toolkit, you both decide to focus on the two most common quality care problems your department experiences. You are now ready to address next steps with the information you have.

1. Apply the AHRQ toolkit to your department and to the two focus areas of concern that you have identified.

2. Describe how you will engage the staff (clinical and nonclinical) in the new initiative.

References

Adler, L., Denham, C., McKeever, M., Purunton, R., Guilloteau, F., Moorhead, D., & Resar, R. (2008). Global trigger tool: Implementation basics. *Journal of Patient Safety, 4*(4), 245–249.

Austin, J., Jha, A., Romano, P., Singer, S., Vogus, T., Wachter, R., & Pronovost, P. (2015). National hospital ratings systems share few common scores and may generate confusion instead of clarity. *Health Affairs, 34*(3), 423–430.

Barach, P., & Johnson, K. (2013). Assessing risk and harm in clinical microsystems. In W. Sollecito & J. Johnson (Eds.), *McLaughlin and Kaluzny's continuous quality improvement in health care* (4th ed., pp. 249–274). Burlington, MA: Jones & Bartlett Learning.

Benton, J., Arm, D., & Flynn, J. (2013). Identifying and minimizing risk exposures affecting nursing practice to enhance patient safety. *Journal of Nursing Regulation, 3*(4), 5–9.

Casey, D. (2006). Fundamentals of outcomes measurement. In D. Nash & N. Goldfarb (Eds.), *The quality solution* (pp. 93–113). Sudbury, MA: Jones & Bartlett Publishers.

Chassin, M., Loeb, J., Schmaltz, S., & Wachter, R. (2010). Accountability measures—Using measurement to promote quality improvement. *The New England Journal of Medicine, 363*(7), 683–688.

CMS Blog. (2016, January 12). Comments of CMS Acting Administrator Andy Slavitt at the J.P. Morgan Annual Health Care Conference. Retrieved from http://blog.cms.gov/2016/01/12/

comments-of-cms-acting-administrator-andy-slavitt-at-the-j-p-morgan-annual-health-care-conference-jan-11-2016/

Donabedian, A. (1980). *Explorations in quality assessment and monitoring, Volume 1: The definitions of quality and approaches to its assessment.* Ann Arbor, MI: Health Administration Press.

Ettinger, W. (2006). Basic tools for quality improvement. In D. Nash & N. Goldfarb (Eds.), *The quality solution* (pp. 115–131). Sudbury, MA: Jones & Bartlett Publishers.

Evans, S., Berry, J., Smith, B., Esterman, A., Selim, P., O'Shaughnessy, J., & DeWit, M. (2006). Attitudes and barriers to incident reporting: A collaborative hospital study. *BMJ Quality Safety in Health Care, 15,* 39–43.

Finkelman, A., & Kenner, C. (2016). *Professional nursing concepts: Competencies for quality leadership* (3rd ed.). Sudbury, MA: Jones & Bartlett Publishers.

Fisher, E., Staiger, D., Bynum, J., & Gottlieb, D. (2007). Creating accountable care organizations: The extended hospital medical staff. *Health Affairs, 26*(1), 44–57.

Gottlieb, J. (2006). Analyzing quality data. In D. Nash & N. Goldfarb (Eds.), *The quality solution* (pp. 73–92). Sudbury, MA: Jones & Bartlett Publishers.

Harrington, L. (2009). Hardwiring nursing quality. *Nurse Leader, 7*(2), 44–46.

Hughes, R. (2008). Chapter 44: Tools and strategies for quality improvement and patient safety. In R. Hughes (Ed.), *Patient safety and quality: An evidence-based handbook for nurses.* Rockville, MD: Agency for Healthcare Research and Quality. Retrieved from http://www.ncbi.nlm.nih.gov/books/NBK2682/

Institute of Medicine (IOM). (2010). *The future of nursing: Leading change, advancing health.* Washington, DC: The National Academies Press.

Institute for Healthcare Improvement (IHI). (2015a). Introduction to trigger tools for identifying adverse events. Retrieved from http://www.ihi.org/resources/Pages/Tools/IntrotoTriggerToolsforIdentifyingAEs.aspx

Institute for Healthcare Improvement (IHI). (2015b). Improvement tip: Focus on harm, not errors. Retrieved from http://www.ihi.org/resources/Pages/ImprovementStories/ImprovementTipFocusonHarmNotErrors.aspx

Institute for Healthcare Improvement (IHI). (2016a). Introduction to trigger tools for identifying adverse events. Retrieved from http://www.ihi.org/resources/pages/tools/intrototriggertoolsforidentifyingaes.aspx

Institute for Healthcare Improvement (IHI). (2016b). IHI global trigger tool for measuring adverse events. Retrieved from http://www.ihi.org/resources/Pages/Tools/IHIGlobalTriggerToolforMeasuringAEs.aspx

Institute for Healthcare Improvement (IHI). (2016c). Transforming care at the bedside. Retrieved from http://www.ihi.org/resources/pages/ihiwhitepapers/transformingcareatthebedsidewhitepaper.aspx

iSixSigma. (2016a). DMAIC versus DMADV. Retrieved from http://www.isixsigma.com/new-to-six-sigma/design-for-six-sigma-dfss/dmaic-versus-dmadv/

iSixSigma. (2016b). Value stream mapping. Retrieved from http://www.isixsigma.com/tools-templates/value-stream-mapping/

Kaiser Family Foundation (KFF). (2014). Mapping marketplace enrollment. Retrieved from http://kff.org/interactive/mapping-marketplace-enrollment/

Kelly, D., Johnson, S., & Sollecito, W. (2013). Measurement, variation, and CQI tools. In W. Sollecito & J. Johnson (Eds.), *McLaughlin and Kaluzny's continuous quality improvement in health care* (4th ed., pp. 77–116). Burlington, MA: Jones & Bartlett Learning.

Keroack, M., & Rhinehart, E. (2013). The investigation and analysis of clinical incidents. In B. Youngberg (Ed.), *Patient safety handbook* (2nd ed., pp. 125–142). Burlington, MA: Jones & Bartlett Learning.

Kizer, K., & Stegun, M. (2014, October). Serious reportable adverse events in health care. In Agency for Healthcare Research and Quality (Ed.), *Advances in patient safety* (pp. 339–352). Retrieved from http://www.ncbi.nlm.nih.gov/books/NBK20598/

Levinson, D. (2012, January). *Hospital incident reporting systems do not capture most patient harm.* Washington, DC: U.S. Department of Health and Human Services.

Li, J., Boulanger, B., Norton, J., Yates, A., Swartz, C., Smith, A., . . . Williams, M. (2015). "SWARMing" to improve patient care: A novel approach to root cause analysis. *Joint Commission Quality Patient Safety, 41*, 494–501.

Mainz, J. (2003, December 6). Defining and classifying clinical indicators for quality improvement. *International Journal for Quality in Health Care.* Published online. doi:http://dx.doi.org/10.1093/intqhc/mzg081

Muhlestein, D. (2015). Growth and dispersion of accountable care organizations in 2015. Retrieved from http://healthaffairs.org/blog/2015/03/31/growth-and-dispersion-of-accountable-care-organizations-in-2015-2/

National Academy of Sciences (NAS), Health and Medicine Division (HMD). (2015). *Vital signs: Core measures for health and health care progress.* Washington, DC: The National Academies Press.

National Committee for Quality Assurance (NCQA). (2016). HEDIS® and Quality Compass®. Retrieved from http://www.ncqa.org/HEDISQualityMeasurement/WhatisHEDIS.aspx

National Patient Safety Foundation (NPSF). (2015). RCA² improving root cause analyses and actions to prevent harm. Retrieved from http://www.npsf.org/?page=RCA2

National Quality Forum (NQF). (2010, October). The ABCs of measurement. Retrieved from http://www.qualityforum.org/Measuring_Performance/ABCs_of_Measurement.aspx

Press Ganey. (2015). National database of nursing quality indicators. Retrieved from http://www.pressganey.com/solutions/clinical-quality/nursing-quality

Regenstein, M. (2013). Understanding the first Institute of Medicine report and its impact on patient safety. In B. Youngberg (Ed.), *Patient safety handbook* (2nd ed., pp. 1–16). Burlington, MA: Jones & Bartlett Learning.

Rosen, A. (2010, November). Are we getting better at measuring patient safety? WebM&M, Agency for Healthcare Research and Quality. Retrieved from http://webmm.ahrq.gov/perspective.aspx?perspectiveID=94

Sadeghi, S., Barzi, A., Mikhail, O., & Shabot, M. (2013). *Integrating quality and strategy in healthcare organizations.* Burlington, MA: Jones & Bartlett Learning.

Shojania, K. (2015, November). In conversation with . . . Kaveh Shojania, MD. *Perspectives on Safety.* Retrieved from https://psnet.ahrq.gov/perspectives/perspective/184

Storme, T. (2013). *Healthcare analytics for quality and performance improvement.* Hoboken, NJ: John Wiley & Sons, Inc.

The Joint Commission. (2012). Quality check facts. Retrieved from http://www.qualitycheck.org/help_qc_facts.aspx

U.S. Department of Health and Human Services (HHS). (2016, March 3). HHS reaches goal of typing 30 percent of Medicare payments to quality ahead of schedule. Retrieved from http://www.hhs.gov/about/news/2016/03/03/hhs-reaches-goal-tying-30-percent-medicare-payments-quality-ahead-schedule.html

U.S. Department of Health and Human Services (HHS), Agency for Healthcare Research and Quality (AHRQ). (2004, July). Frequently asked questions. AHRQ quality indicators. Retrieved from www.qualityindicators.ahrq.gov/FAQs_Support/default.aspx

U.S. Department of Health and Human Services (HHS), Agency for Healthcare Research and Quality (AHRQ). (2012). AHRQ quality indicators toolkits for hospitals. Retrieved from http://www.ahrq.gov/professionals/quality-patient-safety/index.html

U.S. Department of Health and Human Services (HHS), Agency for Healthcare Research and Quality (AHRQ). (2014, October). Toolkit for using the Quality Indicators™ Toolkit: Fact sheet. Retrieved from http://www.ahrq.gov/research/findings/factsheets/quality/qifactsheet/index.html

U.S. Department of Health and Human Services (HHS), Agency for Healthcare Quality and Research (AHRQ). (2015a). AHRQ quality indicators. Retrieved from http://www.quality-indicators.ahrq.gov

U.S. Department of Health and Human Services (HHS), Agency for Healthcare Research and Quality (AHRQ). (2015b, August). Chartbook on effective treatment. Retrieved from http://www.ahrq.gov/research/findings/nhqrdr/2014chartbooks/effectivetx/index.html

U.S. Department of Health and Human Services (HHS), Agency for Healthcare Research and Quality (AHRQ), National Quality Measures Clearinghouse (NQMC). (2015a, June 18). Domain framework and inclusion criteria. Retrieved from http://www.qualitymeasures.ahrq .gov/about/domain-framework.aspx

U.S. Department of Health and Human Services (HHS), Agency for Healthcare Research and Quality (AHRQ), National Quality Measures Clearinghouse (NQMC). (2015b, July 7). Help and about. Retrieved from http://www.qualitymeasures.ahrq.gov/faq.aspx

U.S. Department of Health and Human Services (HHS), Agency for Healthcare Research and Quality (AHRQ), Patient Safety Network (PSNet). (2014a, August). Voluntary patient safety event reporting (incident reporting). Retrieved from https://psnet.ahrq.gov/primers/primer/13/voluntary-patient-safety-event-reporting-incident-reporting

U.S. Department of Health and Human Services (HHS), Agency for Healthcare Research and Quality (AHRQ), Patient Safety Network (PSNet). (2014b, August). Root cause analysis. Retrieved from https://psnet.ahrq.gov/primers/primer/10/root-cause-analysis

U.S. Department of Health and Human Services (HHS), Agency for Healthcare Research and Quality (AHRQ), Patient Safety Network (PSNet). (2015, March). Detection of safety hazards. Retrieved from https://psnet.ahrq.gov/primers/primer/24/detection-of-safety-hazards

U.S. Department of Health and Human Services (HHS), Agency for Healthcare Research and Quality (AHRQ), Patient Safety Organization (PSO). (2016a). Common Formats. Retrieved from http://www.pso.ahrq.gov/common

U.S. Department of Health and Human Services (HHS), Agency for Healthcare Research and Quality (AHRQ), Patient Safety Organization (PSO). (2016b). Frequently asked questions. Retrieved from https://pso.ahrq.gov/faq

U.S. Department of Health and Human Services (HHS), Agency for Healthcare Research and Quality (AHRQ), Healthcare Cost and Utilization Project (HCUP). (2015a). HCUP. Retrieved from http://www.hcup-us.ahrq.gov/

U.S. Department of Health and Human Services (HHS), Agency for Healthcare Research and Quality (AHRQ), Healthcare Cost and Utilizations Project (HCUP). (2015b, December). National (nationwide) HCUP databases. Retrieved from https://www.hcup-us.ahrq.gov/databases.jsp

U.S. Department of Health and Human Services (HHS), Agency for Research and Healthcare Quality (AHRQ), Health Information Technology (HIT). (2013a, May). Flowchart. Retrieved from https://healthit.ahrq.gov/health-it-tools-and-resources/workflow-assessment-health-it-toolkit/all-workflow-tools/flowchart

U.S. Department of Health and Human Services (HHS), Agency for Research and Healthcare Quality (AHRQ), Health Information Technology (HIT). (2013b, May). Root cause analysis. Retrieved from https://healthit.ahrq.gov/health-it-tools-and-resources/workflow-assessment-health-it-toolkit/all-workflow-tools/root-cause-analysis

U.S. Department of Health and Human Services (HHS), Centers for Medicare and Medicaid Services (CMS). (2016). CMS quality strategy, 2016. Retrieved from https://www.cms.gov/

medicare/quality-initiatives-patient-assessment-instruments/qualityinitiativesgeninfo/downloads/cms-quality-strategy.pdf

U.S. Department of Health and Human Services (HHS), Centers for Medicare and Medicaid Services (CMS), Center for Clinical Standards and Quality. (2015, March 2). *2015 national impact assessment of the Centers for Medicare and Medicaid Services (CMS) quality measures report*. Retrieved from https://www.cms.gov/Medicare/Quality-Initiatives-Patient-Assessment-Instruments/QualityMeasures/Downloads/2015-National-Impact-Assessment-Report.pdf

U.S. Department of Health and Human Services (HHS), Health Resources and Services Administration (HRSA). (2010, April). Quality improvement. Retrieved from http://www.hrsa.gov/quality/toolbox/508pdfs/qualityimprovement.pdf

U.S. Department of Health and Human Services (HHS), Health Resources and Services Administration (HRSA). (2011a, April). Developing and implementing a QI plan. Retrieved from http://www.hrsa.gov/quality/toolbox/508pdfs/developingqiplan.pdf

U.S. Department of Health and Human Services (HHS), Health Resources and Services Administration (HRSA). (2011b, April). Managing data for performance improvement. Retrieved from http://www.hrsa.gov/quality/toolbox/methodology/performanceimprovement/index.html

U.S. Department of Health and Human Services (HHS), Health Resources and Services Administration (HRSA). (2011c, April). Performance management and measurement. Retrieved from http://www.hrsa.gov/quality/toolbox/508pdfs/performancemanagementandmeasurement.pdf

U.S. Department of Health and Human Services (HHS), Health Resources and Services Administration (HRSA). (2015). What sorts of metrics assess quality improvement? Retrieved form http://www.hrsa.gov/healthit/toolbox/RuralHealthITtoolbox/PatientQuality/metrics.html

U.S. Department of Health and Human Services (HHS), National Quality Strategy (NQS). (2014, September 17). National quality strategy webinar. Retrieved from http://www.ahrq.gov/workingforquality/nqs/webinar091714/webinar5.htm

U.S. Department of Health and Human Services (HHS), Office of the Inspector General (OIG). (2010, January 5). Memo to Director of the Agency for Healthcare Research and Quality: Adverse events in hospitals: Public disclosure of information about events, OEI-06-09-00360. Retrieved from http://oig.hhs.gov/oei/reports/oei-06-09-00360.pdf

U.S. Department of Health and Human Services (HHS), Office of the Inspector General (OIG). (2012, January). Hospital incident reporting systems do not capture most patient harm. Report No. OEI-06-09-00091. Retrieved from https://oig.hhs.gov/oei/reports/oei-06-09-00091.asp

Wachter, R. (2008). *Understanding patient safety*. New York, NY: McGraw Hill.

Wachter, R. (2016, January 16). How measurement fails doctors and teachers. *NYTimes*. Retrieved from http://www.nytimes.com/2016/01/17/opinion/sunday/how-measurement-fails-doctors-and-teachers.html?action=click&pgtype=Homepage&clickSource=story-heading&module=opinion-c-col-left-region&region=opinion-c-col-left-region&WT.nav=opinion-c-col-left-region&_r=0

Zrelack, P., Utter, G., Cuny, J. & Romano, P. (2012). Using the Agency for Healthcare Research and Quality patient safety indicators for targeting nursing quality improvement. *Journal of Nursing Care Quality, 27*(2), 99–10s8.

Section III

Ensuring the Healthcare Environment Is Focused on Quality

Alice:	**"Would you tell me, please which way I ought to go from here?"**
The Cheshire Cat:	**"That depends a good deal on where you want to get to."**
Alice:	**"I don't much care where."**
The Cheshire Cat:	**"Then, it doesn't matter which way you go."**
Alice...	**"So long as I get SOMEWHERE," Alice added as an explanation.**
The Cheshire Cat:	**"Oh, you're sure to do that, if only you walk long enough."**

Lewis Carroll, *Alice's Adventures in Wonderland* (1865)

© Mopic/Shutterstock

The goal of the maze is to reach a state of quality care. As you find your way to the end of the maze there is a critical aspect that must be considered that you need to care about—your roles and responsibilities as a nurse in the healthcare environment that needs major improvement. Just being there is not enough. You need to care and engage in continuous quality improvement.

Creating and Sustaining Quality Care: Prevention of Quality Care Problems

CHAPTER OBJECTIVES

At the conclusion of this chapter, the learner will be able to:

- Critique methods used to prevent or reduce quality care problems.
- Analyze the role of teamwork and the team in continuous quality improvement (CQI).
- Explain the relationship of technology and informatics in CQI.
- Examine the multiple roles and responsibilities of nurses in preventing or reducing quality care problems.

OUTLINE

KEY TERMS

Bar-code medication administration	Early warning system	Rapid response team
Call-out	Electronic health record (EHR)	Read-back
Case management	Electronic medical record (EMR)	Safe zone
Check-back	Health informatics technology (HIT)	Safety walkarounds
Checklist	Huddle	Signout
Clinical guideline	Interoperability	Situation, background, assessment, recommendation
Coaching	Meaningful use	
Comprehensive Unit-based Safety Program (CUSP)	Medication reconciliation	Spread
Clinical decision support (CDT)	Mentoring	Standard
Computerized physician/provider order entry (CPOE)	Patient-centered rounds	Teach-back
	Patient safety primer	TeamSTEPPS®
Crew resource management (CRM)	Personal health record (PHR)	Time-out
Disease management	Policy	Universal Protocol
	Procedure	Workflow

Introduction

This chapter concludes the content on the measurement process used in quality improvement (QI) programs. It is easy to view continuous quality improvement (CQI) as a process to collect data and then through analysis determine the status of care quality; however, if staff stop the process here, then care is unlikely to improve. What do healthcare organizations (HCOs) do with this information to make changes when needed to improve care? These approaches may be directed at preventing errors and quality problems, applied in response to situations in which errors or problems occur, and then used to prevent future similar situations. Some of the methods discussed in this chapter are also included in other chapters, as they may be used for several purposes during the measurement process. In addition, to critiquing examples of methods used to accomplish this goal, the chapter examines some of the nurse's roles and responsibilities in preventing or reducing quality care problems. **Figure 11-1** describes a process map of performance management, providing a summary of content that has been described in other chapters. In this chapter, the focus is on steps 5 to 6b in the process map.

Examples of Methods to Prevent or Reduce Quality Care Problems

QI programs can be viewed from multiple perspectives. The most common one, and the perspective focused on in most of this text, is a QI program that is developed, implemented, and evaluated within an HCO. In addition, we have broader perspectives, state and national perspectives, and even a global perspective. An important aspect of CQI is sustainability, which means keeping CQI going, developing strategies and changes to improve care. **Figure 11-2** describes factors that influence successful CQI implementation within an HCO.

Spread, or actively disseminating best practice and knowledge gained from the CQI process so that individual HCOs can apply them, is an important part of application at the state and national levels (IHI, 2013). Steps involved in a spread plan include the following (HHS, HRSA, 2011a, pp. 15–16):

- List changes to be spread.
- Evaluate new system against current system. Process mapping is helpful and identifies key differences; these are the areas that the spread team will focus on to make changes.
- Discuss potential impact or challenges that might result from adopting the redesigned system and developing a plan to manage those impacts.
- Create an action plan to make the changes and describe how you will capture information to monitor. Identify those areas you can just change and those areas where it might be better to test changes using methods such as plan-do-study-act methodology.

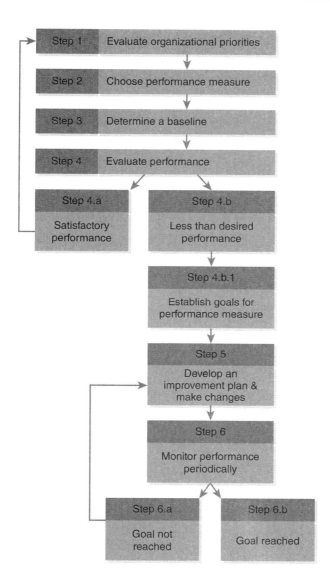

Figure 11-1. Process Map of Performance Management Pathway
Reproduced from U.S. Department Health and Human Services & Health Resources and Services Administration. (April 2011). Performance management and measurement. Retrieved from http://www.hrsa.gov/quality/toolbox/508pdfs/performancemanagementand-measurement.pdf

Spread can lead to consideration of other changes in processes for additional improvement. The CQI team needs to consider what is needed to support spread— to hardwire or ensure that the improvement is part of the work environment and practice. Factors that may be important, although they vary with the improvement focus, are staff levels and mix, expertise, staff roles and responsibilities, staff training, supplies and equipment, health informatics, policies and procedures, organizational structure and culture, management, and so on.

Figure 11-2. Factors Influencing Successful CQI Implementation

Reproduced from Sollecito, W. & Johnson, J. (2013). Factors influencing the application and diffusion in CQI in health care. In W. Sollecito & J. Johnson (Eds.), *McLaughlin & Kaluzny's Continuous quality improvement in health care* (4th ed., pp. 49–73). Burlington, MA: Jones & Bartlett Learning.

After the CQI problem is identified and analyzed, decisions are made about interventions or strategies to resolve or prevent the problem. Development of an implementation plan is discussed in more detail in other chapters but is also relevant here. The focus is on best practice, which is identified by using gap analysis—what is wrong and how can it best be corrected using available evidence (evidence-based practice [EBP] and evidence-based management [EBM]). The plan includes details about the actions or tasks that are needed, team member assignment to tasks, target completion date, tracking of the actual completion date, communication and/or training required with target dates and then actual dates of completion, implementation start date, and comments about completion of implementation (HHS, AHRQ, 2012).

Healthcare Organization and Professional Methods

HCOs and healthcare professions are concerned about CQI and use various strategies to engage in CQI and improve care. Some of these methods are done in collaboration with others, and some focus either on the HCO or a profession. The Connect to Current Information section at the end of the chapter provides links to sites that provide further information or examples for some of the methods described.

Redesigning Systems and Processes

When an HCO recognizes that it has sufficient CQI problems, it may decide to undergo a redesign or transformation to improve. This situation involves the HCO and healthcare professions within the organization, as well as other staff. Some of the common factors that might indicate the need for this step include the following (Gabow, Eisert, Karkhanis, Knight, & Dickson, 2005, p. 3):

- Little application of knowledge from other industries
- Enormous redundancies in care delivery processes
- Numerous patient handoffs
- Major workforce shortages

- Employee dissatisfaction
- Limited involvement of the patients and their families in hospital care
- Patient dissatisfaction

Redesigning the system and processes requires detailed assessment to ensure that the HCO or a specific unit of the HCO is ready to handle change, develop the description of the design or change required and structure for the redesign process, implement data collection, use effective tools to analyze the data and methods to facilitate the change, and continue to evaluate in a consistent manner. This then becomes a change cycle.

According to the Agency for Healthcare Research and Quality (AHRQ) (HHS, AHRQ, 2015c): "**Workflow** is the sequence of physical and mental tasks performed by various people within and between work environments." When you think about workflow, you need to consider that workflow happens in a variety of situations, such as within a unit, clinic, department, or HCO; between HCOs, between healthcare providers and teams, between a healthcare provider and a patient (before, during, and after an encounter); and as you think about your work, often unconsciously. These instances of workflow may occur sequentially or simultaneously. Informatics has a critical role in workflow, and changes to improve workflow often involve use of informatics. Understanding the workflow process may lead to a better understanding of multiple aspects of care delivery. Often workflow is oversimplified and not considered a critical factor in CQI; however, it is important. The AHRQ website includes tools for assessing and improving workflow.

Staffing is another factor, which has been discussed in this text. There is much literature about the need for levels of staffing that provide an effective work environment, reduce nurse fatigue and burnout, and provide nurse–patient time that reduces "rushing" and limits time with patients. Patient satisfaction and reaching patient outcomes have also been connected to staffing. Potter and colleagues (2014) discuss the complexity of meeting staffing needs:

> Certainly understaffing is a threat to patient safety. However, merely increasing the number of RNs on a patient care unit may not be a panacea if the environment in which RNs work is not conducive to clinical decision-making. Better understanding is needed with respect to the conditions in an acute care environment that affect clinical decision-making. (pp. 49–50)

Understanding of workflow and impact on staffing is a critical component of improving work processes.

These authors anticipate greater research into staffing needs in the future:

> The research team will conduct additional observations... so that sufficient data can be compiled to examine the association between cognitive shifts, interruptions, cognitive load, and the incidence of errors and omissions in care. Further work is also needed to explore the relationship of variables such as nurse experience, type of clinical specialty setting, and delivery of care models with clinical decision-making patterns. (Potter et al., 2014, p. 50)

Position Descriptions and Performance Appraisal

HCOs use position descriptions to provide clear descriptions of position responsibilities and requirements to maintain a position, but these descriptions also need to support expected care needs that staff must provide for quality care and a positive work environment. To provide greater support for staff engagement in CQI, CQI responsibilities should be included in all position descriptions for clinical and nonclinical staff. The position description is the first place where the organization demonstrates its commitment to CQI to new employees. During hiring, CQI should be discussed, such as asking about the applicant's viewpoint of CQI and experience with CQI and at the same time providing an opportunity to discuss the relevance of CQI to the HCO and the position responsibilities. This theme is carried through to orientation, both HCO orientation and specific orientation activities per unit assigned and the new employee position.

Performance appraisal is directly related to the HCO's QI program. Using surveys, the HCO performance appraisal form, and individual interviews, performance appraisal can be an important source of CQI data. Performance evaluation includes an evaluation form to ensure that staff are consistently evaluated using the same questions. Recording of this information from the interview may be useful in identifying needs. Self-assessment not only allows staff to identify where they stand at the time of their performance evaluation, but also helps staff improve their self-assessment skills as they provide direct care; when staff work they need to continually assess their performance. This constant self-evaluation has an important impact on CQI in practice, with staff using critical thinking and clinical reasoning and judgment to prevent problems while they provide care.

First, through the position requirements, as noted previously, the expectation of staff engagement in CQI is clear. This is then discussed in performance appraisal—annual and ongoing. Staff need to consider how they have participated in CQI when they complete their self-appraisal, and then the supervisor and employee should discuss this responsibility, adding comments to the appraisal of CQI participation. This assessment should not be a blame session but rather a constructive discussion.

The QI program also uses aggregate information from performance appraisal. For example, a nurse manager should summarize staff performance appraisal information after completing annual reviews. The results should be in aggregate form rather than with individual identifiers. As the nurse manager assesses the unit staff involvement in CQI, the following questions might be considered: What CQI activities are staff involved in? How many staff are involved in CQI, and how many are not? What are the barriers to participation reported by staff? What makes it easier for staff to participate in CQI? Are staff familiar with the unit's CQI data? What CQI problems do staff think are most critical on the unit?

What has improved in the past year? Do staff think they are getting sufficient and clear updates about CQI? Are there methods that should be used to increase this communication, and if so, what methods? This type of aggregate information can then be combined across the HCO to provide important organization-wide CQI data, but efforts should not stop with data sharing—steps need to be taken to change and improve. During performance appraisal, the supervisor and employee should work out a specific plan for employee engagement in CQI or improvement of this area of practice.

Clinical Ladder

Clinical ladders have been used in HCOs for some time. They are used to recognize clinical and professional competence and provide support for career advancement (Donley & Flaherty, 2008). This HCO approach to recognize staff is primarily focused on direct care or bedside nurses, addressing the concern that there is an overemphasis on management and promotion to management positions. Staff who participate in clinical ladders have to demonstrate competencies and provide examples, often referred to as a portfolio. How does this relate to CQI? Nurses need to demonstrate CQI activities as one aspect of professional activities. Using a ladder assists HCOs in emphasizing CQI as a part of staff responsibilities and pushes staff to actively participate in the development of strategies to prevent or respond to quality care concerns.

Policies and Procedures

HCO **policies** and **procedures** serve many purposes, and most of them are connected to CQI. Policies and procedures clarify important communication and consistent processes within an HCO—to ensure care quality, consistency, and other objectives. They also help to communicate critical concerns with the expectation that staff will follow them. Changes in policies and procedures must be communicated to staff in a timely manner, and often the changes are driven by CQI needs. For example, during root cause analysis of medication errors, it is noted that the documentation procedure steps were not clear. This then led to a change in the medication administration documentation procedure, but staff must be informed about changes and then apply the changes. HCOs now use evidence to support policies and procedures whenever best evidence is available, and evidence may also drive changes in current policies and procedures.

Evidence-Based Practice Requirements and Influence on Standardization of Care

EBP is discussed in many sections of this text. Best practice not only impacts policies and procedures, but also implementation of care and, ideally, CQI activities and initiatives (e.g., assisting in identifying measures/indicators that are based on evidence). EBP improves decision-making, and this includes decisions about care as well as management decisions (EBM), many of which are related to CQI. As nurses get involved in EBP and reviewing evidence, they learn more about effective care and apply this evidence to their practice and to management needs in the HCO.

Standards

As discussed in this text, standards are important to healthcare professionals, accreditors, government agencies, and HCOs. Standards are guides and should be based on best evidence. Some **standards** focus on professional issues such as competence, and others focus on patient care by identifying practice expectations. HCOs use standards that are developed by external sources such as the American Nurses Association, but they also develop their own standards, which should not conflict with critical professional or government standards. Standards then guide care, and thus have an impact on the quality of care, and they should be considered during the CQI process as methods for reducing quality care problems or responding to them.

Clinical Guidelines and Protocols

Clinical Practice Guidelines We Can Trust (IOM, 2011) is an important report that examines the need for developing and using effective clinical guidelines. A **clinical guideline** is a written description of care for a specific patient population. It acts as a guide for staff; however, the guidelines should not be used automatically without careful assessment of individual needs, recognizing that recommendations may need to be adapted. Guidelines should be based on evidence whenever possible. Clinical protocols are similar to guidelines but typically are described in a chart so that the information is easy to review and use. The protocol identifies expected assessment data, actual and potential problems, interventions, timelines, outcomes, and responsibilities (Finkelman & Kenner, 2016). Using clinical guidelines or protocols provides a consistent approach that has been reviewed by experts based on evidence. These tools can assist in providing effective care. Data on the use of guidelines and adaptions can then be used in assessing quality, and they can be used to track expected outcomes to determine if they were met and also applied as a strategy to improve.

Patient Safety Primers

Patient safety primers are evidence-based sources of information about patient safety available on the AHRQ website (HHS, AHRQ, PSNet, 2016b). These primers are an example of government-sponsored CQI resources that are easy to access and use. HCOs need current information for their staff as they develop, implement, and evaluate their QI programs and make changes to prevent and/or resolve CQI problems.

Case Management

The purpose of **case management** is to get the right services to patients when needed with the goal of avoiding fragmented and unnecessary care (Finkelman, 2011). Key elements of case management are coordination and collaboration. Case managers work with individual patients, typically patients with complex needs (e.g., chronic illness). Lack of coordination and collaboration is a barrier to effective care and meeting expected outcomes, thus impacting quality care. Case management may then be a strategy used to improve care.

Disease Management

Disease management services are used to better ensure patient-centered care and have an impact on quality care (Finkelman, 2016). Typically, third-party payers implement these services and then collaborate with HCOs to ensure coordinated care for patients with complex needs, such as chronic illness (e.g., diabetes, cardiac conditions, cancer, arthritis, respiratory conditions). The services focus on prevention, early detection and diagnosis, treatment, and care management, including self-management. Health literacy is an important factor for patients receiving disease management services and is discussed in other chapters.

Quality Improvement Committee

HCO committee structure typically includes a QI committee that works closely with the HCO's QI program. These committees carry major responsibility for guiding the development, implementation, and evaluation of the QI program. The committee participates in all levels of CQI planning: strategic, operational, and individual CQI projects. The committee should meet all the HCO committee requirements, such as size, selection of chairperson, documentation of minutes, meeting schedule, and so on. Committee membership should be representative of management, clinical staff, including a variety of healthcare professionals, medical records, admissions/discharge, utilization review and risk management, health informatics, financial, staff education, and community representatives when possible.

HCOs use different titles for committees, and QI committees are no exception. For example, The Joint Commission includes the Environment of Care Committee, which may also be called the Patient Safety Committee. The goal is ensure a patient environment and a work environment that are safe and allow healthcare providers to function effectively. An HCO may choose to use a broader term—*quality*, rather than just *safety*—and many HCOs do this, as safety is a dimension of quality care.

Utilization Review/Management Committee

As mentioned in this text, utilization review is a rich source of data about patients and services. Some HCOs have a committee that assists utilization review staff in the work they do to collect the data, but more importantly the committee may assist in analyzing the data and ensuring that the data are shared and used for multiple CQI purposes. This committee not only is a source of data and analysis, but it also makes decisions that impact improvement—changes and strategies to prevent errors or resolve CQI problems. For example, the utilization review committee might note that data indicate there are long waits for admission from the emergency department to inpatient units; however, its work could stop here. With focus on strategies to improve, the committee might propose some changes in admission process to reduce this wait time—basing its recommendations on the analysis of the data and causes. In doing this, the committee demonstrates how it is part of the measurement process, and it also participates at the next level in the CQI process, intervention.

Staff Education

This text has discussed the importance of staff education. Staff competence has a direct impact on care. The ANA standards (ANA, 2010) emphasize the need for structured staff education that is based on evidence-based standards. Staff education includes orientation and all ongoing education for staff. Staff education specialists need to work with HCO staff and the QI committee to assist in identifying care needs, problems, and errors to improve care. Often staff education is the intervention chosen to respond to a CQI problem to improve care; however, it is important that lack of education or competence be identified as a cause through analysis methods. It is too easy to just say, "Provide an education program to staff and the problem will be solved." Staff education specialists have a lot of contact with staff in many areas of the HCO, and their observations and interactions with staff can help to provide additional CQI. This input can expand understanding of processes and CQI concerns and may be helpful in assessing outcomes for changes that are implemented to prevent errors or resolve CQI problems. In addition, staff education programs include support interventions to improve care, and staff education specialists work with staff throughout the HCO to improve care and staff engagement in CQI. For example, an education program on a new medication procedure may be provided to nursing staff. Then staff education specialists may work with staff on the units as they apply the new procedure.

Mentoring and Coaching

Mentoring is using a role model to assist in career development. A staff member may select a mentor for career guidance. **Coaching** is another related method used to provide career guidance and support. To be effective, it should be ongoing, and the coach should have the necessary expertise and knowledge to provide useful guidance to a nurse. A supervisor may be viewed as a coach, whereas a mentor is not a supervisor. The coach provides constructive feedback, and this then provides informal performance appraisal with self-assessment. Both of these methods include setting goals and working toward meeting them. Why are mentoring and coaching related to CQI? Since both focus on improvement and advancement, they impact individual staff performance and thus impact CQI. Those who act as mentors and coaches should include discussion of CQI responsibilities and QI knowledge and competencies to assist in developing CQI competencies and engagement in CQI.

Structured Communication Methods

As CQI needs were increasingly recognized, it became clear that communication problems are the major cause of quality care concerns and errors. Understanding the need to improve communication by making it more structured and consistent led to methods and strategies to prevent errors or resolve CQI problems. Healthcare delivery systems turned to other industries, such as aviation, to adopt some methods and also developed new approaches. Typically, an HCO will adopt several structured communication methods, and staff are trained in their use and then expected to apply the method(s).

Checklists

Checklists are used in a variety of ways in HCOs to reduce errors. Gawande (2009) identifies two reasons why healthcare providers may fail. The first reason is we do not know enough. Science is not clear, and so we have a partial understanding. Secondly, we fail due to ineptitude, or we have the knowledge but apply it incorrectly. These reasons can be viewed as focused on individuals, but they have system implications. Development of knowledge is not just an individual responsibility. Not applying knowledge correctly can be due to individual staff problems such as not keeping up with current information, not following recommendations such as those found in a procedure, and other personal reasons, but there are also system issues. These issues might be failure of the HCO to provide sufficient information or to do so in a timely fashion, lack of staff education, inadequate staff to handle a change or the job that needs to be done, or lack of HCO knowledge of need to change. Gawande (2009) offers a simple and effective tool for reducing errors:

> We need a different strategy for overcoming failure, one that builds on experience and takes advantage of the knowledge people have but somehow also makes up for our inevitable human inadequacies. And there is such a strategy—though it will seem almost ridiculous in its simplicity, maybe even crazy to those of us who have spent years carefully developing ever more advanced skills and technologies. It is a checklist. (p. 13)

A **checklist** is "an algorithmic listing of actions to be performed in a given clinical setting" (HHS, AHRQ, PSNet, 2014a). The purpose is to make sure all steps are followed in the expected order and to document this process. As discussed in other chapters, checklists may also be used to collect data, but in this chapter we consider the checklist as a tool that helps to focus staff on the required tasks to ensure greater quality care, reducing risk of errors.

Why does the checklist work? Research indicates that for many tasks, we operate reflexively or "on autopilot," or we use attentional behavior, which requires problem solving and planning. For some tasks, lack of concentration, distraction and disruptions, fatigue, and stress may lead us to slips or failure to complete the task. When this happens, error risk increases. So no matter how many times one has done a procedure, the checklist should be followed. The expectation is that everyone will follow the standardized checklist, all steps in the order identified. The list should be developed by stakeholders and agreed upon for effective use. Use of checklists is not appropriate for all care activities, particularly activities that require attentional behavior. In this case, avoidance of diagnostic errors or problems with handoffs requires different approaches and training of staff. However, a checklist might be a component of a handoff, such as a checklist to ensure that discharge steps have been taken, but checklists should not relieve staff from using critical thinking and clinical reasoning and judgment to ensure an effective discharge process.

The checklist is simple and requires limited, if any, training to use, but implementing checklists is not a simple process. A checklist provides a consistent method of checking to make sure what needs to be done is done in a consistent, standardized way; the list helps with memory recall. Even though physicians are pushed by physician leaders (such as Atul Gawande, a surgeon), it is not easy to get staff, particularly physicians, to use checklists. Gawande noticed that nurses used a variety of checklists, such as on rounds, and this tool kept order during rounds, or they used a checklist for a procedure to ensure that all steps were completed. Aviation uses checklists for its pilots and staff on planes, and they are also used to check the mechanical status of the plane. These practices led health care to consider use of checklists. The danger in health care is that some assume that use of a checklist is equivalent to teamwork and team communication, and it is not (Shojania, 2015).

Staff need to understand the purpose of the checklist, its content, and how it may or may not affect other aspects of care. The checklist should be based on the steps in the focused procedure or action and should correspond with what is expected and realistic. Leadership needs to ensure that the culture expects use of checklists and discuss the impact on patient outcomes by providing current data for staff. When the checklist is not used, this needs to be addressed. Data about use and errors that might occur are valuable in understanding the CQI process and care, and they then can be used to plan and implement appropriate changes in care. Checklists are not just a tool, but are also a method to better understand processes, communication, and teamwork. This information should then be used to improve practice and outcomes.

There are two perspectives of surgical checklists: (1) Do they make a difference in care quality? (2) Are they used as recommended (compliance)? A study examined compliance by using remote video auditing with real-time feedback (Overdyk et al., 2015). In the groups that used the auditing, there were improved rates of sign-in, time-outs, and signouts. As a result of this study and other related work, the AHRQ notes that if used during surgery, this type of auditing can make a difference and should be used (Xiao, Mackenzie, & Seagull, 2015). Requiring use of checklists does not ensure that they will be used or that they will reduce all errors. This is similar to the long-term problems with hand washing compliance; just requiring it does not mean it will be done or done effectively.

Situation, Background, Assessment, Recommendation

What types of communication do nurses and physicians primarily learn and use (Narayan, 2013)? Physicians tend to use a communication style that focuses on prioritizing and lists, which appears to apply critical thinking more than does the nurse's approach of using timeline-descriptive narrative as the focus of communication. Due to these differences, there can be clashes in how communication proceeds and what is communicated or not communicated. As mentioned in this text, disruptive behavior or incivility between nurses and physicians is influenced by communication. Nurses frequently have to make decisions about when to ask for more assistance and also when to contact the physician. Given the differences in how communication may be conducted, consideration must be given to how communication can be improved to prevent problems in teamwork and QI. A recommendation is to use more structured, clear communication methods. **Situation, background, assessment, recommendation** (SBAR or ISBAR) is one of these methods. Use of these communication methods typically leads to more "efficient communication that promotes effective collaboration, improves patient outcomes, and increases patient satisfaction with care" and reduces interprofessional communication problems (Narayan, 2013, p. 507). The SBAR/ISBAR elements include the following.

- **I**ntroduction (who you are)
- **S**ituation (what is going on with the patient)
- **B**ackground (information that is critical to better understand the situation)
- **A**ssessment (what you think is the problem)
- **R**ecommendation (what you would do to solve the problem)

SBAR also includes callouts and check-backs. In a **call-out**, you communicate important information to the team so that all hear the same information at the same time, reducing the chance of miscommunication or some team members not hearing the same information. **Check-backs** occur when you ask the team if they heard the information and understood it.

Nurses are involved in many of the situations in which SBAR could improve communication and quality of care (Haig, Sutton, & Whittington, 2006). Understanding, training, and management and staff commitment to its use make a difference in its effectiveness. Care delivery is complex, and many issues arise at the same time, such as complex patient needs; need for supplies, equipment, and medications; documentation requirements; changing staffing and team composition; emergencies that might occur; and typical workday stress and possible problems with coworkers. These dynamics impact how difficult it might be to improve communication and maintain effective communication. Using an approach, such as SBAR, can help with this process.

What should you do as a nurse before you initiate SBAR in a given situation (Narayan, 2013)? You need to consider the patient situation, consider data you have or need, and use critical thinking and clinical reasoning and judgment in the process. Since part of the SBAR is sharing critical information about the patient, it is important to be clear about the information before initiating SBAR. Then you must decide if the situation is emergent (a developing situation), urgent (requiring quick response), or routine; review the patient record and compare data; and organize the information in a concise manner in the SBAR. This information includes primary data or information about the patient's situation that is critical for the physician to know and directly related to the reason for the communication. Secondary data, which represent information that may not be directly related to the specific situation but you consider in your analysis, are also important.

SBAR communication content should be concise; it should take about 60 seconds. In the first 10 seconds, it is important to get the attention of the physician to make your point. There is a tendency for nurses to use the initial contact to explain or apologize for the contact, which is typically a phone call, although it may be done in person. This approach may lead to the listener not listening to the rest of the message, the important parts. The SBAR step that may cause problems for the nurse is recommendations, something that many nurses do not feel comfortable doing or may not know how to do effectively. However, it is critical that you use analysis and provide recommendations based on your work with patients and share your knowledge of patients and experiences in patient care. **Exhibit 11-1** provides an SBAR example.

CUS

When nurses are concerned that their message is not getting across to the physician, the CUS method can be used to assist them in thinking through communication before communicating. CUS is a mnemonic for the following (Leonard, Graham, & Bonacum, 2004, p. 185):

- **C**: I am *concerned* because...
- **U**: I am *uncomfortable* because...
- **S**: The *safety* of the patient is at risk because...

Exhibit 11-1 SBAR Example

This is an example of how SBAR might be used to focus a telephone call between a nurse and a physician. The nurse would not wait for the physician to ask these questions, but rather would routinely provide the information in clear statements as indicated by SBAR.

Situation: *What is going on with the patient?*

A nurse finds a patient on the floor. She calls the doctor: "I am the charge nurse on the night shift on 5 West. I am calling about Mrs. Jones. She was found on the floor and is complaining of pain in her hip."

Background: *What is the clinical background or context?*

"The patient is a 75-year-old woman who was admitted for pneumonia yesterday. She did not complain of hip pain before being found on the floor."

Assessment: *What do I think the problem is?*

"I think the fall may have caused an injury. Her pain is level 9 out of 10."

Recommendation: *What would I do to correct it or respond to it?*

"I think we need to get an x-ray immediately and have her seen by the orthopedic resident."

This type of method, which provides a consistent communication framework, can easily be taught to staff, but there should be discussion about the situations in which it might be used.

Time-out

A **time-out** is a method used to stop work or care when staff are concerned there is risk or an error has occurred. HCOs that actively use time-outs have a designated procedure to follow, and all staff know about the procedure. Typically, any staff member may call a time-out. A common situation in which a time-out is used is in surgery—for example, when using the Universal Protocol for Preventing Wrong Site, Wrong Procedure, or Wrong Person Surgery.

Crew Resource Management

Crew resource management (CRM) is a system that is used in aviation and has been applied to HCOs. CRM focuses on leadership, interprofessional communication, and effective decision-making. It uses all available resources, emphasizes a no-blame culture, and focuses on clear, comprehensive standard operating procedures (HHS, AHRQ, 2015a). CRM can improve the CQI culture within an organization, but it is not an approach that solves problems quickly; nor is it a method that is used alone to improve care.

Signout

Signout occurs when patients are transferred as part of a handoff. The signout is the transmission of information about the patient (HHS, AHRQ, PSNet, 2015a). HCOs should have protocols that describe how the signout should be done. Standardizing this communication better ensures more effective written and verbal signouts or more effective transfers. The environment for this communication should be one of limited interruptions and noise so that staff can focus. I-PASS is one standardized method used for signout. It includes the following:

- *Illness severity.* One-word summary of the patient acuity, such as stable, unstable, observe
- *Patient summary.* Brief summary of the patient's diagnoses and treatment plan
- *Action list.* To-do items to be completed by the healthcare provider receiving the input
- *Situation awareness and contingency plans.* Directions to follow in case of changes in the patient's status, often in an "if-then" format
- *Synthesis by receiver.* An opportunity for the receiver of the message to ask questions and confirm the plan of care

The Joint Commission requires that its accredited HCOs use a standardized method for communication during handoffs, with individual HCOs identifying the methods their staff will use.

Read-Backs and Huddles

Read-backs occur when staff repeat written or oral information; for example, the nurse repeats an order back to a physician to make sure the information is correct. **Huddles** are used to call a team or group of staff together to discuss a critical concern. A huddle is a short meeting with staff focusing on a specific issue; it can be scheduled or unscheduled. HCOs should have a protocol for how and when these methods should be used. Huddles usually include a huddle sheet (checklist or worksheet). The unscheduled huddle may be used when any staff member wants to address a concern or review what needs to be done or has been done with the team. A read-back may be part of the huddle. These brief meetings should be efficient and to the point. A huddle supports CQI by identifying potential risk, near misses, or other quality problems, providing time for staff to discuss what should be done (i.e., actions), and read-back ensures that information is clearly exchanged to avoid errors and missed information.

Change-of-Shift Reports

The nurses' work environment is complex and disorganized, involving multiple staff and other people (patients, family, visitors)—an environment that is high risk for errors. Shift reports are structured methods for exchanging information about the patients and the unit when staff are coming in and going out. It is an extremely important time for handoffs. As noted in this text, these reports may use a variety of methods or combination of methods, such as face-to-face interaction with the unit staff, the team, or individual staff in a meeting format; rounds with exchange of information in verbal and written form; and/or recorded communication. Failure to share information affects consistent care, knowledge of patient status, errors and near misses, and patient satisfaction. Shift report may also be a time to identify CQI concerns and actions that need to be taken. Other information may also be shared, such as a change in procedure or a clinical guideline that would make a difference in care provided. Improving shift reports is an important CQI strategy and not just a method to get more CQI data.

Whiteboards

Whiteboards may seem like an unusual topic for a text on QI. They are a simple, effective method to provide structured communication. Units use them to share critical information for staff, such as staff assignments. It is important to consider patient privacy factors when placing the whiteboards for staff access and the type of data included on the board. Information included may ensure that staff know whom to contact about individual patients or may provide other unit information.

Staff Meetings

Staff meetings are held in various parts of HCOs routinely. For example, they may occur at the level of a unit, a particular department or service, or the HCO as a whole. These meetings offer many opportunities to support and engage in CQI. Sharing information to update staff increases consistency and reduces staff stress in not knowing current information. Both of these factors can limit quality, interfering with effective work. These meetings are also opportunities to identify successes (improvement) and to identify problems. Staff might analyze the problem and move to solutions or set up a process for this to occur. Minutes from meetings provide documentation about issues, problems, solutions, and other details discussed, all of which might apply to CQI. Staff meetings should include time for sharing CQI results and discussing implications for the staff and the unit (e.g., department, service). Providing clear visuals, such as using some of the methods discussed in this text (e.g., dashboards) helps staff to quickly appreciate the data, move to considering implications, develop interventions/strategies, and take actions. Meetings are critical times to develop strategies to respond to quality concerns and to inform staff of changes to resolve concerns.

Other Methods

A variety of other methods, many of them clinically focused, are used to prevent CQI problems and to improve care. The methods discussed in this section provide additional perspectives on CQI activities found in HCOs to prevent errors and/or resolve CQI problems.

Rapid Response Teams

The major purpose of **rapid response teams (RRTs)** is to identify and respond when patients are experiencing deterioration in their condition. This intervention has become an important QI strategy. A systematic review examined whether RRTs could identify preventable factors (Amaral et al., 2015). The results of this review indicated that when RRTs responded, almost 20% of the patients had experienced an adverse event. Out of these patients, 80% of the events were preventable. RRTs may be considered a method to assist a patient who has problems and could also be a trigger to identify potential adverse events. The AHRQ's Patient Safety Network describes their use as follows:

> Patients whose condition deteriorates acutely while hospitalized often exhibit warning signs (such as abnormal vital signs) in the hours before experiencing adverse clinical outcomes. In contrast to standard cardiac arrest or "code blue" teams, which are summoned only after cardiopulmonary arrest occurs, rapid response teams are designed to intervene during this critical period [ideally before a critical event occurs], usually for patients on general medical or surgical wards. (HHS, AHRQ, PSNet, 2014c)

The AHRQ identifies three rapid response system models (HHS, AHRQ, PSNet, 2014c):

- *Medical emergency team.* Personnel include physicians (critical care or hospitalist) and nurses; responsibilities include responding to emergencies.
- *Critical care outreach.* Personnel include physicians and nurses; responsibilities include responding to emergencies, following up on patients discharged from the intensive care unit (ICU), proactively evaluating high-risk unit patients, and educating unit staff.
- *Rapid response team.* Personnel include the critical care nurse, respiratory therapist, and physician (critical care of hospitalist); responsibilities include responding to emergencies, following up on patients discharged from ICU, proactively evaluating high-risk unit patients, and educating and acting as liaison to unit staff.

The triggers for calling any of these teams might be the same, but team members and what they do might vary. In some HCOs, when patients and families are concerned about the patient, they are encouraged to request this support. It is important for HCOs to provide guidelines to staff and to patients and families on the use of RRTs.

The **early warning system** is a "physiological scoring system typically used in general medical-surgical units before patients experience catastrophic medical events" (Duncan, McMullan, & Mills, 2012, p. 40). This system is what triggers the use of the RRT to prevent failure to rescue. The early warning system must be clear and easy to use. Some hospitals use simple charts that integrate color-coding to easily identify risk and response levels (e.g., fall risk, allergies). The rating scale is used, and depending upon the score, the decision is made to request expertise. Staff require training to effectively use the early warning system. Use of this type of rapid assessment and decision-making can lead to positive outcomes for the patient. The AHRQ recommendation is that any staff may initiate the request for calling an RRT, applying, for example, any of the following trigger criteria (HHS, AHRQ, PSNet, 2014c):

- Heart rate over 140/min or less than 40/min
- Respiratory rate over 28/min or less than 8/min
- Systolic blood pressure greater than 180 mm Hg or less than 99 mm Hg
- Oxygen saturation less than 90% despite supplementation
- Acute change in mental status
- Urine output less than 50 cc over 4 hours
- Staff member with significant concern about the patient's condition
- Other criteria used by some HCOs: chest pain unrelieved by nitroglycerin, threatened airway, seizure, uncontrolled pain

The criteria list needs to be clear and concise and shared with staff. Any changes to the list also must be shared in a timely manner. Nurse managers should ensure that staff know about the process and the criteria for calling the RRT. Data from use of RRTs are important to track, but here we are focused on how the data might be used as a strategy to respond to a problem. For example, an HCO identifies an increase in critical care events that could have been prevented and decides to implement an RRT as a strategy to help prevent these events.

Safety Walkarounds

Face-to-face discussion and observations are important in the CQI process, and a critical element is direct contact with frontline staff and management. **Safety walkarounds** are a method used to communicate to staff and patients that the HCO leadership is committed to improvement—engaged in the process. This direct involvement of leadership provides an "information-to-action feedback loop designed to lead to a decrease in adverse events and patient harm" (Graham, Brookery, & Steadman, 2014, p. 225). Safety walkarounds help reduce errors because there is greater reporting of near misses and actual errors; increased information sharing and discussion;

recognition of human factors, particularly those related to communication and teamwork; clarification and support of internal and external patient safety standards; and identification of environmental, equipment-related, or product-related hazards, and possible solutions are discussed (Graham et al., 2014).

Walkarounds should include critical managers (such as the nurse manager), medical director, supervisor, and frontline staff and may also include representatives from higher-level management. It is best to have a briefing before the walkaround to provide time to highlight any concerns the manager may have about the area to be visited and identify other aspects that will be covered. Discussion during the walkaround should be open and nonjudgmental. Standardized questions may be used, which makes it easier to compare information from one unit to another. After the walkaround, there should be a debriefing with all who participated, discussing issues and identifying and prioritizing next steps identified. Follow-up is important, and when relevant, actions taken following previous walkarounds should be reviewed. It is important that there be guidelines for these rounds. The guidelines should be clear about how to discuss issues in front of patients and families that may have negative implications or privacy concerns. A leader for the walkaround should be clearly designated, and some type of documentation method should be used for the briefing, walkaround, and debriefing. This documentation can then be shared with staff and management who would need to know about the information, and the documentation also serves as a record for CQI purposes.

Patient-Centered Rounds

There are many different types of rounds used in HCOs, including administrative, management, safety/quality, and clinical rounds, and also routine rounds that staff make that are not usually structured or set for routine times. Rounds, as noted in other chapters, may be used to collect data, but they are also a strategy used to prevent or resolve quality care problems.

Patient-centered rounds are rounds that can be configured in a number of ways for different purposes, but the critical element is they focus on the patient and patient needs. In reality, all rounds should be patient-centered. A study examined if the use of a standardized hourly rounding process (SHaRP) improved efficiency, patient satisfaction, and quality and safety metrics compared to not using a structured approach (Krepper et al., 2012). Staff were trained to use SHaRP, and the rounds were called "comfort care rounds." Patients were informed that staff would conduct the rounds hourly with a focus on ensuring a clean environment, assessing pain management needs, and assisting the patient to the toilet or in getting up. Units determined which staff would participate in the rounds. The use of this type of rounds demonstrated significant outcomes in all four areas, although the researchers recommend that more research is needed.

Teach-Backs

Teach-backs occur when staff ask patients to repeat something a patient has been told, for example in a patient education session or care directions. This method also helps to reduce health literacy problems and thus has an impact on CQI directed at meeting expected outcomes. If the patient is not able to repeat the information, then this means staff need to further assess how the information is shared and how to improve the communication.

Safe Zones

The use of **safe zones** is an approach adopted from aviation. The goal during certain activities is to better ensure that there are no interruptions and distractions so that staff can meet their responsibilities effectively and safely. Safe zones are particularly helpful in reducing errors during medication administration. In this situation all staff are informed that the space used for the medication preparation procedure or whenever staff are involved in medication administration this is a safe zone or a time period for no interruptions.

Universal Protocol for Preventing Wrong Site, Wrong Procedure, or Wrong Person Surgery

Universal Protocol for Preventing Wrong Site, Wrong Procedure, or Wrong Person Surgery (often referred to simply as the **Universal Protocol**) establishes a step-by-step protocol to prevent wrong site, wrong procedure, or wrong person surgery (HHS, AHRQ, PSNet, 2003). The Joint Commission supports this protocol, as does the AHRQ. The protocol includes a time-out at the beginning of a surgical procedure. The entire surgical team participates. Wrong site, procedure, and person events are considered to be never events or hospital-acquired complications by the Centers for Medicare and Medicaid Services (CMS), and The Joint Commission considers these events to be sentinel events for which there is zero-tolerance. This procedure is a critical strategy used by HCOs. Since 2009, the CMS has not reimbursed for these events when their beneficiaries experience them in the hospital. In addition, focusing on the Universal Protocol, some research has found that actions taken before or after the use of the Universal Protocol need to be examined, as this is when errors may still occur even though staff feel comfortable that they are using the protocol (Paull et al., 2015).

Medication Reconciliation

With the increasing use of medications and many patients taking multiple medications, there is greater risk for errors in HCOs and with patients at home. More than half of patients also have one or more unintended medication discrepancies at the time of hospital admission (Cornish et al., 2005).

Medication reconciliation is formulating a list of medications (e.g., drug name, dosage and frequency, administration method, purpose of the medication, and prescriber) and reviewing the list to ensure that there are no conflicts in the medications. Healthcare providers need a clear policy and procedure for medication reconciliation, and the use of this policy and procedure should be monitored (Ketchum, Grass, & Padwojski, 2005). The Joint Commission requires its accredited HCOs to have a medication reconciliation policy and procedure. Problems that can arise if this is not done are omitted medications, incorrect dosages, incorrect route, incorrect timing, same medications that have different formulations, allergies, and failure to discontinue contraindicated medications (Rozich et al., 2004). Implementing medication reconciliation is not always easy. For some patients it can take time to complete. Some patients may not know or provide accurate information. Asking patients to bring in a written list of their medications does help, but they should be reminded that the list should be an updated list. The AHRQ comments that medication reconciliation done by the hospital pharmacist offers some help preventing this problem, but it is not sufficient. Nurses are also typically involved in medication reconciliation. Greater use of electronic records may make a difference, but more evidence is required. Patient engagement in this process is also important.

Among the most common adverse events after discharge are discrepancies in medication orders, such as medication not listed or change in dose not provided (HHS, AHRQ, PSNet, 2015b). Using medication reconciliation is also important in home care to ensure that patient medications are safe (Marrelli, 2016). Checking a patient's medication storage methods, such as medication boxes, and availability of outdated medications should be included in this process. In addition, it is important to check reasons why patients may not be following a prescribed medication routine (e.g., inability to afford medications, side effects, lack of transportation to get medications). Out-of-date medications may indicate that the patient is "stretching out" use and thus taking less medication over time, skipping doses, and so on. Medication compliance is important to patient outcomes.

Summary of Key Recommended Methods to Prevent or Reduce Quality Care Problems

Identifying high-risk situations that require responses should be based on evidence and reliable sources, as should the strategies/interventions used to respond. In 2013, the AHRQ identified the top 10 patient safety strategies/interventions (Barclay, 2013):

- Preoperative/anesthesia checklists to reduce operative and postoperative events
- Bundles, including checklists, to reduce septicemia associated with central lines

- Catheter reminders, stop orders, nurse-initiated removal protocols, other interventions to limit urinary catheter use
- Bundles to prevent ventilator-associated pneumonia, including head-of-bed elevation, sedation vacations, oral care with chlorhexidine, and subglottic suctioning endotracheal tubes
- Hand hygiene
- Do-not-use list for hazardous abbreviation
- Multicomponent interventions to help prevent pressure ulcers
- Barrier precautions to reduce healthcare-associated infections
- Central line placement guided by real-time ultrasonography
- Strategies to improve venous thromboembolism prophylaxis

Stop and Consider #1

Some methods to prevent or reduce quality problems, such as collecting data, may also be used during the measurement process.

Teams

Teams have not been a major focus in healthcare delivery, particularly interprofessional teams; however, this is changing. How do teams relate to CQI? There are many factors to consider with teams and CQI. As Robichaud and colleagues (2012) explain, "The teamwork that is required for interprofessional collaboration in healthcare is not an inherent attribute of the current system, and must be fostered. Education, training, and role modeling are important enablers" (p. 156). The term "team" does not include "I" (Weinstock, 2010). Teams are not groups of people who do their work alone and then periodically come together to collaborate. Teams also support the critical element for effective CQI—active staff participation. Teams are an important part of today's QI programs and initiatives, and they have an impact on many of the strategies/interventions used to prevent and improve care, as many of these methods require effective staff participation.

How does interprofessional education (IPE) relate to patient and healthcare system outcomes (NAS/HMD, 2015)? IPE is discussed in other sections of this text, but here it is important to remember its relevance to teams and CQI. A critical first step is increased effective collaboration and coordination between education and practice, which is not easy to accomplish. There is also a need for more research evidence on interprofessional collaboration. The National Academy of Sciences, Health and Medicine Division (NAS/HMD, 2015) notes this lack of research-based support for IPE: "Although there is a widespread and growing belief that IPE may improve interprofessional collaboration, promote team-based healthcare delivery, and enhance personal and population health, definitive evidence linking IPE to desirable intermediate and final outcomes does not yet exist" (p. 6). Linking IPE to collaborative behavior changes requires a systematic approach.

High-Performance Teams

HCOs need to assess their use of teams and teamwork. Effective teams require members (healthcare professionals) who do the following (IOM, 2003):

- Learn about other team members' expertise, background, knowledge, and values.
- Learn individual roles and processes required to work collaboratively.
- Demonstrate basic group skills, including communication, negotiation, delegation, time management, and assessment of group (team) dynamics.
- Ensure that accurate and timely information reaches those who need it at the appropriate time.
- Customize care and manage smooth transitions across settings and over time, even when the team members are in entirely different physical locations.
- Coordinate and integrate care processes to ensure excellence, continuity, and reliability of the care provided.
- Resolve conflicts with other members of the team.
- Communicate with other members of the team in a shared language, even when the members are in entirely different physical locations.

What outcomes are evaluated to determine team effectiveness? A systematic review of 6,934 articles primarily used outcomes focused on length of stay, readmission, or mortality rates for general medicine patients (Pannick et al., 2015). However, common outcomes have not been effective in assessing outcomes of interprofessional teams. They recommend that complications and preventable adverse events should be included in assessing interprofessional team outcomes.

It is common when interprofessional teams are discussed to forget that administration/management/leadership need to be part of the team concept in an HCO (Begun, White, & Mosser, 2011). High-performance teams are associated with administrators who support the need for a culture that emphasizes CQI. Administrators facilitate resources, such as budget and staffing, so that care can be improved. In short, they are in the position to be a driver for success. Management needs to demonstrate that teamwork is integrated into all aspects of the HCO, beginning with the HCO's vision, mission, and goals, and the QI program. To do so, administrators must understand the clinical care process and its relationship to CQI. It is also the top administrator who works with the HCO's board of directors; the administrator needs to explain to the board the need for CQI; the CQI process, goals, and outcomes; and the importance of a team approach. The board approves the budget, and developing, implementing, and evaluating a QI program require funding. Achieving these objectives requires collaboration and partnership between management and staff—teamwork.

Interprofessional team education should include teamwork and group processes, reflection and documentation, communication, shared knowledge or general common knowledge base, and ethics. Effective teams need to have members who meet the purpose of the team and can provide knowledge and expertise, and members should be representative of the areas of concern, such as the clinical specialty or the appropriate administrative area, such as financial, documentation, CQI, and health informatics. The typical team size is five to seven members; too many or too few members is a barrier to effectiveness. Each team should strive to do the following (HHS, HRSA, 2011b, p. 4):

- Gain buy-in from the leadership.
- Define roles and responsibilities.
- Recognize stages of team growth: forming, storming, norming, performing.
- Set ground rules.
- Establish an effective team meeting process.
- Set meeting agendas.
- Set meeting outcomes/actions and document.

Teams and QI Projects

HCOs need to assess not only their CQI process but also how their teams function and impact the process and results. This assessment should include the readiness for the team to do its job. For example, a team working on a CQI project should consider the following questions (HHS, HRSA, 2011c, p. 4):

- Has the organization identified and prioritized its desired results?
- Is there an established means to measure progress toward those results or can it be created?
- Is there a process for tracking and measuring progress toward its desired results, which includes effective means to display data?
- Is there a communication plan that includes how individuals working to achieve the desired results can exchange and provide ongoing feedback?
- Is there an established plan to periodically review progress?
- Is there a process to intervene when needed as a means to improve progress?

It is easy for CQI teams to quickly get into a CQI problem without stopping to plan. This is a mistake and often leads to haphazard actions and outcomes. The Health Resources and Services Administration (HHS, HRSA, 2011c) recommends the use of an aim statement when undertaking an improvement process:

An *aim statement* provides a CQI team with a focused target or a goal to achieve through its quality improvement work. An aim statement is a written declaration of what an organization wants to accomplish. An effective aim contains measurable and time-sensitive parameters for the expected results of an improvement process. (p. 7)

Stop to consider planning, as discussed in this text. To improve CQI efforts and team results consider the following questions: (1) What will improve? (2) When will it improve? (3) How much will it improve? (4) For whom will it improve?

Unfortunately, not all dynamics of clinical teamwork can be considered positive. Collective vigilance, as described by Jeffs, Lindgard, Berta, and Baker (2012), "can potentially create risk by eroding individual professional accountability through reliance on other team members to catch and correct their errors" (p. 122). The problem of collective vigilance was observed in a study that also noted a dissimilar finding—when healthcare providers are involved in a near miss, they frequently work in isolation from other staff who might be able catch and correct potentially harmful errors. In other words, working in a team can create overreliance on team members, but working in isolation can leave providers without a support system. Another factor is that "over time, adaptive processes by workers and ongoing transgressions can become accepted, routine practices that are embedded into professional interactions and can erode performance" (Amalberti, Vincent, Auroy, & de Saint Maurice, 2006; Cook & Rasmussen, 2005; Jeffs et al., 2012, p. 125). These examples do not demonstrate high-performance situations in work groups or teams and can interfere with improving care because team members do not intervene when they should. They could improve care by stepping in and noting potential or actual problems. Teams must work together and act effectively.

The Physical Environment and Teamwork

Another aspect of teamwork, which is often forgotten, is the physical environment. Teams work and communicate in a physical space, a simple fact that impacts their work and CQI. A multisite collective case study of three rural hospitals in South Australia examined the collaborative working culture of each hospital. Gum, Prideaux, Sweet, and Greenhill (2012) describe the results as follows:

> Of the cultural concepts examined, the physical design of nurses' stations and the general physical environment were a major influence on an effective collaborative practice. Factors that were important were communication barriers related to poor design, lack of space, frequent interruptions, and a lack of privacy. (p. 21)

Tight space increases staff stress, and lack of space for private conversations or work meetings limits communication and planning. Lack of space for relaxation limits opportunity for team members to rest, impacts care quality and burnout, and limits opportunities for members to have personal dialogue and get to know one another. Work space can be problematic, increasing risk for errors. For example, limited space to move around and get supplies and equipment can be a factor when preparing medications, when providing direct care, or when trying to arrange supplies and equipment in emergencies. Decentralized nurses' stations reduce walking and provide more time for care, but they also may limit team interaction and increase risk of working in silos, providing less time to discuss care and ask questions of peers. Other spaces for staff interaction, as noted above, should be provided. Space is also associated with territory and power; for example, the title "nurses' station" symbolizes the space's function for nurses, not all staff. The unit workstation has long been a place of interprofessional work, but in many HCOs, it is still referred to as the nurses' station. Staff safety is also an important factor associated with physical space, as noted in other sections of this text.

In summary, the following are competencies that better ensure effective collaborative interprofessional teamwork (IPEC, 2011, pp. 19, 21, 23, 25):

- Work with individuals of other professions to maintain a climate of mutual respect and shared values.
- Use the knowledge of one's own role and those of other professions to appropriately assess and address the healthcare needs of patients and populations served.
- Communicate with patients, families, communities, and other health professionals in a responsive and responsible manner that supports a team approach to the maintenance of health and treatment of disease.
- Apply relationship-building values and the principles of team dynamics to perform effectively in different team roles to plan and deliver patient- and population-centered care that is safe, timely, efficient, effective, and equitable.

Accomplishing these competencies requires greater emphasis on IPE for all healthcare profession students.

TeamSTEPPS®

One of the most respected and common methods for team development and team function is **TeamSTEPPS®**, which was developed by the U.S. Department of Defense's Patient Safety Program in collaboration with the AHRQ). The (HHS, AHRQ, 2015b) describes TeamSTEPPS® as follows:

> [TeamSTEPPS® is] an evidence-based teamwork system aimed at optimizing patient care by improving communication and teamwork skills among healthcare professionals, including frontline staff. It includes a comprehensive set of ready-to-use materials and a training curriculum to successfully integrate teamwork principles into a variety of settings.

Figure 11-3 describes this model. The goal for CQI teams should be team ownership of CQI within the HCO. As the HHS, AHRQ (2014a) states, "If a team has tools and strategies, it can leverage to build a fundamental level of competency in

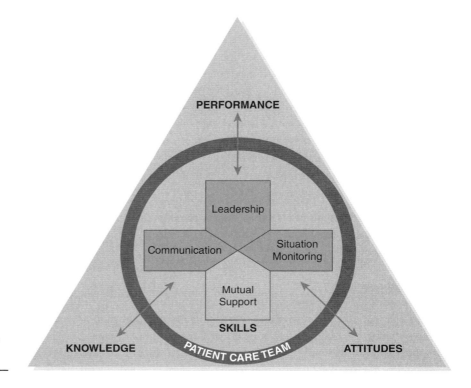

Figure 11-3.
TeamSTEPPS®
Reproduced from Agency for Healthcare Research and Quality. (2014). Pocket guide: TeamSTEPPS®. Retrieved from http://www.ahrq.gov /professionals/education /curriculum-tools/teamstepps /instructor/essentials /pocketguide.html#frame

each of those skills. Research has shown that the team can enhance three types of teamwork outcomes: performance, knowledge, and attitudes." This teamwork system can be described as follows (HHS, AHRQ, 2015c):

- A powerful solution to improving patient safety within [an] organization
- An evidence-based teamwork system to improve communication and teamwork skills among healthcare professionals
- A source for ready-to-use materials and a training curriculum to successfully integrate teamwork principles into all areas of [the] healthcare system
- Scientifically rooted in more than 20 years of research and lessons from the application of teamwork principles

Applying this model provides higher-quality, safer patient care by doing the following: producing highly effective medical teams that optimize the use of information, people, and resources to achieve the best clinical outcomes for patients; increasing team awareness and clarifying team roles and responsibilities; resolving conflicts and improving information sharing; and eliminating barriers to quality and safety.

The model has three phases. The first phase is pretraining to ensure the HCO and its staff are ready to implement TeamSTEPPS®. The training focuses on teamwork skills of leadership, communication, situation monitoring, and mutual support. The second phase focuses on a structured training for trainers in the HCO and for healthcare staff. The final phase is implementation of TeamSTEPPS ® and sustaining it in the HCO. Training materials are evidence-based and provide a structured learning experience using modules, guides, videos of vignettes supporting the model, coaching, and other methods to assist staff in understanding teamwork and implementing this teamwork model. Since this method and all its resources were developed and maintained on the Internet for easy access by the federal government, they are freely available to be used by all HCOs and healthcare providers. **Exhibit 11-2** describes TeamSTEPPS® model in greater detail. The Connect to Current Information section at the end of the chapter provides a link to additional information about TeamSTEPPS®.

Exhibit 11-2   Description of TeamSTEPPS

Three Phases of the TeamSTEPPS Delivery System

The three phases of TeamSTEPPS are based on lessons learned, existing master trainer or change agent experience, the literature of quality and patient safety, and culture change. A successful TeamSTEPPS initiative requires a thorough assessment of the organization and its processes and a carefully developed implementation and sustainment plan.

Phase 1: Needs Assessment

The goal is to determine the HCO's readiness for implementing Team-STEPPS, which requires a training needs analysis. For more information about conducting a needs assessment, visit http://www.ahrq.gov/teamstepps/readiness/index.html.

Phase 2: Planning, Training, and Implementation

Phase 2 focuses on the planning and implementation of the TeamSTEPPS initiative. Because TeamSTEPPS was designed to be tailored to the organization, options in this phase include implementation of all tools and strategies in the entire organization, a phased-in approach that targets specific units or departments, or selection of individual tools introduced at specific intervals (called a "dosing strategy"). As long as the primary learning objectives are maintained, the TeamSTEPPS materials are very adaptable.

Phase 3: Sustainment

The goal is to sustain and spread improvements in teamwork performance, clinical processes, and outcomes resulting from the TeamSTEPPS initiative.

The key objective is to ensure that opportunities exist to implement the tools and strategies taught, practice and receive feedback on skills, and provide continual reinforcement of the TeamSTEPPS principles on the unit or within the department.

Details of an HCO Site Assessment

A site assessment includes identifying opportunities for improvement; determining the readiness of the HCO or unit/department within an HCO, such as leadership support; identifying potential barriers to implementing change; and deciding whether resources are in place to successfully support the initiative. Phase 1 assessment includes the following:

1. *Establish an organizational-level change team.* The organizational-level change team should consist of an interprofessional team that represents the healthcare professionals within the HCO. Successful change teams include organizational leaders who are committed to changing the current culture.
2. *Conduct a site assessment.* A site assessment, also called team training needs analysis, is a process for systematically identifying teamwork deficiencies so training programs can be developed to address those deficiencies. This information is then used to identify critical training and develop training objectives and allows the program to be individualized.
3. *Define the problem, challenge, or opportunity for improvement.* The team must identify the recurring problem that threatens patient safety and then determine how this problem results from existing processes and procedures and devise a flowchart or map of the process during which the problem occurs. With information and processes properly mapped, it becomes clear what interventions are needed, what the objective of these interventions should be, and how ready the organization is to engage in these interventions.
4. *Define the goal of your intervention.* List the goals that will reduce or eliminate the risk to safe patient care. For each goal, state in one sentence what will be achieved, who will be involved (whose behavior will change), and when and where the change will occur. Ideally, a team process goal, a team outcome goal, and a clinical outcome goal will be defined.

Details for Planning, Training, and Implementation of TeamSTEPPS

The tools and strategies needed to address opportunities for improvement in an organization will be determined by the phase 1 assessment. The next step is to develop a customized implementation and action plan, followed by training and implementation. A brief description of the steps for planning, training, and implementation follows.

1. *Define the TeamSTEPPS intervention.* Decide whether "whole training" (all the tools in one sitting) or "dosing" (specific tools targeted to specific interventions) is the best intervention tactic. Whole training optimizes teamwork but does not maximize learning. It can also lead to overload or uncertainty about which tools best fit improvement opportunities. Dosing is the recommended approach because it allows for direct linking of tools and strategies with specific opportunities for improvement to minimize training fatigue and overload.

2. *Develop a plan for determining the intervention's effectiveness.* There are a variety of ways to evaluate the impact of training. The plan should assess whether trainees have acquired new knowledge, skills, or attitudes at the end of training; whether individuals are taking their learning back to the workplace and using it on the job; and whether organizational objectives are being met.

3. *Develop an implementation plan.* Assess what groups will be trained, the order in which they will be trained (if not together and all at once), and what level of training they will receive. Include in the plan who will conduct training and where and when training will take place.

4. *Gain leadership commitment to the plan.* Inform leaders of all facets of the plan, including how much time will be used for training and the desired resources to support it. Leadership commitment often yields plan refinement. The key is to know what elements of the plan cannot be altered.

5. *Develop a communication plan.* Develop a plan for communicating what will be done and how the goal will be achieved. Leaders (both designated and situational) should provide information to all those in their departments or units about the initiative. It is crucial to tie together all activities that will take place with the overall goal for the initiative (i.e., improved patient safety).

6. *Prepare the HCO.* For any initiative to be fully successful, transfer of training must be achieved. Transfer is achieved by ensuring new knowledge or skills are learned and applied in the work environment. The change team must ensure the work environment is prepared to foster transfer of training so new tools and strategies are applied on the job.

7. *Implement training.* The most effective strategy for delivering the training initiative is one that involves teams of trainers that include physicians, nursing staff, and support staff. A combination of the curricula is

recommended when training different sets of staff independently. The TeamSTEPPS system includes three different medical team-training curricula and a complete suite of multimedia course materials:

a. **Train the Trainer.** This 2.5-day training course is designed to create a cadre of teamwork instructors with the skills to train and coach other staff members.

b. **TeamSTEPPS Fundamentals.** This curriculum includes 4 to 6 hours of interactive workshops for direct patient care providers.

c. **TeamSTEPPS Essentials.** This curriculum is a 1- to 2-hour condensed version of the Fundamentals course and is specifically designed for nonclinical support staff.

Details for Sustaining a TeamSTEPPS Intervention

The designated change team manages sustaining interventions through coaching and observing team performance. An effective sustainment plan should account for ongoing assessment of the effectiveness of the intervention, sustainment of positive changes, and identification of opportunities for further improvements.

1. *Provide opportunities to practice.* Any TeamSTEPPS-based initiative will be much more successful if the change team accounts for opportunities to practice these behaviors. It is important to embed opportunities for practice in day-to-day functions.

2. *Ensure leaders emphasize new skills.* Leaders play a critical role in sustainment because they are responsible for emphasizing daily the skills learned in TeamSTEPPS training. The goal is for leaders to engage in activities that will ensure continuous involvement in teamwork.

3. *Provide regular feedback and coaching.* Regular feedback and coaching are key to ensuring interventions are sustained. Change team members, champions from the unit, and leaders should develop and use a coaching and feedback plan that allows for sufficient observation and feedback opportunities.

4. *Celebrate wins.* Celebrating wins bolsters further sustainment and engagement in teamwork. When using a TeamSTEPPS-based initiative, it is critical to celebrate successes for two reasons. First, it recognizes the efforts of those who were engaged from the beginning, and second, it provides detractors or laggards a tangible example of how teamwork has improved the current operations.

5. *Measure success.* The change team should measure success through satisfaction with training, demonstrations of learning, effective use of tools and strategies on the job, and changes in processes and outcomes.

It is useful to ensure that measurement of pre-training factors is parallel with post-training factors so changes can be assessed.

6. *Update the plan.* The final stage in any TeamSTEPPS-based intervention is to revise the plan as the organization's needs change. The change team should determine when organizational needs have changed and ensure the sustainment plan continues to focus on the needs of the organization or unit where the intervention has been implemented.

Modified from Agency for Healthcare Research and Quality (AHRQ). (September 2015). TeamSTEPPS®: Strategies and tools to enhance performance and patient safety. About TeamSTEPPS®. Retrieved from http://www.ahrq.gov/professionals/education/curriculum-tools/teamstepps/about-teamstepps/index.html

Examples of Types of Teams Related to CQI

With the increase in use of teams in clinical care, particularly interprofessional teams, there is greater emphasis on teams in CQI. The following are some examples of specific types of teams used by HCOs to expand their CQI activities and integrate more staff in the process.

CQI Project Teams

The (HHS, HRSA, 2011b) describes the importance teamwork in the CQI process as follows:

> For a CQI project to succeed, an organization must use the knowledge, skills, experiences, and perspectives of a wide range of people. A CQI project requires problem solving, multiple decisions, and effective solutions that involve complex systems. A comprehensive multidisciplinary [interprofessional] approach by a CQI team is preferred over individual decision makers, especially when a task is complex, creativity is necessary, the path to improvement is unclear, efficient use of resources are required, [and] cooperation is essential to implementation. (pp. 1–2)

CQI project teams need to be flexible as they go through the process to improve care focused on a specific concern. Team members must be engaged and have a stake in the outcome. No one person has the knowledge or expertise to resolve a CQI problem; it takes a team representing multiple aspects of knowledge and expertise. Selecting members for a CQI team is critical to successful improvement. The following member attributes should be considered (HHS, HRSA, 2011b, p. 2):

- Respected by a broad range of staff
- Team players
- Excellent listeners

- Good communicators
- Proven problem solvers
- Frustrated with the current situation and ready for change
- Creative and able to offer solutions
- Flexible—demonstrated by their willingness to change and accept new technology
- Proficient in the areas and systems focused for improvement

Crisis Management Teams

Some clinical adverse events are also referred to as sentinel events, which result in a patient(s) experiencing a permanent psychological and/or physical harm (or death) (Conway, Federico, Steward, & Campbell, 2011). Many of the strategies used to address these serious adverse events also apply to all adverse events. Crisis management should be part of the response to serious events, and key leaders in the HCO should be involved as need arises. There should be policies and procedures for coping with sentinel events, including how to apply crisis management. Conway and colleagues (2011) discuss the importance of the crisis management team (CMT) in responding to a crisis event, saying the CMT's role "is to ensure that the priorities of the patients and families, staff, and organization are met, as well as to ensure enhanced communication, support, assessment, resolution, learning, and improvement following the event" (p. 11). This team should include key stakeholders and provide expertise. The purpose of the team is to determine the risk of problems occurring and of potential complications to a problem, creating a response plan, implementing the plan, and evaluating and revising the plan over time. As is true for other adverse events, risk assessment and root cause analysis should be done. The team should consider the following questions when evaluating the implementation of the plan (Conway et al., 2011, p. 13):

- What worked?
- What didn't work?
- What could have been done better?
- What did you learn?

The team's engagement should be timely and transparent. Risk management should be involved if there are concerns about malpractice, which is not an uncommon concern with situations that require crisis management. It is often important to consider not only internal communication but also external communication, such as the media, government agencies, and law enforcement, to effectively manage the response.

An example of a crisis for which a CMT was activated occurred in a university medical center in the fall of 2015 (CBS News, 2015; U.S. & World, 2015). A woman delivered twins; one was stillborn and the second lived an hour. One of the infant's remains was lost, even leading the hospital to search the city dump. This crisis required immediate examination to assist the family and prevent further events like this one. In this case, the media was involved, so managing the media was critical. HCO leadership should have a procedure for response to media, including how to communicate with the media and the police. Staff need to be informed about this procedure. Given the increase in situations in HCOs that involve guns, drugs, suicide, and violence, even murder, all HCOs need to be clear about crisis management to respond to the situation's immediate and long-term demands to better ensure safety for patients, families, visitors, and staff, and ultimately, to ensure quality care.

Comprehensive Unit-Based Safety Program

Comprehensive Unit-based Safety Program (CUSP) was developed by the AHRQ as a framework to improve patient safety at the unit level. **Figure 11-4** illustrates this framework, which considers the implications of change. Teams and teamwork are critical components in CUSP, which uses "sensemaking" by applying the following process (HHS, AHRQ, 2014b):

- Initiate a conversation among members of an organization involved in an event/issue.
- The purpose is to reduce the ambiguity about the event/issue—literally to make sense of it.
- The conversation is the mechanism that combines that knowledge into a new, more understandable form for the members.
- Members develop a similar representation in their minds that allows for action that can be implemented and understood by all who have participated in the conversation.

As situations are examined on a unit, staff teams gain a better understanding about what happened; why it happened; what might be done to decrease risk of reoccurrence; and how staff will know when risk is reduced. The nurse manager and unit staff work together to reduce risk and also to respond to CQI problems that occur. CUSP is commonly associated with the use of TeamSTEPPS®.

Stop and Consider #2

Teamwork is a part of practice and also the CQI process.

Technology and Informatics

Health informatics technology (HIT) is more than technology. Coiera (2003) describes it as follows: "Although definitions vary, informatics involves the study of information and communication systems in health care and the application of these systems for decision-making and other tasks." Solutions are part of technology and informatics,

Figure 11-4.

Comprehensive Unit-Based Safety Program (CUSP)

Reproduced from Agency for Healthcare Research and Quality. (2014). Learn about CUSP. Retrieved from http://www.ahrq .gov/professionals/education /curriculum-tools/cusptoolkit /modules/learn/sllearncusp .html#slide1

involving data collection methods and analysis of data; these solutions are often focused on preventing errors and resolving CQI problems (Kuziemsky & Reeves, 2012). Much of CQI depends on web-based reporting systems; anonymous, automated, integrated systems; reporting consistency; the quality, accessibility, and measurability of data; and survey and detection of adverse events. Effective HIT provides methods for secure, efficient, and effective storage and sharing of information.

In 2009, the federal Health Information Technology for Economic and Clinical Health (HITECH) Act was passed. This legislation has had an impact on health care, with its incentives to implement new technology such as computerized physician/provider order entry (CPOE), which is discussed later in this chapter. The law also emphasizes meaningful use. In 2016, the AHRQ issued a call for more grant proposals to gain more knowledge about HIT safety—focused on safe HIT practices related to design, implementation, usability, and safe use of HIT by all healthcare providers (NIH, 2016). This type of initiative demonstrates the increasing need for research and support for new initiatives to improve HIT.

With the growing recognition of the need for effective HIT, the U.S. Department of Health and Human Services (HHS) developed the Federal Health IT Strategic Plan. This plan provides direction for 2015–2020 focused on national healthcare delivery to ensure effective systems with all types of HCOs. The vision and a description of the plan's goals and objectives are found in **Figure 11-5** and **Table 11-1**.

Healthcare delivery also uses many types of technology that may or may not be associated with informatics and computer systems. Examples of common methods and equipment are unit-dose systems, smart administration pumps, telemetry monitoring, bar coding, telehealth equipment, and robotics in surgery. Effective use requires that healthcare professionals understand the purpose and use the technology effectively. Staff need to know how to use the equipment and participate in any clinical staff required maintenance or equipment checks prior to use, and staff need to complete required procedures for implementation and evaluation of technology use, document as required, and complete required patient assessment while using the technology. The HCO and staff need to identify and respond to CQI needs such as data, errors, and solutions. Equipment must be up to date, maintenance needs must be met, and records must be kept about use and tracking of any problems for CQI purposes.

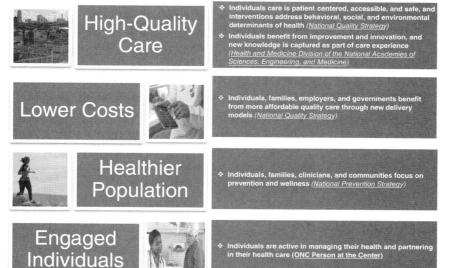

Figure 11-5. The Vision and Expected Results that Guide the Federal Health IT Strategic Plan 2015–2020

Reproduced from U.S. Department of Health and Human Services (HHS) & National Coordinator for Health Information Technology (ONC). (2014). Federal IT strategic plan: 2015–2020. Retrieved from https://www.healthit.gov/policy-researchers-implementers/health-it-strategic-planning

TABLE 11-1 Federal Health IT Strategic Plan 2015–2020 Goals: Quick Reference Guide

	Goal	Objective
Collect	**Goal 1:** Expand Adoption of Health IT	▪ **Objective A:** Increase the adoption and effective use of health IT products, systems, and services ▪ **Objective B:** Increase user and market confidence in the safety and safe use of health IT products, systems, and services ▪ **Objective C:** Advance a national communications infrastructure that supports health, safety, and care delivery
Share	**Goal 2:** Advance Secure and Interoperable Health Information	▪ **Objective A:** Enable individuals, providers, and public health entities to securely send, receive, find, and use electronic health information ▪ **Objective B:** Identify, prioritize, and advance technical standards to support secure and interoperable health information ▪ **Objective C:** Protect the privacy and security of health information
Use	**Goal 3:** Strengthen Healthcare Delivery	▪ **Objective A:** Improve healthcare quality, access, and experience through safe, timely, effective, efficient, equitable, and person-centered care ▪ **Objective B:** Support the delivery of high-value health care ▪ **Objective C:** Improve clinical and community services and population health
	Goal 4: Advance the Health and Well-Being of Individuals and Communities	▪ **Objective A:** Empower individual, family, and caregiver health management and engagement ▪ **Objective B:** Protect and promote public health and healthy, resilient communities
	Goal 5: Advance Research, Scientific Knowledge, and Innovation	▪ **Objective A:** Increase access to and usability of high-quality electronic health information and services ▪ **Objective B:** Accelerate the development and commercialization of innovative technologies and solutions ▪ **Objective C:** Invest, disseminate, and translate research on how health IT can improve health and care delivery

Reproduced from U.S. Department of Health and Human Services (HHS) & National Coordinator for Health Information Technology (ONC). (2015). Federal health IT strategic plan 2015-2020: Quick reference factsheet. Retrieved from https://www.healthit.gov/sites/default/files/FederalHealthIT_Strategic_Plan.pdf

HIT is a rapidly changing area that is influenced by many factors. An example of an initiative to improve medication administration and management of prescriptions is a new system established by the state of New York. It is the first state to require that all prescriptions be created electronically (Otterman, 2016). This change will also increase the state's ability to track use of controlled substances at a time when there is increased concern about the growing problem of addiction. There are some difficulties with the requirement that will mean changes and adjustment; for example, when patients come to a healthcare provider, they need to know the name of the pharmacy they want to use, and if it turns out the medication is too expensive, it will not be easy to make changes. This change in prescription procedure should reduce errors that occur due to handwriting but will require changes in the healthcare delivery system and in preparing patients. It is a system that requires an efficient electronic system for all providers. **Figure 11-6** describes the relationship of HIT to CQI, as noted by the HHS.

HIT is also expanding rapidly in health care, and thus we have greater access to data through many types of digital records, expanding ability to complete effective retrospective reviews and capture more information. Real-time triggers help to catch errors in processes, and these also need to be examined, as they may lead to important information to use in preventing future errors. It is also important to recognize that sometimes HIT acts as a barrier to improvement and may actually lead to errors, just as medical equipment may help improve care but may also be associated with care problems and errors. Other examples of barriers are alarm/alert fatigue, errors made in CPOE, and poor interoperability of different electronic medical/health record systems.

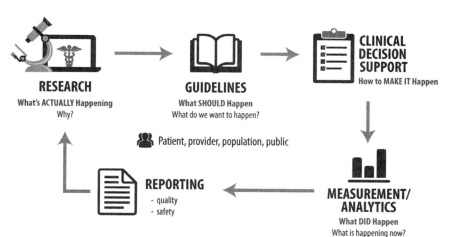

Figure 11-6. Health IT Enabled Quality Improvement Ecosystem

Reproduced from U.S. Department of Health and Human Services & National Coordinator for Health Information Technology. (2014). Health IT enabled quality improvement: A vision to achieve better health and health care. Retrieved from https://www .healthit.gov/sites/default/files /HITEnabledQualityImprovement-111214.pdf

Technology can assist teams, increasing communication, decision-making, and sharing of information in an efficient manner (Kuziemsky & Reeves, 2012). It offers collaborative tools that can increase the team's efforts in care coordination and improve quality. However, just as in nonwork settings, overreliance on technology for communication reduces face-to-face team interaction, which is critical to development and maintenance of team structure and function.

Care transitions and handoffs are discussed elsewhere in this text. Here the focus is on HIT and its potential for improving transitions (Marcotte, Kirtane, Lynn, & McKethan, 2015). If HIT is integrated into plans to reduce transition problems, it then addresses the need to resolve gaps in care and quality. The discharge process requires complete and timely information. HIT can automate this information and ideally share it between HCOs and healthcare providers. Improved information flow can fill the gap and ensure consistency and reduce errors. When medication reconciliation is part of HIT, it can reduce errors. Patient activation is required for patient-centered care. HIT can assist by increasing electronic information sharing with patients, providing patient education opportunities, and offering other resources for patients.

Nurses need to be involved in HIT to support their practice but also to better ensure their own engagement in CQI. The core healthcare professions competencies include "utilize informatics" (IOM, 2003). Emerging technologies are important, requiring nurses to keep up to date and participate in the development, implementation, and evaluation of HIT systems. Nurses have critical roles and responsibilities related to technology; however, to make technology initiatives work effectively, nurses need to be involved in the beginning stages of HIT development within HCOs and continue their involvement through evaluation and improvement. Not only do all nurses need to know about HIT and participate in its application, nursing informatics is also a specialty that supports a nursing role in HIT (ANA, 2014). Certification and graduate programs are available for the specialty, and some HCOs have formal positions for nurses with this specialty. Nursing is also recognized by the Healthcare Information and Management Systems Society as important in leading and should be visible in efforts to achieve healthcare delivery transformation through technology and informatics (HIMSS, 2011).

With the growth of HIT, providers have more opportunities to improve care and reduce costs, although not all HIT meets these goals. When safety is the focus, HIT does not necessarily always demonstrate positive results. As Ehlert and Rough (2013) warn, "Technology can instill a false sense of security, leading to carelessness by healthcare professionals" (p. 470). Some AHRQ-funded researchers suggest that there is need to develop a better model or framework for HIT that focuses on safety and CQI, and this was done in 2015 (HHS, ONC, 2015a). The purpose of this model, as explained by Sitting and Singh (2015), is to

refine the science of measuring health IT-related patient safety, make health IT-related patient safety an organizational priority by securing commitment from organizational leadership, and develop an environment conducive to detecting, fixing and learning from system vulnerabilities... focusing on three related domains: (1) concerns unique and specific to technology; (2) concerns created by the failure to use health IT appropriately or by misuse of health IT; and (3) the use of health IT to monitor risks, health care processes, and outcomes and to identify potential safety concerns before they can harm patients.

In 2015, the HHS published a report, *Connecting Health and Care for the Nation: A Shared Nationwide Interoperability Roadmap, Draft Version 1.0.* This report provides a roadmap supporting **interoperability** or "the ability of a system to exchange electronic health information with and use electronic health information from other systems without special effort on the part of the user" (HHS, ONC, 2015a, p. 18). The key issue is access to information when needed by people. In addition, there is movement to active consideration of the patient to support patient-centered care in HIT. Important principles should be followed when the plan is implemented (HHS, ONC, 2015a, pp. 20–21):

- Build upon the existing health IT infrastructure.
- Recognize that one size does not fit all.
- Empower individuals, giving them more access to information.
- Leverage the market, recognizing the greater need now for seamless flow of electronic clinical health information.
- Simplify.
- Maintain modularity; provide flexibility to the system, as change will be ongoing.
- Consider the current environment and support multiple levels of advancement.
- Focus on value.
- Protect privacy and security in all aspects of interoperability.
- Include scalability and universal access.

Careful planning of use of electronic methods can reduce later planning and implementation problems, such as delays in getting information, duplication, and omissions. If you have a clear understanding and description of the process, then there is greater chance HIT systems will be in sync with real-world processes (Jackson, 2004). Rudman, Bailey, Hope, Garrett, and Brown (2014) describe the benefits of effectively used technology: "Technology has the potential to improve workflow and the fluid transmission of vital information on errors that surface from a system perspective, without placing blame on fallible individuals and institutions" (p. 196).

Recognizing the critical need for access to CQI information and supporting evidence-based resources, the CMS and the Office of the National Coordinator for Health Information Technology introduced a new Internet site, eCQI Resource Center, in January 2016, describing it as a one-stop shop for the most current resources to support electronic clinical QI. The end of chapter *Connect to Current Information* provides a link to this site. **Table 11-2** describes potential benefits and safety concerns of HIT components.

Meaningful Use

A variety of communication devices are also associated with technology. There is greater use of smartphones in clinical areas and use of other devices such as tablets and laptops. These devices can have a positive impact on CQI, as staff have more timely access to information and can search the Internet for information that was not as easily accessible in the past. For all of these devices, a critical concern is patient privacy and confidentiality. HCOs have policies and procedures that must be followed to prevent problems. These requirements should support CQI efforts of using technology and sharing data, when appropriate, with appropriate persons.

Hacking, however, is a growing problem, allowing access of private information to get into the hands of people who might abuse this information. Some HCOs have even been "held hostage" by hackers who gain control of the HCO electronic systems and require that money be paid to regain access (Balakrishnan, 2016). In the future, other types of events may occur. This risk requires HCOs to be extra vigilant and to try to anticipate potential problems so that they can be prevented.

In July 2010, the Office of the National Coordinator for Health Information Technology and the CMS issued significant new rules that have had an impact on HCOs. These rules, **meaningful use**, are criteria that hospitals and CMS-eligible providers must meet to be identified as meaningful users of HIT (HHS, 2016). If HCOs and eligible CMS providers do not meet these criteria, the providers will not receive CMS payment for services. The criteria were developed to better ensure that services and related HIT are meeting the recommendations from the *Quality Chasm* reports. The specific meaningful use purposes are as follows (HHS, 2016):

1. Improve quality, safety, efficiency, and reduce health disparities.
2. Engage patients and their families (through electronic communication).
3. Improve care coordination.
4. Ensure adequate privacy and security protection for personal health information.
5. Improve population and public health through data collection and analysis of data.

HCOs must apply these criteria to their HIT and connect it to their CQI program.

Meaningful use, similar to other initiatives, has changed over time. The Acting Administrator of CMS commented in early 2016 about new changes:

The meaningful use program as it has existed, will now be effectively over and replaced with something better. Since late last year we have been working side

TABLE 11–2 Potential Benefits and Safety Concerns of Health IT Components

Computerized Physician/Provider Order Entry (CPOE)

An electronic system that allows providers to record, store, retrieve, and modify orders (e.g., prescriptions, diagnostic testing, treatment, and/or radiology/imaging orders).

Potential Benefits	Safety Concerns

■ Large increase in legible orders
■ Shorter order turnaround times
■ Lower relative risk of medication errors
■ Higher percentage of patients who attain their treatment goals
	■ Increases relative risk of medication errors
	■ Increased ordering time
	■ New opportunities for errors, such as:
	  ● Fragmented displays preventing a coherent view of patients' medications
	  ● Inflexible ordering formats generating wrong orders
	  ● Separations in functions that facilitate double dosing
	  ● Incompatible orders
	■ Disruptions in workflow

Clinical Decision Support (CDS)

Monitors and alerts clinicians of patient conditions, prescriptions, and treatment to provide evidence-based clinical suggestions to health professionals at the point of care.

Potential Benefits	Safety Concerns

■ Reductions in:
  ● Relative risk of medication errors
  ● Risk of toxic drug levels
  ● Management errors of resuscitating patients in adult trauma centers
  ● Prescriptions of nonpreferred medications
■ Can effectively monitor and alert clinicians of adverse conditions
■ Improve long-term treatment and increase the likelihood of achieving treatment goa
	■ Rate of detecting drug–drug interactions varies widely among different vendors
	■ Increases in mortality rate
	■ High override rate of computer generate alerts (alert fatigue)

(Continued)

TABLE 11-2 Potential Benefits and Safety Concerns of Health IT Components (*Continued*)

Bar Coding

Bar coding can be used to track medications, orders, and other healthcare products. It can also be used to verify patient identification and dosage.

Potential Benefits	Safety Concerns

■ Significant reductions in relative risk of medication errors associated with:
  ● Transcription
  ● Dispensing
  ● Administration errors
	■ Introduction of workarounds; for example, clinicians can:
	  ● Scan medications and patient identification without visually checking to see if the medication, dosing, and patient identification are correct
	  ● Attach patient identification bar codes to another object instead of the patient
	  ● Scan orders and medications of multiple patients at once instead of doing it each time the medication is dispensed

Patient Engagement Tools

Tools such as patient portals, smartphone applications, email, and interactive kiosks, which enable patients to participate in their healthcare treatment.

Potential Benefits	Safety Concerns
■ Reduction in hospitalization rates in children ■ Increases in patients' knowledge of treatment and illnesses	■ Reliability of data entered by patients, families, or unauthorized users

Note: This table is not intended to be an exhaustive list of all potential benefits and safety concerns associated with health IT. It represents the most common potential benefits and safety concerns.

Reproduced with permission from Institute of Medicine. (2012). Health IT and patient safety: Building safer systems for better care. Washington, DC: National Academies Press. Courtesy of the National Academies Press, Washington, DC.

by side with physician organizations across many communities—including with great advocacy from the American Medical Association—and have listened to the needs and concerns of many. We will be putting out the details on this next stage over the next few months, but I will give you themes guiding our implementation. For one, the focus will move away from rewarding providers for the use of technology and towards the outcome they achieve with their patients. Second, providers will be able to customize their goals so tech companies can build around the individual practice needs, not the needs of the government. Technology must be user-centered and support physicians, not distract them. Third, one way to aid this is by leveling the technology playing field for start-ups and new entrants. (CMS Blog, 2016)

This initiative is an example of how CQI is never static and requires nurses to keep up to date with changes. Ideally, nurses should participate in health policy, providing their expertise and sharing their concerns about nursing care and the healthcare delivery system and relationship to CQI-related policy.

Electronic Medical/Health Record

HIT includes the electronic medical/health record, patient engagement tools such as personal health records, and health information exchanges. HIT is not one product but rather multiple products and systems. One has to consider that the use of HIT usually requires interaction with staff and this interaction can then increase risk (IOM, 2012).

The **electronic medical record (EMR)** is a digital record that includes provider medical and clinical data for a patient. The **electronic health record (EHR)** includes the same information plus more comprehensive information about the patient's history. The EMR/EHR is used to share information from one provider to another. **Personal health records (PHRs)** include the same information as the EMR and EHR, but the patient keeps the record and maintains it. These digital records help track data over time, identify patients who are due for preventive visits and screenings, monitor patient measures of certain parameters, and improve overall quality of care in practice (HealthIT.gov, 2015). Selecting, implementing, and evaluating an EMR requires a team approach. In a study reported in 2012, 71% of providers who adopted EHRs indicated they would make the same decision again. These digital systems typically also include "notification of potentially dangerous drug interactions, verify medications and dosages, and reduce the need for potentially risky tests and procedures" (HealthIT.gov, 2015). The HHS identifies the Common Clinical Data Set for electronic records, which includes the following (HHS, ONC, 2015a, p. 12):

- Patient name
- Sex
- Date of birth
- Race
- Ethnicity
- Preferred language
- Smoking status
- Problems
- Medications
- Medication allergies
- Vital signs

- Care plan field(s), including goals and instructions
- Procedures
- Care team members
- Immunizations
- Unique device identifier(s) for patient's implantable device(s)
- Notes/narrative

EMR/EHR development and implementation began in a disorganized manner, and thus the result was great variation in hardware and software used in HCOs with limited early concern about sharing across HCOs. There was little standardization, and now this is a problem, as we need more effective inter-HCO sharing and sharing with government agencies. Using a common set supports records with consistent content and organization within and across HCOs, improving communication, care, and ease of accessibility. The HHS Office of National Coordinator for Health Information Technology coordinates the department's national HIT efforts, focusing on adoption of national standards and support of interoperable exchange of health information (HHS, ONC, 2015b).

The Affordable Care Act (ACA) provides funding to assist with the expansion of EMR/EHR adoption, believing that this technology will greatly assist in transforming and improving health care. These tools can be used to improve care and increase teamwork effectiveness. The following are examples of the potential impact digital records may have on CQI (HealthIT.gov, 2015):

- Quick access to patient information from multiple locations to assist in providing coordinated, efficient care
- Decision support, clinical alerts, reminders, medical information
- Performance-improving tools, real-time quality reporting
- Legible, complete documentation that facilitates accurate coding and billing
- Interface with labs and other sources of information
- Safer, more reliable prescribing
- Error reduction when multiple caregivers are involved in the care (i.e., care coordination)
- Improved care transitions (handoffs) between settings
- Up-to-date information for emergency care (i.e., care coordination)

Patients also benefit directly. There is reduced time to fill out information per visit, as the provider has the information digitally. The patient can receive reminders about care needs and information, and e-prescriptions can be sent to the pharmacy. Referrals can be made electronically. In some cases, patients can access their provider electronically. Digital records also have an impact on risk management by providing timely and detailed documentation and may also help prevent liability actions, as accurate information can be provided about the care provided and use of EBP.

According to the HHS, CMS (2015), the Medicare and Medicaid Electronic Health Record Incentive Programs provide "incentive payments to eligible professionals, eligible hospitals, and critical access hospitals (CAHs) as they adopt, implement, upgrade, or demonstrate meaningful use of certified EHR technology." The CMS incentive program has been a strong driver in getting providers to use digital records, with data reporting that 8 in 10 physicians have adopted or plan to adopt digital records (HHS, 2014). HITECH has helped increase adoption of digital records. Since the passage of HITECH, more nongovernment hospitals have adopted EMR/EHR systems. Charles, Gabriel, and Furukawa (2014) report the following:

> In 2013, nearly six in ten (59%) non-federal acute care hospitals had adopted at least a basic EHR system with clinician notes. This represents a 34% increase from the previous year and a more than five-fold increase in EHR adoption since 2008. In addition, a vast majority of acute care hospitals (93%) possessed EHR technology certified as meeting federal requirements for Meaningful Use objectives.

A recent study examined the adoption of EMR/EHRs and their impact on hospital adverse events (Furukawa et al., 2016; Helwig & Lomotan, 2016). The sample for this retrospective analysis of the Medicare Patient Safety Monitoring System from 2012 through 2013 included 45,235 patients at risk for 347,298 adverse events. The focus was on fully electronic records that included physician notes, nursing assessments, problem lists, medication lists, discharge summaries, and provider orders. Fully electronic record for patients with cardiovascular conditions, surgery, and pneumonia indicated that between 17% and 30% were less likely to experience adverse events in the hospital, indicating a positive outcome when using electronic records, leading to better coordinated care with less risk of harm. There were limitations in the study that require further examination, such as high-alert medications in the system, safety features used, and determination of which methods had greatest influence on adverse events. Although it has long been believed that electronic records improve care, more research is needed.

As many HCOs have updated their EMR/EHRs or plan to do so, a common concern is risk of errors when using electronic documentation systems. This topic is not new, but when changes in systems are made, the introduction of errors needs to be considered; moreover, the change process itself increases risk of errors. It takes about a year for an HCO and its staff to adjust to a new system, and the first year is a high-risk period for errors (Abramson et al., 2013).

Schwiran and Thede (2011) offer valuable insight into the relationship between nursing care and the EMR/EHR:

> Two significant challenges have always faced nursing: (a) how to differentiate nursing's contributions to patient care from those of medicine; and (b) how to incorporate descriptions of nursing care into the health record in a manner that is commensurate with its importance to patients' welfare.

These challenges are even more important with computerized medical records. One of the underlying drivers of the latter challenge is the use (or disuse) of standardized communication among nurses. Standardized nursing terminologies (SNTs) may help in recognizing nursing interventions, improving communication among nurses and with other staff, improving patient care, providing access to data about nursing care interventions and outcomes, increasing compliance with standards of care, and providing data to help to assess nursing competencies. In a study of a survey of 1,268 nurses, the respondents were asked about SNT. A large proportion of the sample had no experience or knowledge of SNTs (Schwiran & Thede, 2011). The SNT that was the most recognizable by one-third of the respondents was that of the North American Nursing Diagnosis Association (NANDA), but these respondents had not used it since graduation. One-quarter said they had not used the Nursing Intervention Classification or the Nursing Outcome Classification since graduation. These findings raise questions about the need for SNT: Why is this type of information important? Is it integrated into electronic records? If there is conflict and lack of nursing participation in using these methods that focus on nursing terminology, what is the value of teaching them to students? Do we then confuse communication, particularly interprofessional communication? There are no clear answers to these questions, but in the future, more examination of this issue is needed in order to arrive at the best approach for nursing and for healthcare delivery.

Computerized Physician/Provider Order Entry

Computerized physician/provider order entry (CPOE) is supported by the HITECH Act of 2009 and by the National Quality Forum as a method to support quality care. When a hospitalized patient receives a medication, there are four steps that occur: (1) ordering, (2) transcribing the order (if handwritten), (3) dispensing the medication by the pharmacists, and (4) administering medication. CPOE was developed to respond to the high rate of errors associated with the first and second steps in the medication process; more than 90% of errors occur at these two steps (HHS, AHRQ, PSNet, 2014b). Using the CPOE, a provider can enter an order directly into a computerized system and then the pharmacist receives the information. This process eliminates some of the problems with the ordering step found in noncomputerized systems such as poor handwriting, inappropriate use of abbreviations, or not using HCO-approved abbreviations, and unclear orders. Transcribing problems may be eliminated; for example, accuracy is not dependent on a staff member's ability to transcribe orders. The order can then be clearly read by a pharmacist who has the knowledge to assess the quality of the order for the patient's needs, clinical status, and required treatment. In addition, software can often identify errors in orders and alert the provider at the time the order is entered.

In 2016, the HHS, AHRQ reported on a review of the use of CPOE systems (HHS, AHRQ, PSNet, 2016a). This report comments on a Food and Drug Administration

(FDA) review of the safety of these systems, which noted major usability problems with all the systems tested. The following are some of the specific problems that were identified:

- Inconsistent medication naming within and across systems
- Poor medication search functions
- Difficulty interpreting displays
- Vulnerability to wrong-patient errors when multiple records were open
- A lack of standardization alerts, an abundance of irrelevant alerts, and a lack of reasons documented for alert overrides among clinical decision support functions
- Medication reconciliation modules lacking standard terms and not easily accommodating team-based reconciliation workflows

Clinical Decision Support

Clinical decision support (CDS) is used to prevent errors and may also have an impact on omissions and act as a solution to improve care. For example, a CDS may alert the healthcare provider of a wrong dosage, inappropriate administration method, incorrect frequency of administration, problem with patient drug allergies, concerns about drug–drug interactions, and conflict with drug–laboratory factors when comparing laboratory results with the medication order (HHS, AHRQ, PSNet, 2016a). If there were a potential problem, this type of system would send out alerts on the computer to the healthcare provider's device. In some cases, the CDS will also send out alerts when orders should be considered for specific diagnoses—treatment that would normally be considered for the diagnosis but is not ordered.

Often CPOE is combined with a CDS; however, combining the two systems requires planning and staff training when it is implemented. One problem that has occurred and may influence how providers respond to alerts is alert fatigue. Just because the provider receives an alert on the computer that something requires attention does not mean the provider will respond or respond with correct action. CPOE and CDS systems are also expensive. HCOs need to select systems that best meet their needs (Nuckols et al., 2015).

Some studies recommend that there be greater evaluation of critical drug–drug interactions on a national professional basis, as there are too many alerts given and then providers override them (Phansalkar et al., 2013). Overusing alert systems may lead to more problems. In a study that examined improvement of usability of drug–drug interaction CDS alerts, researchers identified interventions that they think should be used to improve alerts (Payne et al., 2015). Recommendations include use of consistent terminology; use of visual cues and minimal text; and consideration of formatting, content, and reporting so that usability is improved. Alerts should provide the healthcare provider with the option to reject the alert and then provide an explanation, which should be more than just "will monitor." This option is much better than just ignoring alerts, and it provides CQI data that can be tracked over time.

An example of an error that can occur when using CPOE is wrong patient drug orders. This is thought to be an error that is not routinely reported, particularly if voluntary reporting is the major tool used to get the data. A study that focused on automated surveillance of electronic data "hypothesized that wrong-patient orders are recognized by the healthcare provider who inputted the order shortly after entry, promptly retracted, and then reentered for the right patient" (Adelman et al., 2013, p. 305). This situation is considered to be a near miss, a type of event that happens 100 times more frequently than adverse events (IOM, 2013). The study recommends that all hospitals measure their retract-reorder events to determine if there is a problem and, if so, adjust their software to better ensure alerts and other methods to decrease this near miss.

CDS should include the right information, shared with the right people, via the right channels, in the right formats, and at the right time (HHS, AHRQ, NQS, 2014). Responding to these care aspects should optimize information flow, including communication of what, who, where, when, and how. Effective use of CPOE should include the following (Ehlert & Rough, 2013, p. 475):

- Relevant patient information (e.g., demographic data, laboratory and diagnostic test results) must be readily available at the time of prescribing or order entry.
- Drug–drug interaction, drug allergy, drug–laboratory, drug contraindication, and maximum–minimum dosing alerts for potentially serious mistakes must be provided. (Sensitivity of alerts can be a problem, so they need to be tracked and adjusted as needed.)
- The selection of standard order sets (medication use algorithms and guidelines for high-risk patient populations) should be automated at the point of prescribing.
- The system must be efficient and easy to use. (If too complex, physician compliance will be reduced.)

Bar-Code Medication Administration

Bar-code medication administration is use of bar codes located on the patient's identification to compare with the bar code found on orders or, in case of medications, found on the individual patient drug package. The bar code electronically confirms a patient's identity in the system and provides an alert if not the correct patient, timeline for order, or order. Many HCOs use bar-code medication administration. This technology should reduce errors and adverse events, providing an alert system at the point of care. Bar codes are now used for more than medication administration, as they are also used for many treatment actions that require patient identification. For this electronic identification method to be effective, staff must actively use it. Some systems will block the healthcare provider from moving to next steps if the bar-code procedure is not used; for example, they may be denied access to medication storage.

Tables 11-3 provides guidelines for safe use of decentralized automated dispensing systems and patient safety when using technology during medication administration.

Medical Devices

Medical devices have had a major positive impact on CQI; however, they can also lead to errors and problems with CQI. In a review of studies that examined factors related to recognition, reporting, and resolution of incidents associated with medical devices, it was noted that incidents were not commonly reported due to concern about fear of punishment, uncertainty about what should be reported and how incident reports are used, and limitations of time to complete reporting (Plisena, Gagliardi, Urbach, & Clifford, 2015). Medical device security has also become an important topic that can impact care delivery and CQI. For example, if there are passwords that must be used to access a medical device, how does the staff member know the password? What happens if the password changes? In emergencies, how does requiring a password impact the ability to get care to the patient when needed? Security is important, but it has to be practical for the healthcare delivery system (HIMSS, 2016). The FDA is responsible for approval of many medical devices. In addition, as mentioned earlier, there has been increasing concern about hacking and cybersecurity in computer systems, and these concerns may also apply to medical devices, which may have similar risks compared to computers.

In a recent report to the U.S. Senate Committee on Health, Education, Labor, and Pensions, specific concern about safety and infection risk with a medical device, closed-channel duodenoscopes, was identified. This is, of course, a serious concern, but there is something else in the report that is even more important. The report notes that Congress needs to "fund a national medical device evaluation system, so that the FDA can 'effectively monitor the safety of medical devices on the market rather than relying on adverse event reporting'" (Saint Louis, 2016, p. A13). The report notes that manufacturers do not always report adverse events or report them in the required time frame. The FDA provides MedWatch adverse event reporting program for HCOs and staff to use. The following are examples of possible types of medical device problems that might be reported (Simone, Brumbaugh, & Ricketts, 2014, p. 403):

- Electric beds (e.g., patient entrapment, electric shock)
- Negative pressure wound therapy devices (e.g., bleeding, infection)
- Patient lifts (e.g., falls)
- Infusion pumps (e.g. overdose or underdose, shock, fire)

TABLE 11-3 Guidelines for Safe Use of Decentralized Automated Dispensing Systems

Agree with the vendor on a documented preventive maintenance schedule that does not disrupt workflow.

Any high-risk medications stocked in devices should be accompanied by an alert system for nurses (such as a maximum-dose prompt).

Carefully select stored drugs based on the needs of the patient care unit, patient age, diagnosis, and staff expertise.

Conduct monthly expiration date checks, concomitantly verifying inventory accuracy. Configure devices to provide single-dose (or single-drug) access whenever possible, focusing such control on high-risk medications and controlled substances. Develop an ongoing competency assessment program for all personnel who use or affect the system, including direct observation and random restocking accuracy audits, as well as observation of dispensing accuracy as part of the assessment.

Develop a system to remove all recalled medications.

Develop clear, multidisciplinary system downtime procedures that are included in an ongoing competency program.

Develop strict safety criteria for selecting medications that are (and are not) appropriate for storing in devices.

Develop systems to account for narcotic waste, and routinely audit controlled substance dispenses versus patient orders and medication administration records.

Do not stock look-alike and sound-alike drugs in the same open-access drawer.

Have strict security procedures to limit unauthorized access.

Place allergy reminders for specific drugs such as antibiotics, opiates, and NSAIDs on appropriate drug storage pockets, or have them automatically appear on the dispensing screen.

Require all personnel to attend formal training and demonstrate competency prior to assigning them access to the system.

Require nurses to return medications to a return bin, never back to the original storage pocket or location.

Require pharmacist medication order review and approval before administration of the first dose of medication (profile dispensing), and limit medications in which profile dispensing may be overridden.

Use open-access drawers only for stocking drugs with low potential for causing patient harm if administered in error.

Whenever possible, use bar coding capabilities for restocking medications and for retrieval.

With few exceptions, maximize use of unit-dose medications in ready-to-administer form.

All actions and usage on a system must be reportable in an easily reviewed format, including identification of the user, the medication, the patient for whom the drug was dispensed, and the time of the transaction.

At medication administration, one system must be able to identify and document the medication, person administering the medication, and patient by utilizing bar code technology.

Hospital admit/discharge/transfer and medication order entry computer systems should be interfaced with automation devices to provide caregivers with warnings about allergies, interactions, duplications, and inappropriate doses at the point of dispensing and/or administration.

Information necessary to properly manage patient care must be accurate, accessible, and timely.

Pertinent patient- and medication-specific information and instructions entered into pharmacy and/or hospital information system should be available electronically at the point of care (administration), and the system should prompt the nurse to record pertinent information before administration may be documented.

Real-time systems integration should exist from the point of prescribing (order entry) through dispensing and through documentation of medication administration.

The system must accommodate bar-coded unit-dose medications and utilize the bar code capability for drug restocking, retrieval, and administering medications.

The system should force users to confirm the intention whenever medications are accessed or administration is attempted outside of the scheduled administration time or dosage range. Such events should be signaled visibly or audibly for the user, and all such events should be electronically documented and reported daily for follow-up.

The interface with the pharmacy computer system should allow the nurse to view and access only those medications that have been ordered for the specific patient.

The nurse should be electronically reminded when a medication dose is due (and by a different mechanism when it is past due).

User access should be restricted to a unique user identification code and password, or a unique bar code.

- Peritoneal dialysis machines and components (e.g., increased intraperitoneal pressure, problems with administration sets)
- Glucose meters and strips (e.g., improper storage of strips, false high or low blood glucose values)
- Foley catheters (e.g., infection, breakage, insertion trauma)
- Gastrointestinal tubes and feeding pumps (e.g., fluid contamination, cessation of infusion)

The FDA expects staff to complete their HCO incident reports in addition to reporting to the FDA. The FDA (2014) gives the following guidelines for reporting:

Product problems should be reported to the FDA when there is a concern about the quality, authenticity, performance, or safety of any medication or device for the following reasons: suspect counterfeit product, product contamination, defective components, poor packaging or product mix-up, questionable stability, device malfunction, and labeling concerns.

Many problems or adverse events are not reported; for example, staff may not think a problem/event is important or may think reporting will make no difference. This failure to report then may lead to greater problems, as the FDA can do nothing to the resolve these problems, such as addressing the problem with the device manufacturer. The FDA has the expertise to decide if a problem should be examined and to determine actions that may need to be taken, but without report of problems, changes are not possible.

Stop and Consider #3

Health informatics may help improve care and may also act as a barrier to quality care.

Multiple Roles of Nurses in Preventing or Reducing Quality Care Problems

Nurses are responsible for the daily monitoring and management of the quality of health care delivered to patients. The nurse's responsibilities include immediate detection and intervention when patients' clinical conditions change, although not all nurses are prepared for or demonstrate this responsibility. Expert nursing practice requires not only psychomotor and affective skills, but also complex thinking processes such as making inferences and synthesizing information to choose a course of action. Nurses constitute the surveillance system for early detection of patient complications and problems, and they are in the best position to choose a course of action. Their responsibilities include the following (Potter et al., October 2014, p. 39; Benner et al., 2002; Higuachi & Donald, 2002; Clark & Aiken, 2003):

- Understand the need for and demonstrate complete participation in the medication process, including knowledge about medications.
- Assist in collecting CQI data.
- Participate in root cause analysis.
- Participate in incident reporting as required by your HCO.
- Recognize the importance of sentinel events and participate in reporting and analysis of these events.
- Use standardized, structured communication methods such as SBAR.
- Participate actively on teams; collaborate and coordinate care.
- Participate actively in the HCO accreditation process.
- Use tools provided by your HCO such as checklists, protocols, and clinical guidelines to improve care and participate in their selection and/or development.
- Use methods such as failure mode and effects analysis effectively.
- Attend and actively participate in clinical rounds and safety rounds.
- Recognize the negative impact of failure to rescue, and implement methods to reduce it.
- Consider documentation a critical component of care and take care when documenting.
- Engage with other staff and managers to develop and maintain a culture of safety.
- Recognize the need for a healthy work environment and the impact of human factors on CQI. Apply this knowledge to yourself, such as recognizing risks that increases when you are tired, work long hours, and are stressed.
- Follow all required infection control protocols.
- Ask management to share CQI data, analysis, and conduct routine discussion of outcomes with staff.
- Ensure that the workspace for clinical care and medication administration is as free as possible from disruptions and noise.
- Use EBP and EBM.
- Apply medication reconciliation as needed.
- Recognize the importance of near misses and how this type of error impacts your practice, and take action.
- Request that information and resource access be accurate and timely (e.g., receipt of lab test results, delivery of medications and supplies to the unit).
- Participate in CQI-related committees and task forces.
- Keep patient-centered care in focus at all times, and remain mindful of how can you improve it.
- Work to improve your participation in handoffs and use HCO-required methods such as checklists and standardized, structured communication methods.

- Respect all members of the staff—clinical and nonclinical.
- Participate in staff education and peer evaluation.

Healthcare professionals must participate in self-regulation and self-improvement (Malloch, Benner, Sheets, Kenward, & Farrell, 2010). In 2007, the National Council of State Boards of Nursing (NCSBN) began an initiative to better understand nursing practice and quality care and to develop a national database of nursing errors, referred to as the Taxonomy of Error, Root Cause Analysis, and Practice Responsibility (TERCAP) (Benner, Malloch, & Sheets, 2010; NCSBN, 2015). The TERCAP® database includes data on patient profile, patient outcome, setting, systems issues, healthcare team, nurse profile, intentional misconduct or criminal behavior, safe medication administration, documentation, and practice breakdown. This database is different from the National Database of Nursing Quality Indicators (NDNQI), which is also discussed in this text. The NDNQI focuses on specific nursing indicators, whereas the TERCAP database is focused on nursing errors that are reported prospectively online to state boards of nursing and then analyzed and shared with the NCSBN, although not all states participate (as of 2015, 26 states participate).

Why is TERCAP® important to the discussion in this chapter? It recognizes the need to track nursing errors nationally and by state and in doing so recognizes that there must be something unique in identifying a nursing error. The work done to develop the TERCAP® database system provides information about nursing care, nursing education, errors, and quality care (Benner et al., 2010). We need to understand more about how nursing practice impacts care and how we can learn from errors. The intent of TERCAP® is not to move backwards toward a "blame" culture within nursing education, but rather forward toward a culture of safety and a better understanding of the root cause of errors from a system view, both education and practice, and from an individual view. This extensive examination of nursing practice based its framework on the five healthcare professions core competencies and the Quality and Safety Education for Nurses six core competencies for nurses. As noted earlier in this text, these two sets of competencies do not completely agree, although they are very similar.

TERCAP led to the identification of three major standards of nursing practice that are integral to CQI (Malloch et al., 2010, p. 12):

- *Safe medication administration.* The nurse administers the right dose of the right medication via the right route to the right patient at the right time and for the right reason.
- *Documentation.* Nursing documentation provides relevant information about the patient and the measures implemented in response to the patient's needs.
- *Attentiveness/surveillance.* The nurse monitors what is happening with the patient and staff. The nurse observes the patient's clinical condition; if the

nurse has not observed a patient, then he or she cannot identify changes and/or make knowledgeable discernments and decisions about the patient.

Table 11-4 describes the TERCAP nursing practice breakdowns in greater detail.

TABLE 11–4 Overview of the TERCAP Database	
Nursing Practice Breakdown	**Description**
Medication administration	To safely and effectively administer drugs, the nurse must assess the patient's status, actions needed, medication side effects, other medications the patient is taking, the patient's environment, and other care activities provided to the patient. If the patient is able, then the patient should be involved in the administration process. The nurse must be knowledgeable about the drug to be administered. Prevention of errors and improvement require assessment of system design and how to support effective, safe medication administration, particularly avoiding the approach of the "status quo"—doing things the way we always have.
Communicating patient data	Nurses have multiple ways to communicate/share patient data and assessment to others—the care team. Documentation is the primary method used, and today it has moved more to digital methods, though some HCOs still use non-digital methods. Digital methods require effective collaboration with health informatics.
Attentiveness/ surveillance	Nurses use surveillance to gather information and assess what is happening to the patient. This should be an active part of nursing practice. At the same time that better surveillance is needed, it can also be a burden and increase work, and many factors can negatively impact surveillance, such as fatigue, stress, workload, lack of expertise for the situation, and so on. The Institute of Medicine particularly addresses the nurse's role in surveillance in its significant report *Keeping Patients Safe: Transforming the Work Environment* (2004).
Clinical reasoning/ judgment	Nurses need to use clinical reasoning and judgment in their practice as they assess patients and outcomes based on data that they obtain. If a nurse does not select and use the best intervention, this is clinical reasoning/judgment breakdown.

(Continued)

TABLE 11-4 Overview of the TERCAP Database *(Continued)*	
Prevention	The nurse uses interventions to prevent or reduce risks, hazards, or complications that may be related to illness or treatment. It is easier to identify lack of prevention, as one can use the outcomes of complications as the measure that prevention was not done or ineffective. Engaging the patient is a critical factor in prevention.
Intervention	Intervention refers to the nurse acting on behalf of the patient—an act made by the nurse. If the nurse does not execute an intervention correctly or the timing is not what it should be, then this is an intervention breakdown. Intervention does not include assessment, surveillance, and monitoring, even though these efforts do provide important information for interventions. Interventions are visible and invisible (related to surveillance).
Interpretation of orders	Communication of orders is an important part of care delivery, and nurses must guard against the risk of misinterpretation (e.g., incomplete orders, illegible writing, problems in transcribing orders, and now digital errors).
Professional responsibility and patient advocacy	Nurses must speak up for their needs to provide quality care (e.g., staffing levels and mix), and they also speak for the patient to ensure patient needs are understood and met when possible. As nurses meet this practice area, they must consider professional boundaries as described by the National Council of State Boards of Nursing.

Data from Benner, P., Malloch, K., & Sheets, V. (Eds.). (2010). *Nursing pathways for patient safety.* St. Louis, MO: National Council State Boards of Nursing and Mosby.

As CQI measures are considered, one approach for HCOs to take when considering nursing practice within the HCO is to use the practice breakdowns that are part of TERCAP®: medication administration, communicating patient data, attentiveness/surveillance, clinical reasoning/judgment, prevention, intervention, interpretation of orders, and professional responsibility. This type of initiative provides more opportunities for nurses to meet their CQI responsibilities as a profession and within the healthcare delivery system.

Stop and Consider #4

In the course of a nurse's daily practice, there are many opportunities for the nurse to prevent or reduce quality care problems.

Conclusions

Information in this chapter ties together the content on CQI measurement by discussing multiple methods/strategies/interventions used to prevent and reduce quality care problems and respond to problems. Nurses need more knowledge not only about CQI but also about how to engage in the CQI process and change. Nurses need "opportunities to pose nursing practice questions, identify process flow, implement and monitor change, and then evaluate and chart related outcomes" (Beckel & Wolf, 2013, p. 648). Appendix B provides a list of examples of major HCOs and agencies, governmental and nongovernmental, that provide CQI resources for HCOs and healthcare professions.

Apply CQI

Chapter Highlights

- HCOs use multiple methods/strategies/interventions to assist in preventing or reducing quality care problems—to intervene and to improve. These methods/strategies/interventions are chosen by the HCO and staff, but in some cases are influenced by requirements from accreditors, third-party payers, and government agencies (state and federal).
- HCOs and healthcare professional organizations may develop and/or use the following methods/strategies/interventions: redesign of systems and processes, position descriptions and performance appraisal, clinical ladders, policies and procedures, evidence-based practice (EBP) requirements, standardization of care, clinical guidelines and protocols, case management, disease management, QI committees, utilization review/management committees, staff education, and mentoring and coaching.
- Documentation of CQI data, analysis, and solutions are an important part of preventing or reducing quality care problems and improving care.
- Structured communication methods are used by many HCOs to reduce problems with ineffective communication. Examples are SBAR (situation, background, assessment, recommendation), time-outs, crew resource management, signouts, read-backs, huddles, worksheets, change-of-shift reports, whiteboards, and staff meetings.
- Other methods/strategies/interventions that are more patient-centered are rapid response teams; safety walkarounds; patient-centered rounds; teach-backs; safe zones; the collaborative care model; CUSP (Comprehensive Unit-based Safety Program); the Universal Protocol for Preventing Wrong Site, Wrong Procedure, or Wrong Person Surgery; and medication reconciliation.
- Teams and teamwork are critical to all aspects of CQI.

- TeamSTEPPS, developed by the federal government, is an evidence-based approach to staff team training that is used by many HCOs.
- Technology and informatics are important in providing care. They also are used to prevent or reduce quality care problems; for example, they are used for data collection and analysis and for providing alerts to providers.
- Common health informatics technology (HIT) are the electronic medical record/electronic health record (EMR/EHR), computerized physician/ provider order entry (CPOE), clinical decision support (CDS), and bar-coding medication administration.
- Medical devices require maintenance and correct use to prevent errors and safety concerns with their use. Nurses and other staff with technology experience work together to ensure that devices are used effectively.
- Nurses need to be more actively involved in preventing or reducing quality care problems. These responsibilities require that nurses be prepared to meet them.

Critical Thinking and Clinical Reasoning and Judgment: Discussion Questions and Learning Activities

1. Select one of the examples of methods/strategies/interventions used to prevent or reduce quality care problems, and discuss the method and how it impacts care. Do this in a team, with each member selecting a different method/strategy/intervention. When possible, provide examples from practice. In the team discussion, consider the pros and cons of using the method/strategy/intervention.
2. Why are teams and teamwork important to CQI? Provide three examples to support your response.
3. What is the purpose of meaningful use?
4. Ask a staff member from a local HCO's HIT department to speak to the class about HIT. Students should prepare questions based on chapter content.
5. Provide two examples of how a nurse can prevent or reduce quality care problems. Support your example with references.

Connect to Current Information

- AHRQ: PocketGuide—TeamSTEPPS
  http://www.ahrq.gov/professionals/education/curriculum-tools/teamstepps/
  instructor/essentials/pocketguide.html#frame
- AHRQ: Organizational Readiness Assessment Checklist
  http://www.ahrq.gov/professionals/education/curriculum-tools/teamstepps/
  readiness/index.html

- FDA: Medical Device Safety
  http://www.fda.gov/medicaldevices/safety/default.htm
- HealthIT.gov
  https://www.healthit.gov/
- eCQI Resource Center Sponsored by the CMS
  https://ecqi.healthit.gov/
- AHRQ: CUSP Toolkit
  http://www.ahrq.gov/professionals/education/curriculum-tools/cusptoolkit/
     index.html
- The Joint Commission: Universal Protocol
  http://www.jointcommission.org/standards_information/up.aspx
  http://www.jointcommission.org/assets/1/18/up_poster1.pdf
- AHRQ, PSNet: Patient Safety Primers
  https://psnet.ahrq.gov/primers

EBP, EBM, and Quality Improvement: Exemplar

Wittie, M., Ngo-Metzger, Q., & Lebrun-Harris, L. (2016). Enabling quality: Electronic health record adoption and meaningful use readiness in federally funded health centers. *Journal of Healthcare Quality, 38*(1), 42–51.

This large study is a major examination of the adoption and use of electronic health records.

Questions to Consider:

1. What is the design used for this study, including research question(s), sample, interventions, data collection, and analysis?
2. What are the results of the study?
3. How might you apply these results to a clinical setting to improve care?

Evolving Case Study

The QI program in a hospital with 250 beds is examining its use of teams and how teams might impact the ability to improve care. You are an expert on teams and CQI and have been invited to speak to the group. Prior to your presentation, you are told that teams are used sporadically throughout the hospital, and more effectively in medical units. Staff have had little education about teams, and some staff see no value in them, including a variety of professions such as nurses, physicians, and some pharmacists. The nonclinical staff often feel as though they are not part of the teams in the hospital, so they ignore the topic.

Case Questions:

1. Prepare a PowerPoint slide presentation that you will use to explain the importance of teams and teamwork to CQI. Provide three examples to demonstrate the relationship.

2. Select three of the methods/strategies/interventions to prevent or reduce quality care problems discussed in this chapter. Prepare a clear plan to describe the implementation of each method/strategy/intervention along with rationale for use with a specific quality care problem. Discuss how teams would be used.

3. What does a hospital need to do to prepare staff in the use of the methods/strategies/interventions and application to team and team process?

References

Abramson, E., Malhotra, S., Osorio, S., Edwards, A., Cheriff, A., Cole, C., & Kaushal, R. (2013). A long-term follow-up evaluation of electronic health record prescribing safety. *Journal of American Medical Informatics Association, 20*, e52–e53.

Adelman, J., Kalkut, G., Schechter, C., Weiss, J., Berger, M., Reissman, S.,... Southern, W. (2013). Understanding and preventing wrong-patient drug electronic orders. *Journal of American Informatics Association, 20*(2), 305–310.

Amalberti, R., Vincent, C., Auroy, Y., & de Saint Maurice, G. (2006). Violations and migrations in health care: A framework for understanding and management. *Quality and Safety in Health Care, 15*(Suppl. 1), i66–i71.

Amaral, A., McDonald, A., Coburn, N., Xiong, W., Shojania, K., Fowler, R.,... Adhikari, N. (2015). Expanding the scope of critical care response teams: A feasible approach to identify adverse events. *BMJ Quality Safety.* Retrieved from http://qualitysafety.bmj.com/content/early/2015/06/22/bmjqs-2014-003833.abstract?sid=7588baee-666c-4b2d-98c3-026cb23fe0ba

American Nurses Association (ANA). (2010). *Nursing professional development: Scope and standards of practice.* Silver Spring, MD: Author.

American Nurses Association (ANA). (2014). *Nursing informatics: Scope and standards of practice* (2nd ed.). Silver Spring, MD: Author.

Balakrishnan, A. (2016, February 16). The hospital held hostage by hackers. Retrieved from http://www.cnbc.com/2016/02/16/the-hospital-held-hostage-by-hackers.html

Barclay, L. (2013, March 4). AHRQ identifies top 10 patient safety strategies. Medscape Medical News. Retrieved from http://www.medscape.com/viewarticle/780237

Beckel, J., & Wolf, G. (2013). Identification of potential barriers to nurse-sensitive outcome demonstration. *JONA, 43*(12), 652.

Begun, J., White, K., & Mosser, G. (2011). Interprofessional care teams: The role of the healthcare administrator. *Journal of Interprofessional Care, 25*(2), 119–123.

Benner, P., Malloch, K., & Sheets, V. (Eds.). (2010). *Nursing pathways for patient safety.* St. Louis, MO: National Council of State Boards of Nursing and Mosby.

Benner, P., Sheets V., Uris, P., Malloch, K., Schwed, K., & Jamison, D. (2002). Individual, practice and system causes of errors in nursing: A taxonomy. *JONA, 32*(10), 509–523.

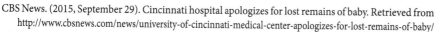

CBS News. (2015, September 29). Cincinnati hospital apologizes for lost remains of baby. Retrieved from http://www.cbsnews.com/news/university-of-cincinnati-medical-center-apologizes-for-lost-remains-of-baby/

Charles, D., Gabriel, M., & Furukawa, M. (2014, May). Adoption of electronic health record systems among U.S. non-federal acute care hospitals: 2008-2013. ONC Data Brief, No. 16. Washington, DC: Office of the National Coordinator for Health Information Technology.

Clark, S., & Aiken, L. (2003). Failure to rescue. *American Journal of Nursing, 103*, 42–47.

CMS Blog. (2016, January 12). Comments of CMS Acting Administrator Andy Slavitt at the J.P. Morgan Annual Health Care Conference. Retrieved from http://blog.cms.gov/2016/01/12/comments-of-cms-acting-administrator-andy-slavitt-at-the-j-p-morgan-annual-health-care-conference-jan-11-2016/

Coiera, E. (2003). *Guide to health informatics* (2nd ed.). Boca Raton, FL: CRC Press.

Cook, R., & Rasmussen, J. (2005). "Going solid": A model of systems dynamics and consequences of patient safety. *Quality and Safety in Health Care, 14*(2), 130–134.

Conway, J., Federico, F., Stewart, K., & Campbell, M. (2011). *Respectful management of serious clinical adverse events* (2nd ed.). Institute for Health Improvement Innovation Series white paper. Cambridge, MA: Institute for Health Improvement. Retrieved from http://www.ihi.org/resources/Pages/IHIWhitePapers/RespectfulManagementSeriousClinicalAEsWhitePaper.aspx

Cornish, P., Knowles, S., Marchesano, R., Tam, V., Shadowitz, S., Juurlink, D., & Etchells, E. (2005). Unintended medication discrepancies at time of hospital admission. *Archives of Internal Medicine, 165*(4), 424–429.

Donley, R., & Flaherty, M. (2008). Promoting professional development: Three phases of articulation in nursing education and practice. *Online Journal of Nursing, 13*(3). Retrieved from http://www.nursingworld.org/MainMenuCategories/ANAMarketplace/ANAPeriodicals/OJIN/TableofContents/vol132008/No3Sept08/PhasesofArticulation.aspx

Duncan, K., McMullan, C., & Mills, B. (2012). Early warning. *Nursing 2012, February*, 38–44.

Ehlert, D., & Rough, S. (2013). Improving the safety of the medication use process. In B. Youngberg (Ed.), *Patient safety handbook* (2nd ed., pp. 461–493). Burlington, MA: Jones & Bartlett Learning.

Finkelman, A. (2011). *Case management.* Upper Saddle River, NJ: Pearson Education.

Finkelman, A. (2016). *Leadership and management for nurses: Core competencies for quality care* (3rd ed.). Upper Saddle River, NJ: Pearson Education.

Finkelman, A., & Kenner, C. (2016). *Professional nursing concepts: Competencies for quality leadership* (3rd ed.). Burlington, MA: Jones & Bartlett Learning.

Furukawa, M., Eldridge, N., Wang, Y., & Metersky, M. (February 6, 2016). Electronic health record adoption and rates of in-hospital adverse events. *Journal Patient Safety*, doi:10.1097/PTS.0000000000000257. Retrieved from http://journals.lww.com/journalpatientsafety/Abstract/publishahead/Electronic_Health_Record_Adoption_and_Rates_of.99605.aspx

Gabow, P., Eisert, S., Karkhanis, A., Knight, A., & Dickson, P. (2005). A toolkit for redesign in health care. Prepared for the Agency for Healthcare Research and Quality. AHRQ Publication No. 05-0108-EF. Retrieved from http://archive.ahrq.gov/professionals/quality-patient-safety/patient-safety-resources/resources/toolkit/index.html

Gawande, A. (2009). *The checklist manifesto.* New York, NY: Metropolitan Books.

Graham, S., Brookery, J., & Steadman, C. (2014, October). Patient safety executive walkarounds (pp. 223–235). Agency for Healthcare Research and Quality (AHRQ). *Advances in patient safety*. Retrieved from http://www.ahrq.gov/professionals/quality-patient-safety/patient-safety-resources/resources/advances-in-patient-safety/index.html

Gum, L., Prideaux, D., Sweet, L., & Greenhill, J. (2012). From the nurses' station to the health team hub: How can design promote interprofessional collaboration? *Journal of Interprofessional Care, 26*, 21–27.

Haig, K., Sutton, S., & Whittington, J. (2006). SBAR: A shared mental model for improving communication between clinicians. *Journal of Quality and Patient Safety, 32*(3), 167–175.

Healthcare Information and Management Systems Society (HIMSS). (2011). *Share the vision: Transforming nursing practice through technology and informatics.* Retrieved from http://www.himss.org/library/nursing-informatics/position-statement

Healthcare Information and Management Systems Society (HIMSS). (2016). Medical device security. Retrieved from http://www.himss.org/resourcelibrary/TopicList.aspx?MetaDataID=1581

HealthIT.gov. (2015). What is an electronic medical record (EMR)? Retrieved from http://www.healthit.gov/providers-professionals/electronic-medical-records-emr

Helwig, A., & Lomotan, E. (2016, February 9). Can electronic health records prevent harm to patients? Retrieved from http://www.ahrq.gov/news/blog/ahrqviews/020916.html

Higuchi, K., & Donald, J. (2002). Thinking processes used by nurses in clinical decision-making. *Journal of Nursing Education, 41*(4), 145–150.

Institute for Healthcare Improvement (IHI). (2013). How-to Guide: Sustainability and spread. Retrieved from http://www.ihi.org/resources/Pages/Tools/HowtoGuideSustainabilitySpread.aspx

Institute of Medicine (IOM). (2003). *Health professions education: A bridge to quality.* Washington, DC: The National Academies Press.

Institute of Medicine (IOM). (2011). *Clinical practice guidelines we can trust.* Washington, DC: The National Academies Press.

Institute of Medicine (IOM). (2012). *Health IT and patient safety: Building safer systems for better care.* Washington, DC: The National Academies Press.

Institute of Medicine (IOM). (2013). *Patient safety: Achieving a new standard for care.* Washington, DC: The National Academies Press.

Interprofessional Education Collaborative Expert Panel (IPEC). (2011). *Core competencies for interprofessional collaborative practice: Report of an expert panel.* Washington, DC: Interprofessional Education Collaborative.

Jackson, K. (2004). Shedding light on medication errors. *For the Record, 16*(4), 27–29.

Jeffs, L., Lingard, L., Berta, W., & Baker, R. (2012). Catching and correcting near misses: The collective vigilance and individual accountability trade-off. *Journal of Interprofessional Care, 26*, 121–126.

Ketchum, K., Grass, C., & Padwojski, A. (2005). Medication reconciliation: Verifying medication orders and clarifying discrepancies should be standard practice. *American Journal of Nursing, 105*(11), 78–79.

Krepper, R., Vallejo, B., Smith, C., Lindy, C., Fullmer, C., Messimer, S., ... Myers, K. (2012). Evaluation of a standardized hourly rounding process (SHaRP). *Journal for Healthcare Quality, 36*(2), 62–69.

Kuziemsky, C., & Reeves, S. (2012). The intersection of informatics and interprofessional collaboration. *Journal of Interprofessional Care, 26*, 437–439.

Leonard, M., Graham, S., & Bonacum, D. (2004). The human factor: The critical importance of effective teamwork and communication in providing safe care. *Quality and Safety in Healthcare, 13*(Suppl. 1), 185–190.

Malloch, K., Benner, P., Sheets, V., Kenward, K., & Farrell, M. (2010). Overview: NCSBN practice breakdown initiative. In P. Benner, K., Malloch, K., & V. Sheets, V. (Eds.), *Nursing pathways for patient safety* (pp. 1–29). St. Louis, MO: National Council of State Boards of Nursing and Mosby.

Marcotte, L., Kirtane, J., Lynn, J., & McKethan, A. (2015). Integrating health information technology to achieve seamless care transitions. *Journal of Patient Safety, 11*(4), 185–190.

Marrelli, T. (2016). Home care nursing. Surviving in an ever-changing care environment. Indianapolis, IN: Sigma Theta Tau International.

Narayan, M. (2013). Using SBAR communications in efforts to prevent patient rehospitalizations. *Home Healthcare Nurse, 31*(9), 504–516.

National Academy of Sciences (NAS), Health and Medicine Division (HMD). (2015). *Measuring the impact of interprofessional education on collaborative practice and patient outcomes.* Washington, DC: The National Academies Press.

National Council of State Boards of Nursing (NCSBN). (2015). Practice errors and risk factors (TERCAP®). Retrieved from https://www.ncsbn.org/113.htm

National Institutes of Health (NIH). (2016). AHRQ announces interest in research in health IT safety. Retrieved from http://grants.nih.gov/grants/guide/notice-files/NOT-HS-16-009.html

Nuckols, T., Asch, S., Patel, V., Keeler, E., Anderson, L., Buntin, M., & Escarce, J. (2015). Implementing computerized provider order entry in acute care hospitals in the United States could generate substantial savings to society. *Joint Commission Quality Patient Safety, 41*, 341–350.

Otterman, S. (2016, March 15). Law changes prescriptions: Paper out, computers in. *New York Times*, pp. A22–A23.

Overdyk, F., Dowling, O., Newman, S., Glatt, D., Chester, M., Armellino, D.,... DiCapua, J. (2015, December 11). Remote video auditing with real-time feedback in an academic surgical suite improves safety and efficiency metrics: A cluster randomized study. *BMJ Quality Safety*, doi:10.1136/bmjqs-2015-004226. Retrieved from http://qualitysafety.bmj.com/content/early/2015/12/11/bmjqs-2015-004226.full?sid=814261de-5a53-485c-a48e-c2210ec6de02

Pannick, S., Davis, R., Ashrafian, H., Byrne, B., Beveridge, I., Athanasiou, T.,... Sevdalis, N. (2015). Effects of interdisciplinary team care interventions on general medical wards: A systematic review. *JAMA Internal Medicine, 175*(8), 1288–1298.

Payne, T., Hines, L., Chan, R., Hartman, S., Kapusnik-Uner, J., Russ, A.,... Malone, D. (2015, March 30). Recommendations to improve the usability of drug-drug interaction clinical decision support alerts. *Journal of the American Medical Informatics Association*. Retrieved from http://jamia.oxfordjournals.org/content/jaminfo/early/2015/03/30/jamia.ocv011.full.pdf

Paull, D., Mazzia, L., Neily, J., Mills, P., Turner, J., Gunnar, W., & Hemphill, R. (2015). Errors upstream and downstream to the universal protocol associated with wrong surgery events in the Veterans Health Administration. *American Journal of Surgery, 210*(1), 6–13.

Phansalkar, S., van der Sijs, H., Tucker, A., Desai, A., Bell, D., Teich, J., ... Bates, D. (2013). Drug-drug interactions that should be non-interruptive in order to reduce alert fatigue in electronic health records. *Journal of American Medical Informatics Association, 20*, 489–493.

Plisena, J., Gagliardi, A, Urbach, D., & Clifford, T. (2015). Factors that influence recognition, reporting, and resolution of incidents related to medical devices and other healthcare technologies: A systematic review. *Systematic Review, 4*, 37. Retrieved from http://www.ncbi.nlm.nih.gov/pmc/articles/PMC4384231/

Potter, P., Wolf, L., Boxerman, S., Grayson, D., Sledge, J., Dunagan, C., & Evanoff, B. (2014, October). An analysis of nurses' cognitive work: A new perspective for understanding medical errors (pp. 39–50). Agency for Healthcare Research and Quality (AHRQ). *Advances in patient safety*. Retrieved from http://www.ahrq.gov/professionals/quality-patient-safety/patient-safety-resources/resources/advances-in-patient-safety/index.html

Robichaud, P., Saari, M., Burnham, E., Omar, S., Wray, R., Baker, R., & Matlow, A. (2012). The value of a quality improvement project in promoting interprofessional collaboration. *Journal of Interprofessional Care, 26*(2), 158–160.

Rozich, J., Howard, R., Justeson, J., Macken, P., Lindsay, M., Resar, R. (2004). Standardization as a mechanism to improve safety in health care. *Joint Commission Journal Quality and Safety, 30*(1), 5–14.

Rudman, W., Bailey, J., Hope, C., Garrett, P., & Brown, C. A. (2014, October). The impact of web-based reporting system on the collection of medication error occurrence data (pp. 195–205). Agency for Healthcare Research and Quality (AHRQ). *Advances in patient safety*. Retrieved from http://www.ahrq.gov/professionals/quality-patient-safety/patient-safety-resources/resources/advances-in-patient-safety/index.html

Saint Louis, C. (2016, January 14). Medical scope is linked to infections, Senate says. *New York Times*, A13.

Schwiran, P., & Thede, L. (2011). Informatics: The standardized nursing terminologies: A national survey of nurses' experiences and attitudes. *OJIN, 16*(2). Retrieved from http://www.nursing-world.org/MainMenuCategories/ANAMarketplace/ANAPeriodicals/OJIN/TableofContents/Vol-16-2011/No2-May-2011/Standardized-Nursing-Terminologies.aspx

Shojania, K. (2015, November). In conversation with... Kaveh Shojania, MD. *Perspectives on Safety.* Retrieved from https://psnet.ahrq.gov/perspectives/perspective/184

Simone, L., Brumbaugh, J., & Ricketts, C. (2014). Medical devices, the FDA, and the home health-care clinician. *Home Healthcare Nurse, 32*(7), 402–408.

Sitting, D., & Singh, H. (2015, July 21). The health IT safety center roadmap: What's next? Health Affairs Blog. Retrieved from http://healthaffairs.org/blog/2015/07/21/the-health-it-safety-center-roadmap-whats-next/ http://healthaffairs.org/blog/2015/07/21/the-health-it-safety-center-roadmap-whats-next/

U.S. & World Report. (2015, September 29). Ohio hospital loses newborn's remains, trash searched. Retrieved from http://www.necn.com/news/national-international/Infant-Remains-Lost-University-of-Cincinnati-Medical-Center-329958311.html

U.S. Department of Health and Human Services (HHS). (2016). Meaningful use regulations. Retrieved from https://www.healthit.gov/policy-researchers-implementers/meaningful-use-regulations March 2, 2011.

U.S. Department of Health and Human Services (HHS). (2014, August 7). More physicians and hospitals are using EHRs than before. Retrieved from http://www.hhs.gov/news/press/2014pres/08/20140807a.html

U.S. Department of Health and Human Services (HHS), Agency for Healthcare Research and Quality (AHRQ). (2012). AHRQ quality indicators toolkits for hospitals. Retrieved from http://www.ahrq.gov/qual/qitoolkit/

U.S. Department of Health and Human Services (HHS), Agency for Healthcare Research and Quality (AHRQ). (2014a). Chapter 3: Care coordination measurement framework. Retrieved from http://www.ahrq.gov/professionals/prevention-chronic-care/improve/coordination/atlas2014/chapter3.html

U.S. Department of Health and Human Services (HHS), Agency for Healthcare Research and Quality. (AHRQ). (2014b). Identify defects through sensemaking. Retrieved from http://www.ahrq.gov/professionals/education/curriculum-tools/cusptoolkit/modules/identify/index.html

U.S. Department of Health and Human Services (HHS), Agency for Healthcare Research and Quality (AHRQ). (2015a, March). Plenary: TeamSTEPPS in Crisis Situations. Retrieved form http://www.ahrq.gov/professionals/education/curriculum-tools/teamstepps/national-meeting/2013-conference-materials/ts-crisis-situations.html

U.S. Department of Health and Human Services (HHS), Agency for Healthcare Research and Quality (AHRQ). (2015b, September). TeamSTEPPS®: Strategies and tools to enhance performance and patient safety. Retrieved from http://www.ahrq.gov/professionals/education/curriculum-tools/teamstepps/index.html

U.S. Department of Health and Human Services (HHS), Agency for Healthcare Research and Quality (AHRQ). (2015c). What is workflow? Retrieved from https://healthit.ahrq.gov/health-it-tools-and-resources/workflow-assessment-health-it-toolkit/workflow

U.S. Department of Health and Human Services (HHS), Agency for Healthcare Research and Quality (AHRQ), National Quality Strategy (NQS). (2014, September 17). National Quality Strategy Webinar. Retrieved from http://www.ahrq.gov/workingforquality/nqs/webinar091714/webinar5.htm

U.S. Department of Health and Human Services (HHS), Agency for Healthcare Research and Quality (AHRQ), Patient Safety Network (PSNet). (2003, January). Universal protocol for preventing wrong site, wrong procedure, wrong person surgery. Retrieved from https://psnet.ahrq.gov/resources/resource/3643/universal-protocol-for-preventing-wrong-site-wrong-procedure-wrong-person-surgery

U.S. Department of Health and Human Services (HHS), Agency for Healthcare Research and Quality (AHRQ), Patient Safety Network (PSNet). (2014a, August). Checklists. Retrieved from http://psnet.ahrq.gov/primer.aspx?primerID=14

U.S. Department of Health and Human Services (HHS), Agency for Healthcare Research and Quality (AHRQ), Patient Safety Network (PSNet). (2014b). Computerized provider order entry. Retrieved from http://psnet.ahrq.gov/primer.aspx?primerID=6

U.S. Department of Health and Human Services (HHS), Agency for Healthcare Research and Quality (AHRQ), Patient Safety Network (PSNet). (2014c, December). Rapid response systems. Retrieved from https://psnet.ahrq.gov/primers/primer/4/rapid-response-systems

U.S. Department of Health and Human Services (HHS), Agency for Healthcare Research and Quality (AHRQ), Patient Safety Network (PSNet). (2015a, November). Handoffs and signouts. Retrieved from https://psnet.ahrq.gov/primers/primer/9/handoffs-and-signouts

U.S. Department of Health and Human Services (HHS), Agency for Healthcare Research and Quality (AHRQ), Patient Safety Network (PSNet). (2015b, March). Medication reconciliation. Retrieved from https://psnet.ahrq.gov/primers/primer/1/medication-reconciliation

U.S. Department of Health and Human Services (HHS), Agency for Healthcare Research and Quality (AHRQ), Patient Safety Network (PSNet). (2016a, February). Computerized provider order entry and patient safety. Retrieved from https://psnet.ahrq.gov/perspectives/perspective/191

U.S. Department of Health and Human Services (HHS), Agency for Healthcare Research and Quality (AHRQ), Patient Safety Network (PSNet). (2016b). Patient safety primers. Retrieved from https://psnet.ahrq.gov/primers

U.S. Department of Health and Human Services (HHS), Centers for Medicare and Medicaid Services (CMS). (2015, September). The official web site for the Medicare and Medicaid electronic health records (EHR) incentive programs. Retrieved from https://www.cms.gov/Regulations-and-Guidance/Legislation/EHRIncentivePrograms/index.html?redirect=/ehrincentiveprograms

U.S. Department of Health and Human Services (HHS), Health Resources and Services Administration (HRSA). (2011a, April). Redesigning a system of care to promote QI. Retrieved from http://www.hrsa.gov/quality/toolbox/methodology/redesigningasystemofcare/

U.S. Department of Health and Human Services (HHS), Health Resources and Services Administration (HRSA). (2011b, April). Improvement teams. Retrieved from http://www.hrsa.gov/quality/toolbox/methodology/improvementteams/part4.html

U.S. Department of Health and Human Services (HHS), Health Resources and Services Administration (HRSA). (2011c, April). Readiness assessment and developing project aims. Retrieved from http://www.hrsa.gov/quality/toolbox/methodology/readinessassessment/

U.S. Department of Health and Human Services (HHS), The office of National Coordinator for Health Information Technology (ONC). (2015a). Connecting health and care for the nation: A shared nationwide interoperability roadmap draft version 1.0. Retrieved from https://www.healthit.gov/policy-researchers-implementers/interoperability

U.S. Department of Health and Human Services (HHS). The office of National Coordinator for Health Information Technology (ONC). (2015b). Health IT enabled quality improvement: A vision to achieve better health and health care. Retrieved from https://www.healthit.gov/sites/default/files/HITEnabledQualityImprovement-111214.pdf

U.S. Food and Drug Administration (FDA). (2014). Product problems. Retrieved from http://www.fda.gov/Safety/MedWatch/HowToReport/ucm053091.htm

Weinstock, M. (March 3, 2010). There's no "I" in team. *H&HN.* Retrieved from http://www.hhnmag.com/

Xiao, Y., Mackenzie, C., & Seagull, J. (May 2015). Video to improve patient safety: Clinical and education uses. Agency for Healthcare Research and Quality, Patient Safety Network. Retrieved from https://psnet.ahrq.gov/perspectives/perspective/177/

CHAPTER 12

Nursing Leadership for Quality Improvement

CHAPTER OBJECTIVES

At the conclusion of this chapter, the learner will be able to:

- Examine the current progress of the *Future of Nursing* report.
- Explain the importance of transformational leadership to nursing's role in continuous quality improvement (CQI).
- Critique the need for effective decision-making to ensure quality care.
- Summarize the need for effective communication in leading CQI.
- Formulate a clear statement supporting the need for staff education and improving care.
- Examine the best approach to nursing leadership that supports CQI.
- Explain how the examples of nursing initiatives to improve care are important in supporting nursing leadership and nursing engagement in CQI.

OUTLINE

KEY TERMS

Accountability	Empowerment	Responsibility
Clinical judgment	Leadership	Shared governance
Clinical reasoning	Management	Supervision
Clinical reflection	Micromanaging	Transformational leadership
Critical thinking	Power	
Delegation	Powerlessness	

Introduction

Throughout this text there is content about nurses and the need for more nursing leadership in continuous quality improvement (CQI) at all staff levels and in all settings. This chapter focuses on highlighting some of the aspects that nurses need to consider as they develop their own competencies in CQI and lead efforts to improve care.

The American Nurses Association (ANA) has long been active in pursuing improved care and supporting the need for a more active nursing role in CQI through education, research, publications, lobbying to improve care, collaboration with other organizations, and development of and participation in many other initiatives. In 2016, The ANA designated its theme for 2016 as "Safety 360—Taking Responsibility." The ANA website offers multiple resources on the culture of safety (ANA, 2016). Some of the topics include the culture of safety, healthy nurses, fatigue and shift work, infections, transitions of care, data and systems thinking, and other related topics, all topics discussed in this text. It is significant that this healthcare professional organization recognized the critical need to improve care and the nursing leadership required to support this improvement.

Progress Toward Meeting *The Future of Nursing: Leading Change, Advancing Health* Recommendations

The Future of Nursing: Leading Change, Advancing Health (IOM, 2010) is discussed throughout this text. The focus now is on the status of this report's evidence-based recommendations—what has been accomplished since 2010 and how does this impact nursing and its role in CQI? In 2016, a progress report was published (NAS/HMD, 2016). If we support the need for improvement in healthcare delivery, then it is important to assess our own professional progress and outcomes and then develop and implement strategies/interventions to continue our efforts as a profession to improve. Since the publication of the 2010 report, the Affordable Care Act (ACA) was passed and its implementation process began. The ACA, too, has had an impact on healthcare delivery, CQI, and nursing. Appendix A provides a summary of some of the quality improvement provisions in the ACA.

After the publication of the 2010 nursing report, a major initiative was undertaken, supported by the Robert Wood Johnson Foundation, to support change based on *The Future of Nursing* recommendations. This initiative is The Future of Nursing: Campaign for Action (referred to here simply as the Campaign) (Campaign for Action, 2016). AARP is also now a partner with the Robert Wood Johnson Foundation in supporting the Campaign. Despite all the work that has been done, we do know we continue to have major problems with healthcare quality. For example, a recent study noted that if death due to error were listed with the major causes of death in the United States, it would rank third (Makary, 2016). News like this emphasizes the challenges we face in healthcare delivery to improve care and health of patients.

The following list summarizes some of the key issues in the progress report by commenting on each of the 2010 recommendations and outcomes. As discussed in many chapters in this text, since 1999 and the first *Quality Chasm* reports, we have moved to a greater concern about quality, diversity and disparities, teams and interprofessional teamwork, cost, collaboration, care coordination, patient-centered care, and integration of the triple aim (better care, healthy people/healthy communities, affordable care) in our view of the healthcare delivery system. The progress report recommendations are related to all of these issues, and even more so than in 2010, as there is greater understanding of the CQI problem. For the focus of this text and chapter, the following list identifies The Future of Nursing report's recommendations, summary of some of the progress report's data, and relevance to CQI:

1. *Remove scope of practice barriers.* In 2010, 13 states met the criteria for full practice authority, and since then, 8 more states have been added. Some states have made some changes but still do not fully meet the criteria. The Centers for Medicare and Medicaid Services (CMS) has expanded the scope of practice for CMS payment; however, medical staff membership and hospital privileges for advanced practice registered nurses (APRNs) continue to be based on state laws and business preferences rather than federal law.

   Relevance to CQI: This outcome is not met, with only 13 states improving since 2010 and more than 50% of the states not meeting the recommendation. How does scope of practice impact CQI? It impacts nursing practice—what nurses do. In the case of this report, the focus was on APRNs. What APRNs and also registered nurses (RNs) can do in their practice is directed by state nurse practice acts. Scope of practice is part of each state's Nurse Practice Act. The CMS as a federal program can determine what services and whom it will cover in its payment system, but it cannot dictate state law regarding nurse practice acts. Healthcare organizations (HCOs) need to then ensure that clinicians of all professions follow the requirements to meet the standards.

2. *Expand opportunities for nurses to lead and diffuse collaborative improvement efforts.* The National Academy of Medicine (NAS/HMD, 2016) explains the need to expand nursing care models to meet the changing demands of health care: "The ACA provisions include development of new models of care to accommodate the large numbers of people previously without access to health insurance. These models focus on teamwork, care coordination, and prevention—models in which nurses can contribute a great deal of knowledge and skill" (p. 15). Some of these new models are accountable

care organizations, nurse managed clinics, and others. These new models support and assist in meeting this recommendation.

Relevance to CQI: Collaboration is a critical component of care today, and it is important to effective interprofessional teamwork, one of the healthcare professions core competencies identified in the *Quality Chasm* reports (IOM, 2003). Effective CQI requires care coordination and collaboration from many stakeholders (clinical and nonclinical), including many professional organizations, professional education programs, accrediting organizations, government agencies, and third-party payers. The new models provide new opportunities for nurses, and in the future it is hoped other models will be developed—and nursing roles and responsibilities will expand.

3. *Implement nurse residency programs.* At the time of the publication of *The Future of Nursing* report, there was concern about staff turnover and retention, and these continue to be concerns. Residency programs are one method that may reduce this problem, and the report focused on these programs for new graduates. The progress report notes that there is also need for these programs for nurses transitioning to new settings and for APRNs. In 2011, the National Council of State Boards of Nursing (NCSBN) engaged in research about transition-to-practice programs (NCSBN, 2016b). Residency programs vary, but the progress report notes that they do have value in helping nurses develop competencies important to improving practice and self-confidence in practice. There is also need for similar programs for nurses in outpatient settings.

Relevance to CQI: This result indicates there has been some progress, although more programs are needed. These programs are costly to develop and implement. The American Association of Colleges of Nursing provides a model and standards for nurse residency programs focused on baccalaureate graduates (BSN), although not all existing residency programs are accredited (AACN, 2016). The programs can be particularly helpful in encouraging nurses to participate in CQI by including nurse residency content and experiences related to evidence-based practice (EBP), CQI, and evidence-based management (EBM).

4. *Increase the proportion of nurses with a baccalaureate degree to 80% by 2020.* The progress report (NAS/HMD, 2016) reports on the improved enrollment in nursing programs: "Baccalaureate program enrollment has increased substantially since 2010: Entry-level baccalaureate enrollment increased from 147,935 in 2010 to 172,794 in 2014; accelerated baccalaureate enrollment increased from 13,605 to 16,935; and baccalaureate completion enrollment (so-called RN [registered nurse] to

bachelor of science in nursing [BSN]) increased from 77,259 to 130,345" (p. 6). There are other important improvements, such as the number of 4-year nursing (BSN) programs increased and more employers are requiring BSN degrees. However, the progress report indicates a need to continue to focus on improving nursing education programs and also that funding for degrees has been relatively flat, which is a barrier to increasing enrollment.

Relevance to CQI: Leaders are needed in all types of healthcare settings to improve care. Education is needed to prepare competent nurses who can assume roles that include CQI activities, meeting the healthcare core competency related to quality improvement (IOM, 2003). Nurses with BSN degrees typically have a positive impact on the quality of care. There are now more opportunities for nurses who do not have BSN degrees to obtain the degree, and many more HCOs are requiring BSNs and supporting nurses to expand their education. This trend will likely continue.

5. *Double the number of nurses with a doctorate by 2020.* The recommendation does not specify details as to type of doctorate (e.g., doctor of nursing practice [DNP], PhD in nursing, PhD in another field) and number of degrees per type. Enrollment in total has increased 15% in 5 years. Major barriers are funding and number of faculty and their experience.

Relevance to CQI: This level of increase makes it difficult to meet this recommendation by 2020. It is expected that nurses with the highest degree would serve in leadership positions in HCOs, on faculty, and in other positions such as policy making and leadership in the government at local, state, and federal levels. All would need to guide nursing engagement in CQI.

6. *Ensure that nurses engage in lifelong learning.* The progress report (NAS/HMD, 2016) states the following: "Continuing education and competence have not kept pace with the needs of the increasingly complex, team-based healthcare system. Nurses and other providers will increasingly need to update skills for providing care in both hospital and community-based settings" (p. 7). We need more data about continuing education, particularly about its impact on patient outcomes. As noted in other chapters, there have been greater efforts to understand and support interprofessional continuing education (IOM, 2009). In addition, we need to better understand the implications of the relationship between nurse certification and credentialing and lifelong learning, and we need to understand the impact of these efforts on practice and patient outcomes as well as on collaboration and leadership.

Relevance to CQI: Education, including lifelong learning, is discussed in other chapters, and it is critical to maintaining and developing knowledge and competencies. Lifelong learning should include content and experiences related to CQI, as this is a rapidly changing area and one in which nurses must actively participate. If we expect staff to engage in interprofessional teams within the context of CQI and practice, interprofessional initiatives are particularly important.

7. *Prepare and enable nurses to lead change to advance health.* There has been progress with the Campaign and the development of the Interprofessional Education Collaborative supported by the Josiah Macy Jr. Foundation. In 2013, the Campaign noted that more work needs to be done to increase interprofessional collaboration. Leadership continues to lag. For example, the percentage of nurses who serve on hospital boards is still too low: In a 2011 survey of 1,000 hospitals, nurses held 6% of the positions and physicians 20%, and in 2014, physicians held the same percentage, and nurses' share had decreased by 5%.

   Relevance to CQI: This is not a positive outcome. There are, of course, many other types of leadership, and nurses are involved or need to be more involved in leadership. Hospital boards direct the vision and goals of the hospitals, including CQI, and thus are important. Nurses need to actively participate in all types of leadership activities. Communicating the need for nursing leadership and what nurses can offer has progressed, but this effort has primarily focused on nurses. More needs to be done to inform other healthcare professionals, patients, families, and other relevant parties about the roles of nurses, and not just during the annual National Nurses Week.

8. *Build an infrastructure for the collection and analysis of interprofessional healthcare workforce data.* This text discusses measurement—how it works and barriers to success. The progress report notes similar concerns in assessing *The Future of Nursing* recommendations. Data must be collected and analyzed to drive decisions. The ACA included a provision to establish the National Healthcare Workforce Commission, focused on all healthcare professions, including nursing. This commission could be considered an important resource for gathering workforce data and analysis; however, there have been problems with funding it. The goal was for this commission to be a source of information and provide guidance to healthcare professions to ensure sufficient number and competent healthcare providers entering the healthcare delivery system, a problem noted in the *Quality Chasm* reports (IOM, 2003).

   One workforce problem that *The Future of Nursing* report noted was nursing workforce diversity, and it continues to be a problem identified in the progress report. Some data about diversity in nursing have been collected. The progress report, however, notes that a review of 5 years is not a sufficient period to effectively evaluate these outcomes. The progress report notes, "African Americans make up 13.6 percent of the general population aged 20 to 40, but 10.7 percent of the RN workforce, 10.3 percent of associate's degree graduates, and 9.3 percent of baccalaureate graduates. The disparity is even greater for Hispanics/Latinos, who make up 20.3 percent of the general population aged 20 to 40, but only 5.6 percent of the RN workforce, 8.8 percent of associate's degree graduates, and 7.0 percent of baccalaureate graduates. Men make up just 9.2 percent of the RN workforce, 11.7 percent of baccalaureate nursing students, and 11.6 percent of graduates" (NAS/HMD, 2016, p. 9). Important focus points are recruitment, retention, and success in nursing education programs. Diversity needs to be a workforce priority.

The progress report identifies barriers to data collection that need to be addressed: lack of consistent national indicators to provide consistent state-to-state data, lag time in data collection and reporting, lack of standardized databases, and need to use proxy measures to assess progress toward *The Future of Nursing* recommendations. The lack of a national infrastructure (the commission) to meet this recommendation continues to be a major problem.

Relevance to CQI: Workforce data are important to CQI. This information provides greater understanding of the current status of problems related to staffing levels and mix and competent staff (for all healthcare professions, not just nursing). This information can then be used to develop strategies to address these problems and also address problems with recruitment and retention as a component of ensuring quality care and reducing errors. This information can also be used to support funding for health professions education and identify improvements that might be needed in health professions education programs.

The progress report concludes with the following remarks:

Continued work is needed to remove scope-of-practice barriers; pathways to higher education need to be strengthened, with specific emphasis on increasing diversity; avenues for continuing competence need to be strengthened; and data on a wide range of outcomes are needed—from the education and makeup of the workforce to the services nurses provide and ways in which they lead. A major and overarching need is for the nursing community, including the Campaign, to build and strengthen coalitions with stakeholders outside of nursing. Nurses need to practice collaboratively; continue to develop skills and competencies in leadership and innovation; and work with other professionals, as no one profession alone can meet the complex needs of the future of health care. (NAS/HMD, 2016, p. 16)

Progress has been made, but not enough. For some of the original report's recommendations, a 5-year time span is not sufficient to determine if recommendations are met, but this is enough time to identify some weaknesses in reaching recommendations that require more effort.

Stop and Consider #1

Five years after the publication of *The Future of Nursing* report, we still have much work to do to meet its recommendations.

Transformational Leadership

Leadership is required in all healthcare settings, such as hospitals, clinics, home care, long-term care, and community or public health services. Today, managers must make more complex decisions and carry more accountability. Ideally, all managers should be leaders, but this is not always the case. This chapter focuses on the nature of leadership and how it can improve care for patients and also improve the HCO work environment. Some staff are in formal management positions, and others are not, but all, including staff nurses, need to understand leadership to work effectively in the healthcare environment. **Transformational leadership** has been identified in various reports and by professional organizations as an important leadership approach for healthcare delivery and nursing leadership and management (Finkelman, 2016; Finkelman & Kenner, 2016). The *Quality Chasm* reports, particularly *Leadership by Example* (IOM, 2002), *Keeping Patients Safe* (IOM, 2004), and *The Future of Nursing* (IOM, 2010) support use of transformational leadership.

Description

Leadership is a term that is formally defined, but it is also a term that requires individuals to apply their own views of leadership—what it means to them and how they view it in others. Concepts that relate to leadership include the following:

- *Advocacy*. The act of speaking for another and providing support
- *Authority*. The power to act
- *Autonomy*. The capacity to determine one's own action
- *Motivate*. To get another person to do something that may require extra effort

Leadership is the ability to influence, inspire, and guide others. It may be confused with **management**, which ensures that the structure and resources exist to accomplish the job. Management focuses on four functions:

1. *Planning*. Identify the short- and long-term objectives and related actions with a timeline.
2. *Organizing*. Arrange resources needed to accomplish the work that needs to be done. Examples of resources are competent and sufficient staff, supplies, equipment, space, and budget.

3. *Leading.* Guide the process of work, which may require directing, delegating, coordinating, influencing, ensuring a positive work environment, and applying other methods to ensure that work is done effectively.
4. *Controlling.* Ensure that outcomes are met, evaluating and adapting as need.

Managers hold specific positions in an organization, such as nurse manager, director of health informatics, director of quality improvement program, pharmacy supervisor, or laboratory manager. The position description for a manager position integrates the four functions.

Value of Transformational Leadership Style

As is true for CQI and change models, leadership theories and models have changed and adapted, and new ones have been added. Moving from autocratic, bureaucratic, and laissez-faire approaches, the more current emphasis is on transformational leadership. There are other types of models, and many of them incorporate elements of transformational leadership. Transformational leaders are better able to transform the system. As we recognize the need to consider redesigning and improving the status of care quality in the United States, this approach is important to nursing and to the discussion about CQI. **Figure 12-1** describes one perspective of transformation.

Leadership Characteristics, Knowledge, and Competencies

Leaders are found in all types of HCOs. Some are in formal management positions, and some are not. There are myths about leadership, such as the following that are commonly mentioned when leadership is discussed (Goffee & Jones, 2000):

- *Everyone can be a leader.* People may have leadership potential, but not everyone can be an effective leader.
- *Leaders deliver business results.* Leaders do not always deliver expected outcomes.

Figure 12-1. Perspectives for Transformation
Reproduced from Agency for Healthcare Research and Quality (AHRQ). (2004). A toolkit for redesign in health care. AHRQ Publication No. 05-0108-EF. Retrieved from http://archive.ahrq.gov/professionals/quality-patient-safety/patient-safety-resources/resources/toolkit/index.html

- *People who get to the top are leaders.* There are many people in high positions in HCOs who do not function as leaders, although they may have been more effective leaders when in lower positions.
- *Leaders are great coaches.* Not all leaders are great coaches. Some leaders are better at inspiring and influencing, and some are less able to share important competencies for development of staff.

Why is it important to identify myths? We sometimes make assumptions that then lead to poor leadership working relationships, and often management and staff mention these myths. Leaders can be developed with additional education and mentoring, but leaders are not perfect and may function at different levels of effectiveness. Leaders make mistakes, and some leaders may be better at different aspects of leadership than others. We have all encountered managers whose behavior made us wonder how they reached their position. They are promoted to the point where they are not effective. With clinical staff, the assumption often is made that if you are a competent nurse, then you would be an effective manager. This is not always the case. Different characteristics and competencies are required for a management position compared to a clinical staff position. A question commonly asked is, Is a manager a leader? The manager holds a formal leadership position and should be a leader, demonstrating leadership competencies; however, many managers are not leaders or viewed by others as leaders.

Successful leaders and managers should also be able to assess staff mood, morale, and the work environment to effectively guide staff and ensure a positive work environment. Staff often recognize managers who are also leaders, although they may not mention leadership to describe the manager. They might say the manager is interested in more than just "getting the job done" or that the manager seems to care, understands the work processes and impact on staff and outcomes, and engages staff in the process of improving. Staff would not say this manager abstains from decision-making or is not available and leaves them on their own, but rather the manager is there in the workplace for them. The effective manager uses knowledge management by bringing together staff with a variety of knowledge levels and expertise and makes the whole greater than any individual staff member—focusing on teamwork. Whenever possible, a proactive approach prevents problems, improves communication and problem solving, and demonstrates more concern for staff and outcomes. Facilitating staff engagement is a critical method for reaching outcomes. The manager also considers what staff are doing and whether the work can be done more effectively, improving performance. They determine resources that are needed and identify changes in processes to reach better productivity. To accomplish this, the manager requires feedback from staff and staff participation in the change process.

Leaders exhibit a number of important characteristics. They need to have self-understanding, or self-awareness. This trait enables them to understand and assess others and to influence others. Trusting oneself is a critical characteristic. Rigidity does not help a leader; rather, the ability to be flexible at appropriate times results in more effective leadership. Leaders often challenge the status quo. Leaders care about people. Honesty is an important characteristic. Staff usually recognize leaders who are not honest with them. Leaders use advocacy effectively. Just as is true with managers, there are ranges of effective leaders; some are more effective than others. Leaders also focus on staff strengths, not staff weaknesses. This approach develops staff self-confidence.

The term *transformational* in transformational leadership emphasizes change, and this is a critical aspect of this leadership style. Change and improvement are considered critical aspects of successful organizations. HCOs require leaders and managers who appreciate that change is needed and also know how to engage in change and bring staff into the process. Effective leadership does not mean staff are always told what they must do and there is no flexibility (as in autocratic and bureaucratic styles of leadership). Nor does it mean that the leader or manager turns all decision-making and planning over to the staff (as in a laissez-faire style of leadership). The transformational leader is very involved in the process of work and change, but this leader knows how to assess staff and their needs, how to guide them, reward staff, provide constructive criticism, and create and maintain a positive work environment. Transformational leaders guide staff in developing a vision that provides a perspective of the organization in the future—this is where we want to be. The mission statement then connects to the vision and establishes goals and purpose—how we will get to the vision. Issues and factors that drive the need to change the view of HCO leadership include the following:

- Greater need for teams and effective teamwork, including team leaders and members (followers)
- Greater recognition that the specific characteristics of a situation impact leaders and managers
- Increased use of collaboration and coordination
- Need to improve communication
- Increased recognition of need to engage all staff
- Emphasis on change and how to use it as opportunity
- Recognition that factors such as feelings, self-esteem, and listening and responding impact leadership, staff, and work outcomes
- Need for understanding and development of the knowledge worker
- Need for effective use of EBP and EBM

Related to all of these issues and factors is CQI, which cannot be effectively managed without considering how nurses will respond to them. Establishing and maintaining a culture of safety is now an important part of HCO leadership.

To better understand leadership and its relationship to CQI, it is important to identify the areas in which managers must be knowledgeable to be effective and meet their responsibilities:

- Clinical practice
- Communication and relationship building
- Collaboration
- Coordination
- Change process
- Planning and decision-making (strategic and short-term)
- Teams and teamwork
- Guiding and teaching staff
- Delegation
- Budgeting and healthcare financing
- Problem solving and use of critical thinking
- Crisis management
- Performance appraisal
- CQI planning, measurement, and process
- Evidence-based practice and evidence-based management
- Accreditation
- Staffing, including recruitment and retention
- Risk management and utilization management
- Health informatics
- Ethics and legal concerns
- Conflict resolution and negotiation
- Diversity and disparities
- Regulatory compliance
- Policy and procedures, including development and implementation

The competencies required of a leader are the same as those of a manager, although the degree of emphasis placed on each competency may vary depending on the leader's position. The following competencies are required for effective leadership.

- Analyze information and the environment to understand current status, respond to current status and problems, and project future problems.
- Use collaboration and coordination.
- Plan effectively (strategic, operational, project).
- Communicate clearly and in a timely manner.
- Influence and motivate others.
- Create and innovate.
- Ask staff for feedback routinely and apply as appropriate.

- Share information with staff so they can understand decisions and recognize progress.
- Apply the CQI process, including effective measurement.
- Engage staff in CQI.
- Empower others.
- Work effectively on leadership teams and in leading teams.
- Recognize success in others.
- Advocate for patients and their families and for staff.
- Work toward consistent transparency and ethical decision-making.

Effective leadership requires that the leader step back and see the "big picture," and this must be an ongoing process. This is a critical element of transformational leadership.

Leaders and managers gain their leadership knowledge and competencies from a variety of sources. Many have completed formal academic work and may have graduate degrees. Some managers had management content integrated into their professional degree programs, such as leadership and management content in prelicensure programs. The third source is staff education and continuing education. This education should include leadership development, methods to improve management such as time management, priority setting, using the change process effectively, planning methods, budgeting, quality improvement and measurement, and current trends and issues related to health policy and standards.

Staffing, which includes selecting, orienting, and retaining staff, is a key management function. A manager who is a leader will ensure that at the beginning of the process every potential job candidate knows about the leadership style of the manager and how this impacts staff. It is not easy to retain staff. Staff turnover is disruptive and costly, and it often negatively impacts quality care. The more that staff are involved in the work processes and decision-making, the more committed they will be to the organization and the work unit. Involving staff requires a culture that allows for open staff communication. The effective leader knows this and makes efforts to establish and maintain such a culture and supports a culture of safety. Engaging potential staff in CQI even during the selection and hiring process can be very beneficial to the potential employee and the HCO.

Power and Empowerment

Power and empowerment are critical aspects of effective leadership and also important to CQI. **Power** is about "influencing decisions, controlling resources, and affecting behavior. Power can be used constructively or destructively" (Finkelman, 2016, p. 327). To empower is to enable to act (Finkelman & Kenner, 2016). **Empowerment**, however, means that some may gain power and some may lose power and prestige. In organizations that truly practice shared participation in decision-making, middle management tends to lose the most, turning over power and authority to teams. Not only does power mean you can influence others and decisions, but you can often get things done more effectively. When the HCO or its leaders/managers empower staff to work in teams, the teams have authority to make and implement decisions. Management provides guidance but does not dictate. Empowerment does not mean staff make all decisions and that there are no guidelines and boundaries, but these are limited.

Powerlessness also occurs in organizations. Staff feel like they have no influence and cannot influence decisions. This situation is very negative and impacts staff morale and productivity. There are some managers who prefer that staff do not have power, but this situation is not effective leadership and management. It represents destructive use of power.

There are various types of power, and each is based on the source of the power (Finkelman, 2016; Finkelman & Kenner, 2016). Most power is legitimate, originating from a formal position such as a manager position. Some staff gain power due to their experience and/or knowledge, special qualities, or ability to influence others, or as a reward. Another type of power originates when one is in a position to punish someone, which is a negative type of power. A manager may have all or some of these types of power. Staff do not, however, have to be in a formal management position to have some of these types of power. Within a work unit, staff will have different types of power; for example, nurses on a unit may go to one particular nurse whom they consider the nurse to be an expert to ask questions or to get information (expert and information power). Other staff may go to a staff member for advice because that staff member seems to care about the team members and responds quickly (referent power). Nurse managers in a hospital may pick one nurse manager to represent them with upper management because this nurse manager seems to be able to influence or persuade others.

Staff Engagement

Transformational leaders encourage staff to be active in work processes and decision-making. This type of leadership supports "moving a profession, an institution, or some aspect of health care down a new path with different expectations, structures, and ways of conceptualizing how the mission can be achieved in light of changing conditions" (McBride, 2011, p. 179). This leader collaborates with staff to develop the vision by considering the question: Where do we want to be? Staff need to be brought into the process of asking the following: (1) How do we get there? (2) How do we know we have reached our outcomes? Change is a critical and ever-present situation in transformational leadership. The leader knows this and needs to communicate to staff the value of the change process. Staff need to view the work team and their own team membership as critical to success. What can the leader do to engage staff and establish a positive work environment that supports CQI (Finkelman, 2016; Finkelman & Kenner, 2016; IOM, 2002b, 2010; McBride, 2011)?

- Recognize the value of knowledge; provide staff with opportunities to expand knowledge through staff education and other methods such as access to academic programs.
- Ensure that staff have the information and resources they need to do their work.
- Encourage staff to share information and knowledge with the team and through other methods such as presentations at professional meetings, publishing articles, and so on.
- Avoid micromanaging; include staff in decision-making process.
- Listen and respond to staff.
- Recognize staff, team, and individual successes.
- Provide mentoring and coaching opportunities for staff.
- Engage staff in decision-making at all levels.
- Apply standards, policies and procedures, EBP, and EBM.
- Engage staff in evaluation of outcomes at all levels and in CQI.
- Use performance appraisal as a time to recognize accomplishments and provide constructive feedback. Support staff self-assessment.
- Support effective teamwork and expand team competencies.
- Reinforce positive feedback throughout the work processes; do not just wait to do this at the annual performance appraisal.
- Ask staff for feedback about leaders' abilities and outcomes; use this information to improve leadership.
- Recognize that disagreement and conflict may occur; negotiate to meet outcomes.
- Be flexible whenever possible.
- Recognize differences/diversity as opportunities.

Stop and Consider #2

Transformational leadership requires engagement of both the leader and the staff.

Decision-Making

Decision-making is part of daily practice for every nurse in all settings and positions. Effective decision-making, however, is a problem for many nurses. CQI requires effective decisions. Sometimes these decisions need to be made quickly, and sometimes they are made after data collection and data analysis. This text discusses CQI measurement. For nurses to participate in CQI decisions, they need to understand measurement and participate in the process. In this way, nurses can be more active and more effective in making decisions about strategies/interventions to improve care and in working toward their implementation.

Shared governance is used more often today in HCOs because it supports transformational leadership and greater use of shared decision-making—engaging the staff. It may be applied to the entire organization, or it could be used primarily in one department, such as nursing or patient services. Shared governance means that staff have more input into decision-making and there is a structure to facilitate this process. Accountability and responsibility is important at all levels in shared governance, though staff may have different accountability and responsibilities in their daily work to change or improve work processes and outcomes. In this type of organization, there is more collaboration among all levels of staff. There are councils and committees where much of the planning and decision-making occurs. The structured top-down chain of command is then reduced. Communication is critical in this type of organization. It must be clear, timely, and shared with appropriate staff members. This system might be called decentralized decision-making because decisions are made at levels of the organization other than the top. Most decisions are made at the lower levels, where work is done. This structure does not mean that organization-wide decisions are not made or that high-level leaders do not make decisions. It does mean there is more two-way communication and decision-making flow.

Leaders need to have self-confidence, which impacts their decision-making. They often work in situations that are high stress that negatively impact self-confidence. The leader has to reassure others that he or she is able to lead and will be there when needed. This requires self-confidence. How can self-confidence be developed and maintained? Leaders must be able to convince themselves that their ability to lead is effective. When times get tough, and they will, leaders need to be able to talk themselves back into a feeling of self-confidence. Using a mentor may help during these times. Participation in activities outside work that provide release of stress is important. Working 24/7 is not helpful. Staff do not want an exhausted, stressed leader. Being a leader can be lonely, particularly if one is in a high position or in an organization in which there are few managers—for example, a clinic that may have one or just a few managers compared to an acute care or long-term care facility with several layers of managers.

Process: Critical Thinking and Clinical Reasoning and Judgment

Nursing has traditionally emphasized critical thinking; however, more needs to be done to focus on clinical reasoning and judgment (Benner, Hughes, & Sutphen, 2008; Benner, Sutphen, Leonard, & Day, 2010). **Critical thinking** is concerned with questioning, looking at knowledge, intuition, and application of knowledge. Practice and CQI, however, also require use of clinical reasoning and judgment, creative thinking, evaluation of evidence, and application of standards of practice. **Critical reflection** is also important component of critical thinking and "requires that the thinker [the nurse] examine the underlying assumptions and radically question or doubt the validity of arguments, assertions, and even facts of the case" (Benner et al., 2008, p. 3). This type of thinking is important when one examines practices that may require improvement. **Clinical judgment**, staff making decisions about clinical concerns and treatment, requires use of **clinical reasoning**. As Benner and colleagues (2008) describe clinical reasoning as follows:

> Clinical reasoning stands out as a situated, practice-based form of reasoning that requires a background of scientific and technological research-based knowledge about general cases, more so than any particular instance. It also requires practical ability to discern the relevance of the evidence behind general scientific and technical knowledge and how it applies to a particular patient. (p. 4)

Not only are critical thinking and clinical reasoning and judgment important to effective practice, thus helping to ensure quality care, but they also are necessary to implementing an effective CQI process. We tend to focus on collecting data, but analysis is what makes the final difference and provides direction for decisions and development of strategies to improve. Nurses need to use these methods of thinking and their expertise in the analysis phase of the CQI process.

Leadership: Risk and Success

Sometimes effective leaders have to take risks; however, risks need to be considered very carefully. Leaders are able to evaluate pros and cons or costs and benefits and then arrive at a decision. They are not naive about risks, recognizing that some decisions will fail. When they do, leaders use these experiences to learn more about how they lead and make decisions to improve care and their leadership and management. Collecting the best data possible, using effective analysis, and including others in the process may reduce risk in decision-making when guiding CQI activities. In regard to this final point—including others in the decision-making process—Rath and Conchie (2008) offer the following insights:

> Effective leaders surround themselves with the right people and build on each person's strengths. Yet in most cases, leadership teams are a product of circumstances more than design . . . . Executive team members are selected or promoted primarily on knowledge or competence . . . . Rarely are people recruited to an executive team because their strengths are the best complement for those of the existing team members . . . . What's worse, when leaders do recruit for strength, they all too often pick people who act, think, or behave like themselves, albeit unintentionally in most cases. (p. 21)

Selecting team members poorly can lead to ineffective work teams and problems; however, sometimes teams must learn to work together effectively regardless of member characteristics or competencies. This type of situation requires even more effective team leadership.

There is no perfect world. Although much can be said about the importance of effective leadership, finding one person who has all the needed knowledge and competencies can prove impossible. In addition, people and situations change. A person could be a very effective leader in situations that require long-term planning and in-depth analysis, but the same leader may not be so effective in a crisis situation. In the first situation, the leader may have the ability to work with staff and influence them over a long period, building confidence and motivating staff. In the second situation, leadership is needed quickly to understand the problem, engage staff, meet outcomes and take actions, and handle stress. The leader may not be able to do this effectively.

There are times when a manager or leader makes the wrong decision. How these instances are handled with staff says a lot about the manager or leader and can have an impact on the leader's self-confidence and ability to function effectively. The best approach is to admit to staff that an error was made and not focus on excuses. Be clear about the reason(s) for the mistake, and explain the steps that will be taken to resolve the issue and prevent future similar mistakes. This is not easy to do, but staff have greater respect for this type of response. The leader will gain credibility and support through honesty. Staff want to believe in their managers—that they can lead and manage, that they can guide staff and the organization, that they will be there when needed. The process of decision-making is a key time when staff observe and experience leader competencies and may be a time of high stress, particularly if staff do not trust the leader's decision-making ability.

Sometime leaders encounter times when plans do not go as they planned or as they explained to staff. Often, these situations are beyond the control of the leaders, but in some situations, managers higher up in the HCO may be in control, depending on factors in the HCO or the healthcare environment, such as laws and standards that must be followed. Despite this loss of control, the leader must still implement the CQI activities as planned by the quality improvement (QI) program. The best approach with staff is to be honest and transparent, and then collaborate with staff to make the situation as positive as it can be (O'Neil & Chow, 2011). The quality of responses to unexpected change may or may not support trust and open communication. In many situations, it is easier to blame others or even deny that the situation is not going as expected, but these approaches do not provide effective leadership. Self-awareness helps all leaders identify their own strengths and weaknesses. Each leader has a unique combination of strengths and weaknesses; knowing what these are helps the leader be even more effective. However, this is an ongoing challenge as the leaders develop over time and encounter difficult, complex situations. CQI may present as this type of situation for some leaders/managers.

Delegation and Quality Improvement

It may seem unusual to discuss delegation in content about QI, but they are related. What is delegated, by whom, to whom, and when all impact patient and HCO outcomes. Delegation applies to all staff, even nonclinical staff. Work is delegated in all parts of an HCO, including clinical, laboratory, radiology, dietary, physical therapy, clinics, medical records, healthcare informatics, human resources, staff education, admissions, administration, and other areas. **Delegation** involves transferring a specific task to be performed by another person, or empowering another to act. This process gives someone the responsibility and authority to complete a task. The person to whom a task is transferred should be competent, demonstrating required knowledge, skills, and experience to complete a task. Accountability is also part of the delegation process. When delegating responsibility, the person doing the delegating (the delegator) must answer for the subsequent actions taken or decisions made.

Accountability occurs when a person assumes ownership for his or her work. In doing so, outcomes become more important to the person, and it is clearer to others whom is answerable for the work. **Responsibility** is the acceptance of or obligation to do something. It is a two-way process—one person allocates responsibility and the other accepts it. Responsibility cannot be totally delegated, as the delegator has ultimate responsibility for the task. Effective responsibility includes reliability, dependability, and obligation (Marthaler & Kelly, 2008). **Supervision** is an integral part of ensuring CQI and involves directing, guiding, and evaluating performance.

The decision to delegate is the critical issue. It requires the delegator to follow the steps in the delegation process (ANA, 2005). The Connect to Current Information section at the end of the chapter provides a link to this site. This process integrates the five rights of delegation (ANA, 2005; Finkelman & Kenner, 2016):

- *Right task.* The task that is delegatable for the specific patient or situation
- *Right circumstances.* Appropriate setting, available resources, and other factors relevant to the task's completion
- *Right person.* Right person delegating the right task to the right person, who then performs the task
- *Right directions/communication.* Clear, concise description of the task, including the objective(s), limits, and expectations
- *Right supervision.* Appropriate monitoring, evaluation, intervention (as needed), and feedback

CQI requires use of effective delegation as staff make clinical and management decisions to meet patient and HCO outcomes. Delegation should not be a barrier to effective work practice, but rather it is another strategy used to improve care and outcomes.

Stop and Consider #3
Effective decision-making requires ongoing improvement.

Communication: Impact on Leadership in Quality Care

Information is a critical part of leadership and CQI. Interpretation of information may lead to clear understanding, but it also may lead to confusion, poor decision-making, increase in staff frustration, and poor CQI outcomes. Effective leaders are interested in people, and communicating with people is critical to the work environment. This is not to say that they are all overly social, but rather that they are focused on people, like to work with people, and can assess where people stand on issues. They know which people should be involved in the change process and in decision-making, including awareness of who should not be left out and why. They are effective communicators with a variety of types of people and in a variety of situations, even difficult or negative situations. In HCOs communication is a critical element in stressful situations, requiring understanding of stress and need to manage stress for effective communication. It is accepted that communication problems are a common cause of errors, so anything that can be done to improve communication is important to CQI. Other chapters in this text discuss structured communication methods now used in many HCOs, such as SBAR (situation, background, assessment, recommendation). Nurse leaders/managers need to ensure that staff understand these methods and apply them when required.

Stop and Consider #4
Nurse leaders can impact staff and HCO communication.

Leadership: Ensuring That Staff Are Up to Date and Engaged in Quality Care Status

As noted in other chapters, pre-licensure, graduate, and lifelong education (e.g., continuing education) are important to the nursing profession as well as to all HCOs. Nursing leaders in education, whether this is in nursing education programs or in staff education programs, need to ensure that CQI is part of the content and learning experiences. There is no doubt that we need more of this content in all educational experiences for nurses and for nursing students at all levels. It should be integrated throughout the curriculum and also include focused content on CQI so that students recognize its importance. It is also clear, as discussed in this text, that to develop effective interprofessional teams, we need more effective and routine interprofessional education (IPECEP, 2011; NAS/HMD, 2015).

Stop and Consider #5
Staff education needs to be ongoing.

Nursing Leadership and CQI

The American Organization of Nurse Executives (AONE) has long supported CQI and nurses' roles in the process to improve care. Its Guiding Principles include principles that are directly related to CQI. In addition, the AONE integrates into its resources the need to develop leadership and also CQI competencies for clinical nurses and nurse managers. **Exhibit 12-1** describes principles for collaborative relationships between clinical nurses and nurse managers. Effective collaboration is critical to improving care. When clinical nurses and nurse managers work together, communicate, respect one another, and turn to one another for assistance, patient-centered care will be more effective and the quality of care will be a top priority. Goals are established to meet outcomes for patients, and clinical nurses and nurse managers work toward these goals and not against one another. In addition, the AONE describes the role of the nurse executive in patient safety, noting that the nurse executive needs to lead cultural change, provide shared leadership so that staff at all levels are engaged and assume responsibility, build external partnerships for collaboration, and develop leadership competencies around patient safety that focus on safety technology, leadership, culture of safety, and a practice environment of safety (AONE, 2007).

It is important to understand the connection between the microsystem (unit level) and patient quality. **Table 12-1** describes the key characteristics that clinical nurses and nurse managers need to consider when they evaluate the unit's culture and care improvement. **Table 12-2** provides a list of critical questions they should ask as they work to improve.

Effective nurse leadership leads to positive outcomes for HCOs. Staff retention is higher, and through word of mouth, people often apply for positions that allow them to work with a known effective leader. Leadership impacts work outcomes such as productivity, budget goals met, and higher-quality care. When staff morale is higher, all aspects of the work environment, productivity, and quality are positively affected.

Micromanaging, or being overly involved in the details of others' s everyday work functions, limits a person's views and understanding about processes and outcomes. For effective strategic thinking, it is important to consider the entire HCO and its

Exhibit 12-1 ANA/AONE Principles for Collaborative Relationships Between Clinical Nurses and Nurse Managers

Effective Communication Principles

- Engage in active listening to fully understand and contemplate what is being relayed.
- Know the intent of a message, and the purpose and expectations of that message.
- Foster an open, safe environment.
- Whether giving or receiving information, be sure it is accurate.
- Have people speak to the person they need to speak to, so the right person gets the right information.

Authentic Relationships Principles

- Be yourself. Be sure actions match words, and those around you are confident that what they see is what they get.
- Empower others to have ideas, to share those ideas, and to participate in projects that leverage or enact those ideas.
- Recognize and leverage each others' strengths.
- Be honest 100% of the time—with yourself, and with others.
- Respect others' personalities, needs, and wants.
- Ask for what you want, but stay open to negotiating the difference.
- Assume good intent from others' words and actions, and assume they are doing their best.

Learning Environment and Culture Principles

- Inspire innovation and creative thinking.
- Commit to a cycle of evaluating, improving, and celebrating, and value what is going well.
- Create a culture of safety, both physically and psychologically.
- Share knowledge, and learn from mistakes.
- Question the status quo. Ask "what if" rather than saying "no way."

Data from American Nurses Association (ANA) & American Organization of Nurse Executives (AONE). (May 2012). ANA/AONE principles for collaborative relationships between clinical nurses and nurse managers. Retrieved from http://www.nursingworld .org/MainMenuCategories/ThePracticeofProfessionalNursing/NursingStandards /ANAPrinciples/Principles-of-Collaborative-Relationships.pdf

TABLE 12–1 Linkage of Microsystem Characteristics to Patient Safety

Microsystem Characteristics	What This Means for Patient Safety
1. Leadership	▪ Define the safety vision of the organization ▪ Identify the existing constraints within the organization ▪ Allocate resources for plan development, implementation, and ongoing monitoring and evaluation ▪ Build in microsystems participation and input to plan development ▪ Align organizational quality and safety goals ▪ Engage the board of trustees in ongoing conversations about the organizational progress toward achieving safety goals ▪ Recognition for prompt truth-telling about errors or hazards ▪ Certification of helpful changes to improve safety
2. Organizational support	▪ Work with clinical microsystems to identify patient safety issues and make relevant local changes ▪ Put the necessary resources and tools in the hands of individuals
3. Staff focus	▪ Assess current safety culture ▪ Identify the gap between current culture and safety vision ▪ Plan cultural interventions ▪ Conduct periodic assessments of culture ▪ Celebrate examples of desired behavior, for example, acknowledgment of an error
4. Education and training	▪ Develop patient safety curriculum ▪ Provide training and education of key clinical and management leadership ▪ Develop a core of people with patient safety skills who can work across microsystems as a resource
5. Interdependence of the care team	▪ Build PDSA* cycles into debriefings ▪ Use daily huddles to debrief and to celebrate identifying errors

(Continued)

TABLE 12–1 Linkage of Microsystem Characteristics to Patient Safety (*Continued*)

Microsystem Characteristics	What This Means for Patient Safety
6. Patient focus	▪ Establish patient and family partnerships ▪ Support disclosure and truth around medical error
7. Community and market focus	▪ Analyze safety issues in community, and partner with external groups to reduce risk to population
8. Performance results	▪ Develop key safety measures ▪ Create feedback mechanisms to share results with microsystems
9. Process improvement	▪ Identify patient safety priorities based on assessment of key safety measures ▪ Address the work that will be required at the microsystem level
10. Information and information technology	▪ Enhance error-reporting systems ▪ Build safety concepts into information flow (e.g., checklists, reminder systems)

*PDSA: Plan Do Study Act

Reproduced from Barach, P. & Johnson, J. (2013). Assessing risk and harm in the clinical microsystem. In W. Sollecito & J. Johnson (Eds.), *McLaughlin & Kaluzny's Continuous quality improvement in health care,* (4th ed., pp. 249–274). Burlington, MA: Jones & Bartlett Learning.

TABLE 12–2 Questions Senior Leaders Could Ask About Patient Safety

What information do we have about errors and patient harm?
What is the patient safety plan?
How will the plan be implemented at the organizational level and at the microsystem level?
What type of infrastructure is needed to support implementation?
What is the best way to communicate the plan to the individual microsystems?
How can we foster reporting—telling the truth—about errors?
How will we empower microsystem staff to make suggestions for improving safety?
What training will staff need?
Who are the key stakeholders?
How can we build linkages to the key stakeholders?
What stories can we tell that relate the importance of patient safety?
How will we recognize and celebrate progress?

Reproduced from Barach, P. & Johnson, J. (2013). Assessing risk and harm in the clinical microsystem. In W. Sollecito & J. Johnson (Eds.), *McLaughlin & Kaluzny's Continuous quality improvement in health care,* (4th ed., pp. 249–274). Burlington, MA: Jones & Bartlett Learning.

components (departments, units, and so on) and also the external environment—connecting aspects of all to arrive at an understanding of the organization, its structure and function, vision and mission, and expected outcomes. HCO strengths and weaknesses should also be part of this understanding. Maintaining a broad perspective is very important when involved in CQI; data and details are important, but ignoring the "big picture" and system are critical weaknesses of relying too much on micromanaging. Sometimes leaders have to use intuition or their gut reaction to step outside the box and broaden their perspective even when engaged in the CQI measurement process. In many cases, if this is not done, then effective strategic planning may not be as effective. Strategic planning requires understanding of multiple systems and how they interact.

A critical leadership role is the role of advocate, a role that all staff should demonstrate. Advocacy includes supporting rights of patients and focusing on patient-centered care but also making sure rights are actually protected. Advocacy is implemented by sharing information with patients, ensuring informed consent is complete, providing privacy during care, and ensuring that ethical principles are followed. When staff advocate for the patient, they are demonstrating leadership. A staff member who demonstrates leadership works with others collaboratively, works to motivate others just as the staff member would want to be motivated, understands the organization and need to meet outcomes, and strives to improve practice and functions of the organization. When staff engage in CQI, they are advocating for the patient in daily practice (clinical or management) and in CQI activities within the HCO.

Healthy, positive work environments are the responsibility of the HCO, leadership and management, and staff. This type of work environment has a positive impact on quality care, productivity, staff satisfaction and retention, and organization outcomes. It promotes staff engagement and innovation in problem solving. As discussed in other chapters, staff problems such as incivility or even the extreme of violence impact CQI. Nurse leaders need to address the problems, but staff also need to assume responsibility and participate in resolving problems. Nurses at all levels in HCOs should be involved and guide others to improve the work environment. As Davis (2011) states, "Leaders set the tone for the organization . . . . This translates into ensuring that the clinical environment enables staff to practice in a setting whereby their mutual interactions are one of respect and support" (p. 26). The following list identifies some strategies that the leader or manager may use to address or prevent incivility and support a healthy work environment; however, for these strategies to be effective, staff must also commit to resolving the problem (Pearson & Porath, 2005, pp. 9, 12–14).

- *Set zero-tolerance expectations.* These expectations must come from top leadership and be communicated throughout the organization, and then implemented. Management needs to provide a method for reporting problems in applying these expectations.

- *Take an honest look in the mirror.* Leaders/managers must be role models. If there is incivility in the management team, then zero tolerance is not practiced and staff will follow the lead of managers, increasing staff incivility.
- *Weed out trouble before it enters the organization.* It is best to hire civil employees, although employers may not always know whether an applicant is or is not civil when hiring. Employers should check references and find out as much as possible.
- *Teach civility.* Common competencies needed for effective civility are communication, conflict resolution, negotiation, ability to deal with difficult people, stress management, listening, and coaching.
- *Put your ear to the ground and listen carefully; pay attention to warning signals.* Leadership must avoid limiting staff input and must prevent feelings of staff hopelessness and fear of repercussion.
- *When incivility occurs, hammer it.* Leadership should not wait for incivility to get worse. It needs to be dealt with as soon as it is recognized.
- *Heed warning signals.* Common signals are situations in which staff are not allowed to provide input, feelings of hopelessness among staff that problems will be resolved, and fearfulness among staff that if they report an instance of incivility, they will suffer repercussions.
- *Don't make excuses for powerful instigators.* Do not overlook those who stimulate incivility. Managers need to be held accountable for dealing with incivility.
- *Invest in postdeparture interviews.* Most staff that leave positions because of incivility do not report it prior to leaving. Routine postdeparture interview may get to this information, which is very valuable for the manager.

Stop and Consider #6

Nurse leaders, both formal and informal, impact CQI, but lack of leadership is a barrier to effective care.

Examples of Nursing Initiatives to Improve Care

Nurses and nursing organizations have a long history of involvement in various QI initiatives. Several of the current important initiatives are described in this section, and additional examples are discussed in other chapters.

The Magnet Recognition Program® is the only recognition program focused on the nursing service (ANCC, 2016). It provides standards of excellence that many HCOs follow today. When these HCOs meet the Magnet standards, the HCO may be given this recognition. The Magnet standards expect the use of effective leadership and staff engagement in these activities. Structural and process factors, such as adequate staffing, nurse education, collaboration and interprofessional relationships and teams, and nurse autonomy and responsibility, are also considered important. As has been discussed in this text, patient-centered care is critical to effective outcomes. The Magnet Recognition Program® is an example of a program that strongly emphasizes engagement of nurses in CQI (Beard & Sharkey, 2013). The expectation is that Magnet hospitals will excel in CQI and EBP.

The National Database of Nursing Indicators® (NDNQI) is the only nursing database that tracks specific nursing-sensitive indicators related to nursing structure, processes, and patient outcomes, emphasizing the key concepts noted in QI models (Press Ganey®, 2016). The original database was developed with ANA support and administered through several university nursing programs, but now it is administered through Press Ganey®. HCOs voluntarily participate in the database, and thus not all HCOs are involved; currently an estimated 2,000 U.S. hospitals and 98% of Magnet®-recognized HCOs participate in the NDNQI (Press Ganey, 2016). The database provides a monitor for relationships between its specific indicators and outcomes, including hospital-acquired conditions. When the NDNQI® is used, it should be integrated into the HCO's CQI plan.

Transforming Care at the Bedside (TCAB) is another example of a nursing initiative focused on CQI. In 2003, the Institute for Healthcare Improvement in collaboration with the Robert Wood Johnson Foundation developed TCAB (IHI, 2016). TCAB is discussed in other chapters; however, it is important to recognize it as an example of nursing participation at the CQI direct care level. It also provides opportunities to expand nursing engagement at all levels in an HCO's CQI activities. Publications that describe TCAB projects support the need for EBP and EBM to improve care.

The Interdisciplinary Nursing Quality Research Initiative (INQRI) supports interdisciplinary studies. Its website states the following:

These studies comprise the first effort of this size and scope to identify both the ways in which nurses can improve patient care quality and the contributions nurses can make every day that keep patients safer and healthier. INQRI has built a base of knowledge that demonstrates nursing's unique contributions to patients, families, and communities across a diverse range of settings and has created a community of scholars committed to advancing interdisciplinary research to continue to build that knowledge. (INQRI, 2016)

The Robert Wood Johnson Foundation created and continues to support INQRI. Supported studies are indirectly and directly related to CQI concerns and are discussed on the INQRI website. The Connect to Current Information section at the end of the chapter provides a link to this site.

In summary, the AONE's guiding principles provide guidelines about quality and safety for the nurse in future care delivery (AONE, 2010). Given the need to develop competencies related to CQI, it is critical that all nurses be included now and in the future in improving their own practice, whether that practice is in the clinical area or management. **Exhibit 12-2** describes the AONE principles focused on future needs. Nurses should understand and participate in the application of the National Quality Strategy, which is discussed in many chapters of this text (HHS, AHRQ, 2015).

Exhibit 12-2 American Organization of Nurse Executives (AONE) Guiding Principles for the Role of the Nurse in Future Patient Care Delivery: Quality and Safety

- Nurses serve as boundary spanners, ensuring continuity of care when handoffs and transfers are necessary (Gittell, 2009).
- Nurses drive reshaping of healthcare policy in a manner that results in better outcomes for patients and communities.
- The nurse acts as a synergist, integrating complexity science principles, assuming the need to encompass a nonlinear approach to problem solving given the web of interactions embedded in patient care.
- The nurse directs the continual improvement of quality, safety, and value of health care by knowing how to identify good care from the scientific evidence, knowing the actual measured performance in the context where the health professional is learning/practicing and the nature of the gaps, and knowing what activities are necessary—if any—to close the gap(s) (Batalden & Davidoff, 2007).
- Nurses are accountable to steer nursing's professional "identity" to include not only caring, knowledge, honesty, and integrity, but also knowledge and commitment to quality and safety (Cronenwett et al., 2007).
- Nurses drive the identification and mitigation of non-value-added interruptions (Sitterding & Ebright, 2010).
- The nurse guides design of technology that is nurse friendly, supportive of nursing work, accessible, and mobile (Sitterding & Ebright, 2010).
- Nurses lead the shift from an emphasis on critical thinking in practice to an emphasis on clinical reasoning and reasoning in transition (Benner, Sutphen, Leonard, & Day, 2009).
- The nurse demonstrates mindful attention of regulatory and accreditation requirements.
- Nurses spearhead the selection, development, implementation, evaluation, and modification of the electronic medical record and other technologies such as bar coding of medications, blood transfusions, and laboratory specimens.
- Nurses lead interdisciplinary teams with knowledge of the integration of the six Institute of Medicine aims for improvement: safe, timely, effective, efficient, equitable, and patient-centered (STEEEP).

- Nurses accelerate evidenced-based practice (EBP) capacity, such as by reviewing and integrating EBP model, developing active and innovative journal clubs, and requesting and obtaining access to nursing research or EBP experts and mentors (Stetler, Ritchie, Rycroft-Malone, Schultz, & Charns, 2009).
- The nurse integrates EBP into practice, policy, and procedure (Stetler et al., 2009).

References

Batalden, P., & Davidoff, F. (2007). What is "quality improvement" and how can it transform health care? *Quality and Safety in Health Care, 16*, 2–3.

Benner, P., Sutphen, M., Leonard, V., & Day, L. (2009). *Educating nurses: A call for radical transformation*. San Francisco, CA: Jossey-Bass.

Cronenwett, L., Sherwood, G., Barnsteiner, J., Disch, J., Johnson, J., & Mitchell, P. (2007). Quality and safety education for nurses. *Nursing Outlook, 55*(3), 122–131.

Gittell, J. (2009). *High performance healthcare*. New York, NY: McGraw-Hill.

Sitterding, M., & Ebright, P. (2010, April). Patient safety and the cognitive work of nursing: Advances in nursing science and implications for organizational support. Session presented at the 43rd Annual Meeting. American Organization of Nurse Executives. Indianapolis, IN.

Stetler, C., Ritchie, J., Rycroft-Malone, J., Schultz, A., & Charns, M. (2009). Institutionalizing evidence-based practice: An organizational case study using a model of strategic change. *Implementation Science, 4*, 78.

In summary, nurse leaders need to consider the following important elements if they want to develop and maintain a culture of excellence (Sollecito & Johnson, 2013, p. 64):

- *Customer focus.* Emphasizing the importance of both internal and external customers
- *Systems thinking.* Maintaining a goal of optimizing the systems as a whole and thereby creating synergy
- *Statistical thinking.* Understanding causes of variation and the importance of learning from measurement; having the ability to use data to make decisions
- *Teamwork.* Teams of peers working together to ensure empowerment, thereby creating the highest levels of motivation to ensure alignment of the organization, the team, and the individual around the CQI vision
- *Communication and feedback.* Maintaining open channels of communication and feedback to make adjustments as needed, including

modifying the vision to achieve higher levels of quality in a manner consistent with a learning organization, including feedback that is fact based and given with true concern for individuals' organizational success

Sharing these elements with all staff establishes expectations that all staff need to be committed to effectively meeting these elements and leads to improve care.

Stop and Consider #7
Nursing initiatives may impact CQI and require ongoing innovation.

Conclusions

Nursing leadership is not focused solely on nurses in formal management positions such as nurse executives, supervisors, and nurse managers. Nursing leadership must be part of every nurse's practice, whether this is clinical, management, education, or research. For nurses to become active and positive leaders in CQI, each nurse must be knowledgeable about CQI, engage in the CQI process, and commit to quality care for all patients in all types of settings and healthcare situations. This requires that the profession commit to this goal and collaborate within the profession and externally.

In 2008, an article on the role of nurses in hospital CQI noted the importance of this role and related challenges such as

scarcity of nursing resource, difficulty engaging nurses at all levels—from bedside to management, growing demands to participate in more, often duplicative, QI activities; the burdensome nature of data collection and reporting; and shortcomings of traditional nursing education in preparing nurses for their evolving role in today's contemporary hospital setting. (Draper, Felland, Liebhaber, & Melichar, 2008, p. 1)

We continue to face these challenges, although there is now more recognition that we must resolve them.

There is no doubt that nurses are involved in CQI, and this involvement has increased. There is, however, great need for more involvement. Quality care is not just about medical care. With nurses providing 24/7 care in hospitals, they have major responsibilities in hospitals and in other types of HCOs, and nurses should have greater influence over CQI. They are directly involved in ensuring that care meets the aims of safety, timeliness, effectiveness, efficiency, equity, and patient-centeredness (STEEEP) (Sandford, 2011). Nurse leaders need to work toward more effective linkage of nursing, quality, and finance.

The ANA social policy statement states, "Each nurse remains accountable for the quality of care within his or her scope of nursing practice" (ANA, 2015a, p. 191). Competence is a critical element of professional practice, and competence is directly related to quality care. The standards of professional practice provide a clear guideline for practice expectations (ANA, 2015a). The profession's code of ethics emphasizes that nurses have a social contract with the public, and this relates to nursing's relationships and communication with patients (ANA, 2015b). The nursing process includes steps that focus on quality and CQI, particularly outcomes identification and evaluation. EBP is also a critical component of nursing practice, supporting best practice to achieve outcomes, as is the use of EBM to respond effectively to management and CQI issues.

In addition, the major nursing reports that have examined nursing and its role in the healthcare delivery system have had an impact. *Keeping Patients Safe* even focuses on quality in its title, and in this report, as noted earlier, nurses are recognized for what they do to ensure quality care, but also what they could do if they were better prepared in CQI (IOM, 2004). *The Future of Nursing* report focuses mostly on degrees and expansion of scope of practice, but it also discusses the need for nursing leadership in QI (IOM, 2010). The role of nurses and nursing leadership are threaded throughout this text.

Kennedy, Murphy, and Roberts (2013) discuss the National Quality Strategy (NQS) and its implications for nursing, noting particularly that nurses need to be more involved in supporting and applying the NQS (HHS, AHRQ, 2015). The ANA and other nursing professions have long been engaged in healthcare policy development by providing expert testimony to state and federal legislative bodies, serving on committees, lobbying, and working with regulatory bodies such as the NCSBN and individual state boards of nursing. Further, they have assisted in the accreditation of HCOs and nursing education programs. These efforts require ongoing work, work that is really never completed. How can NQS be integrated into nursing? Other chapters also expand on this critical question. Kennedy and colleagues (2013) advocate for the role of effective leadership:

> Leadership makes a difference. If nurses do not engage in discussions about quality in healthcare, their ideas and opinions will not be heard. Nurses can take on leadership roles to influence healthcare delivery, improving quality, safety, and efficiency, and bring evidence for decision-making to the point of care to empower patients as partners. Collectively, nurses must respond to the challenges and opportunities.

APPLY CQI

Chapter Highlights

- *The Future of Nursing* report is a significant report that discusses critical aspects of nursing practice, including leadership and CQI.
- The progress report on *The Future of Nursing* report indicates that after 5 years more work needs to be done to reach the recommendations.

- Transformational leadership is the recommended model for leadership today in HCOs. Nurses need to develop their leadership knowledge and competencies to support this model of leadership. This duty applies to all nurses, not just nurses in management positions.
- Decision-making has a direct impact on CQI—from the perspective of making the best clinical decisions to better ensure quality care and from the perspective of the CQI process when decisions are made to address QI problems.
- Ineffective communication is one of the major causes of quality care problems and errors. Effective communication needs to be part of all CQI efforts and leadership. Ongoing efforts must be made to maintain effective communication through the care and management process.
- Staff need to be prepared to assume roles in CQI. This should begin in academic programs (pre-licensure and graduate) and continue in staff education and continuing education. Nurse leaders and managers need to ensure this preparation occurs. Each nurse must assume responsibility for his or her own lifelong learning, including content and experience related to CQI.
- Nursing leadership can make a difference in effective CQI, but it requires leadership knowledge and competencies.
- Accountability and responsibility are critical elements of CQI and leadership, impacting decision-making, power and empowerment, teams, delegation, and effectiveness of nurses in their practice and in their CQI activities.
- Examples of nursing initiatives that assist in improving care are the Magnet Recognition Program®, National Database of Nursing Indicators (NDNQI), Transforming Care at the Bedside (TCAB), Interdisciplinary Nursing Quality Research Initiative (INQRI), and work done by the American Nurses Association (ANA) and the American Organization of Nurse Executives (AONE).

Critical Thinking and Clinical Reasoning and Judgment: Discussion Questions and Learning Activities

1. Review the summary of the progress report related to *The Future of Nursing* report at http://www.nationalacademies.org/hmd/Reports/2015/Assessing-Progress-on-the-IOM-Report-The-Future-of-Nursing.aspx. Discuss the following questions with your team:
   a. What is the importance of the original report and the progress report?
   b. Which of the recommendations do you think is particularly important, and why?
   c. Do you think anything is missing from the progress report, and if so, what is missing?

(You might want to review the original report, *The Future of Nursing: Leading Change, Advancing Health*. It can be found at the same website.)

2. Describe in your own words the meaning of transformation leadership. Include your view of its relationship to nursing. Provide three examples of when you have observed this type of leadership in the practice setting. How do the examples relate to CQI?

3. Ask three nurse managers to come to a class session. Each should be asked to present a short commentary on his or her view of leadership and its relationship to CQI. Students should prepare questions for the question and answer session.

4. Review the document found at www.ncsbn.org/Joint_statement.pdf. You can download this document as a PDF. This document describes a delegation decision tree. Consider the following in your review by identifying a task you want to delegate. Then apply this task to the decision tree as you answer the questions in the decision tree and consider the key points. You will see in the decision tree that if you answer "no" to a question, the tree takes you in a different direction. This tree has four steps. Consider your own experiences when you have been the delegator or the delegatee. Write down your answers to the following questions:
   a. What was the situation?
   b. How did the process relate to what you are learning about in this chapter?
   c. Was it effective or not? Why?
   d. What would you have done differently?
   e. Which do you prefer to be, the delegator or the delegatee, and why?
   Review your answers. Develop a list of steps you will take to improve when you are either the delegator or a delegatee. Periodically use this process to improve.

5. Describe in writing the relationship of decision-making to CQI and incorporate the relationship of accountability, responsibility, and communication. Provide two examples to support your description.

6. Consider how you will demonstrate leadership as a staff nurse. Write a two-page description and then share it in a discussion group in class or online.

Connect to Current Information

- American Organization of Nurse Executives (AONE)
  http://www.aone.org/
- Nursing Alliance for Quality Care (NAQC)
  http://www.naqc.org/
- Campaign for Action
  http://campaignforaction.org/

- National Council of State Boards of Nursing (NCSBN): Delegation
  https://www.ncsbn.org/1625.htm
- National Database of Nursing Quality Indicators® (NDNQI)
  http://www.pressganey.com/solutions/clinical-quality/nursing-quality
- NCSBN: Transition to Practice (TTP)
  https://www.ncsbn.org/transition-to-practice.htm
- NCSBN: Taxonomy of Error, Root Cause Analysis, Practice-Responsibility (TERCAP)
  https://www.ncsbn.org/113.htm
- Institute for Healthcare Improvement: Transforming Care at the Bedside (TCAB)
  http://www.ihi.org/engage/initiatives/completed/TCAB/Pages/default.aspx
- American Nurses Credentialing Center: Magnet Recognition Program®
  http://www.nursecredentialing.org/Magnet/ProgramOverview
- Interdisciplinary Nursing Quality Research Initiative (INQRI)
  http://www.inqri.org/

EBP, EBM, and Quality Improvement: Exemplar

Goeschel, C. (2011). Defining and assigning accountability for quality care and patient safety. *Journal of Nursing Regulation, 2*(1), 28–33.

    This article discusses the relationship of accountability in health care to quality care and how this relationship impacts professional issues.

Questions to Consider

1. How is accountability described in this article?
2. How is accountability related to quality care and leadership?
3. What does the article say about *The Future of Nursing* report and its application to accountability and need for change to improve care?

Evolving Case Study

The HCO administration has concluded an extensive staff survey about CQI. The results indicate that staff, particularly nursing staff, are not engaged in CQI. Many do not see it as their responsibility. In describing their view of CQI activities, nurses say it is their job to provide "good" care and someone else takes care of the "administrative stuff." There is also a notable decrease in the number of incident report submissions. The Chief Nurse Executive called a special meeting of her administrative staff and all nurse managers.

Case Questions A

You are asked to present background information as found in this chapter at the special meeting.

1. What would you present? (Prepare PowerPoint slides.)

2. Based on the content of your presentation, what are three questions you would ask the group to consider?

Case Questions B

To give the group time to consider the presentation and discussion, the group schedules a second meeting for a week later. The agenda will address the following questions:

1. What do you think should be done to improve leadership for all nursing staff? Be specific.

2. What specific strategies might be used to engage nurses in CQI?

3. How would you assess outcomes of these two efforts? Be specific.

References

American Association of Colleges of Nursing (AACN). (2016). Nurse residency program. Retrieved from http://www.aacn.nche.edu/education-resources/nurse-residency-program

American Nurses Association (ANA). (2005). *Principles of delegation.* Silver Spring, MD: Author.

American Nurses Association (ANA). (2015a). *Scope and standards of practice.* Silver Spring, MD: Author.

American Nurses Association (ANA). (2015b). *Guide to the code of ethics with interpretative statements.* Silver Spring, MD: Author.

American Nurses Association (ANA). (2016). 2016 culture of safety. Retrieved from http://www.nursingworld.org/MainMenuCategories/ThePracticeofProfessionalNursing/2016-Culture-of-Safety

American Nurses Credentialing Center (ANCC). (2016). Magnet Recognition Program® overview. Retrieved from http://www.nursecredentialing.org/Magnet/ProgramOverview

American Organization of Nurse Executives (AONE). (2007). AONE guiding principles for the role of the nurse executive in patient safety. Retrieved from http://www.aone.org/resources/role-nurse-executive-patient-safety.pdf

American Organization of Nurse Executives (AONE).(2010). AONE guiding principles for the role of the nurse in future patient care delivery: Quality and safety principle, pp. 2–3. Retrieved from http://www.aone.org/resources/role-nurse-future-patient-care.pdf

Beard, E., & Sharkey, K. (2013). Innovation amidst radical cost containment in health care. *Nursing Administration Quarterly, 37*(2), 116–121.

Benner, P., Hughes, R., & Sutphen, M. (2008). Clinical reasoning, decision-making, and action: Thinking critically and clinically. In R. Hughes (Ed.), *Patient safety and quality: An evidence-based handbook for nurses* (Chapter 6). Washington, DC: Agency for Healthcare Research and Quality. Retrieved from http://archive.ahrq.gov/professionals/clinicians-providers/resources/nursing/resources/nurseshdbk/index.html

Benner, P., Sutphen, M., Leonard, V., & Day, L. (2010). *Educating nurses: A call for radical transformation*. San Francisco, CA: Jossey-Bass.

Campaign for Action (2016). Campaign for action. Retrieved from http://campaignforaction.org/

Davis, C. (2011). Creating a safe work environment, a plan for success. *Nurse Leader, 9*(8), 25–27.

Draper, D., Felland, L., Liebhaber, A., & Melichar, L. (2008). The role of nurses in hospital quality improvement. Retrieved from http://www.hschange.org/CONTENT/972/?words=Draper

Finkelman, A. (2016). *Leadership and management for nurses: Core Competencies for quality care*. (3rd ed.). Upper Saddle River, NJ: Pearson Education, Inc.

Finkelman, A., & Kenner, C. (2016). *Professional nursing concepts: Competencies for quality leadership* (3rd ed.). Burlington, MA: Jones & Bartlett Learning.

Goffee, R., & Jones, G. (2000). Why should anyone be led by you? *Harvard Business Review*, Sept.–Oct., 63–71.

Institute for Healthcare Improvement (IHI). (2016). Transforming Care at the Bedside. Retrieved from http://www.ihi.org/engage/initiatives/completed/TCAB/Pages/default.aspx

Institute of Medicine (IOM). (2002). *Leadership by example: Coordinating government roles in improving healthcare quality*. Washington, DC: The National Academies Press.

Institute of Medicine (IOM). (2003). *Health professions education: A bridge to quality*. Washington, DC: The National Academies Press.

Institute of Medicine (IOM). (2004). *Keeping patients safe: Transforming the work environment of nurses*. Washington, DC: The National Academies Press.

Institute of Medicine (IOM). (2009). *Redesigning continuing education in the health professions*. Washington, DC: The National Academies Press.

Institute of Medicine (IOM). (2010). *The future of nursing: Leading change, advancing health*. Washington, DC: The National Academies Press.

Interdisciplinary Nursing Quality Research Initiative (INQRI). (2016). About INQRI. Retrieved from http://www.inqri.org/about-inqri

Interprofessional Professional Education Collaborative Expert Panel (IPECEP). (2011). *Core competencies for interprofessional collaborative practice*. Retrieved from www.aacn.nche.edu/education-resources/IPECReport.pdf

Kennedy, R., Murphy, J., & Roberts, D. (2013). An overview of the National Quality Strategy: Where do nurses fit? *OJIN: The Online Journal of Issues in Nursing, 18*(3). Retrieved from http://www.nursingworld.org/MainMenuCategories/ANAMarketplace/ANAPeriodicals/OJIN/TableofContents/Vol-18-2013/No3-Sept-2013/National-Quality-Strategy.html

Makary, M. (2016). Medical error—the third leading cause of death in the U.S. *BMJ*, (May 3). Retrieved from http://www.bmj.com/content/353/bmj.i2139/rr-40

Marthaler, M., & Kelly, P. (2008). Delegation of patient care. In P. Kelly (Ed.), *Nursing leadership and management* (2nd ed., pp. 340–367). Clifton Park, NY: Delmar.

McBride, A. (2011). *The growth and development of nurse leaders*. New York, NY: Springer Publishing Company.

National Academies of Sciences (NAS), Health and Medicine Division (HMD). (2015). *Measuring the impact of interprofessional education on collaborative practice and patient outcomes*. Washington, DC: The National Academies Press.

National Academies of Sciences (NAS), Health and Medicine Division (HMD). (2016). *Assessing progress on the Institute of Medicine report* The Future of Nursing. Washington, DC: The National Academies Press.

National Council of State Boards of Nursing (NCSBN). (2016). Transition to practice. Retrieved from https://www.ncsbn.org/transition-to-practice.htm

O'Neil, E., & Chow, M. (2011). Leadership action for a new American health system. *Nurse Leader, 9*(12), 34–36.

Pearson, C., & Porath, C. (2005). On the nature, consequences and remedies of workplace incivility: Not time for "nice"? Think again. *Academy of Management Executive, 30*(2), 7–18.

Press Ganey®. (2016). NDNQI. Retrieved from http://www.pressganey.com/solutions/clinical-quality/nursing-quality

Rath, T., & Conchie, B. (2008). *Strengths based leadership.* New York, NY: Gallup Press.

Sandford, K. (2011). Making the business case for quality and nursing. *Nurse Leader, 9*(1), 28–31.

Sollecito, K., & Johnson, J. (2013). Factors influencing the application and diffusion of CQI in health care. In W. Sollecito & J. Johnson (Eds.), *McLaughlin and Kaluzny's continuous quality improvement in health care* (4th ed., pp. 49–74). Burlington, MA: Jones & Bartlett Learning.

U.S. Department of Health and Human Services (HHS), Agency for Healthcare Research and Quality (AHRQ). (2015). About the National Quality Strategy (NQS). Retrieved from http://www.ahrq.gov/workingforquality/about.htm

Examples of Affordable Care Act of 2010 Provisions Related to Quality Care

- Establish nonprofit Patient-Centered Outcomes Research Institute (PCORI) focused on comparative effectiveness research
- Improve care coordination for beneficiaries covered by Medicare and Medicaid
- Establish a National Workforce Commission
- Require nonprofit hospitals to use community needs assessments to determine needs
- Increase access via increase in reimbursement options and funding for new programs
- Develop a national quality improvement strategy, which is now called the National Quality Strategy (NQS)
- Improve collection of data about factors that impact disparities on care
- Develop methods to improve coordination of care, such as collaborative care initiatives (e.g., accountable care organizations [ACOs])
- Improve and develop uniform standards for health plans and electronic exchange of health information
- Increase prevention and health promotion initiatives
- Implement pay for performance, value rather than quantity
- Provide additional funding for nursing education programs
- Provide funding (e.g., grants and loans) for students and faculty
- Provide education and training funds focused on geriatrics
- Improve primary care—advanced practice traineeships
- Provide funding for nurse-managed clinics
- Improve health prevention and public health
- Increase workforce diversity
- Create community-based transition programs
- Improve nondiscrimination in health care
- Continue support for the Preventive Services Task Force
- Create the National Health Care Workforce Commission; offer grants and analysis of data related to workforce needs

Examples of Major Healthcare Organizations and Agencies, Governmental and Nongovernmental, Related to Quality Improvement

- Agency for Healthcare Research and Quality (AHRQ)
- AHRQ QI
- AHRQ Safety Primers
- Alliance for Home Health Quality and Innovation (AHHQI)
- Alliance for Pediatric Quality
- Ambulatory Quality Alliance (AQA)
- American Association of Colleges of Nursing (AACN)
- American Health Informatics Community (AHIC)
- American Nurses Association (ANA)
- American Nurses Association National Center for Nursing Quality
- Association for Prevention Teaching and Research (APTR)
- Baldridge Performance Excellence Program
- Center for Studying Health System Change (HSC)
- Consumers Advancing Patient Safety (CAPS)
- Future of Nursing: Campaign for Action
- Healing Environment
- Healthcare Cost and Utilization Project (HCUP)
- Healthcare Information and Management Systems Society (HIMSS)
- Healthcare Effectiveness Data and Information Set (HEDIS)
- Health Resources and Services Agency (HRSA)
- Health Research and Educational Trust (HRET) (Disparities Toolkit)
- Hospital Compare (Medicare)
- Hospital Consumer Assessment of Healthcare Providers and Systems (HCAHPS)
- Improvement Science Research Network (ISRN)

- Initiative on The Future of Nursing: Campaign for Action
- Interdisciplinary Nursing Quality Research Institute (INQRI)
- Institute for Healthcare Improvement (IHI)
- Institute for Safe Medication Practices (ISMP)
- The Joint Commission
- Joint Commission International
- Kaiser Family Foundation (KFF)
- Leapfrog Group
- Magnet Recognition Program
- National Center for Nursing Quality (NCNQ)
- National Committee for Quality Assurance (NCQA)
- National Council of State Boards of Nursing (NCSBN)
- National Database of Nursing Quality Indicators (NDNQI)
- National Guideline Clearinghouse
- *National Healthcare Quality Report and Disparities Reports* (QDR)
- National Institutes of Health (NIH)
- National Institute of Nursing Research (NINR)
- National Institute for Occupational Safety and Health (NIOSH)
- National League for Nursing (NLN)
- National Patient Safety Goals (The Joint Commission)
- National Patient Safety Foundation (NPSF)
- National Priorities Partnership (part of NQF)
- National Quality Forum (NQF)
- National Quality Measures Clearinghouse
- National Quality Strategy (NQS)
- Nursing Alliance for Quality Care (NAQC)
- Occupational Safety and Health Administration (OSHA)
- Partnership for Patients
- Patient-Centered Outcomes Research Institute (PCORI)
- Patient Safety Indicators (PSIs)
- Patient Safety Network (PSNet)
- Quality Interagency Coordination Task Force (QuIC)
- Quality and Safety Education for Nurses (QSEN)
- Six Sigma
- Transforming Care at the Bedside (TCAB)
- Taxonomy of Error Root Cause Analysis and Practice Responsibility (TERCAP)
- Transition Into Practice (TIP)
- U.S. Department of Health and Human Services (HHS)
- U.S. Department of Health and Human Services (HHS), **Centers for** Medicare and Medicaid Services (CMS)

- U.S. Department of Health and Human Services (HHS), Centers for Disease Control and Prevention (CDC)
- U.S. Department of Health and Human Services (HHS), Food and Drug Administration (FDA)
- VA Nursing Outcomes Database (VANOD)
- VA National Center for Patient Safety
- World Health Organization (WHO)
- World Health Organization (WHO), World Health Alliance for Patient Safety
- World Health Organization (WHO), Taxonomy for Patient Safety
- World Health Organization (WHO), Interprofessional Teams

Glossary

accountability A person's responsibility for his or her actions and the outcomes of those actions.

accreditation A method used to assess organizations and determine if they meet minimum established standards.

active error An error that results from noncompliance with a procedure that involves a frontline worker (i.e., direct care worker).

adverse event An injury resulting from a medical intervention, not from the patient's underlying condition.

advocacy Support of a cause or action on another's behalf.

alarm/alert fatigue Failure of the staff to quickly respond to or a tendency to ignore alarms that occur too frequently or that are often false.

autonomy The principle that patients have the right to determine their own rights.

bar code medication administration Use of bar codes located on the patient's identification to compare with the bar code found on orders or, in the case of medications, found on the individual patient drug package.

baseline data Data collected prior to a change has occurred in order to compare conditions after the change.

benchmarking The act of comparing a situation before a change is implemented to the situation after a change is implemented.

beneficence The principle that nurses should not inflict harm and should safeguard the patient.

blame culture A professional environment in which errors are examined with a focus on assigning blame to individuals.

brainstorming A method used to identify as many ideas as possible so that the ideas can then be assessed to determine if they can be used or should be eliminated.

bullying Harmful, deliberate actions intended to embarrass, offend, or distress another person.

call-out A communication approach in which the person communicates important information to the team so that everyone hears the same information at the same time, reducing the chance of miscommunication or some team members not hearing the same information.

case management A patient care effort designed to get the right services to patients when needed with the goal of avoiding fragmented and unnecessary care.

certification Authorization to provide care in a given capacity. Through standardized examination, nurses can demonstrate expertise in a specialty area and validate knowledge for certification as determined by the American Nurses Credentialing Center.

change A difference in some aspect of the care dynamic, involving the patient, system, healthcare services, and so on.

change agent An individual or team who focuses on the problem or change issue and possible approaches to take.

check sheet A simple form used to collect and document data that allows staff to quickly indicate whether an expected action or observation occurred.

check-back A communication approach in which the person asks the team if they heard the information and understood it.

checklist A list designed to indicate the order in which steps are to be followed and to document this process.

clinical decision support (CDT) A method used to prevent errors and omissions by monitoring situations and alerting clinicians of patient conditions, prescriptions, and treatment to provide evidence-based clinical suggestions to health professionals at the point of care.

clinical guideline A written description of care for a specific patient population based on evidence.

clinical judgment The process of making decisions about clinical concerns and treatment.

clinical reasoning The application of experience and research in reasoning through clinical scenarios.

coaching A method used to provide career guidance and support.

code of ethics A set of ethical standards that guide a care provider's behavior.

code of silence A professional environment in which staff do not feel safe in speaking up, even when they know something is wrong, and thus do not help effect change.

collaboration The act of partnering with another qualified provider to bring about optimal patient care.

collaborative care model An initiative to increase patient engagement by focusing on managing the health of a population rather than on treating a specific diagnosis.

common format A set of definitions and reporting formats developed by the Agency for Healthcare Research and Quality that offer healthcare organizations consistency across one another when reporting data external to the healthcare organization.

comparative effectiveness research The review of evidence-based practice to provide healthcare providers with state-of-the-science information to make the best quality and cost decisions for patients.

compassion fatigue A type of cumulative stress experienced by nurses through repeated exposure to emotionally difficult situations.

competency A level of performance that is expected within the nursing profession.

comprehensive unit-based safety program (CUSP) A program developed by the Agency for Healthcare Research and Quality to consider the implications of change. Teams and teamwork are critical components in CUSP.

computerized physician/provider order entry (CPOE) A computerized method to support quality care in which four steps occur when a hospitalized patient receives a medication: (1) ordering, (2) transcribing the order (if handwritten), (3) dispensing the medication by the pharmacists, and (4) administering medication.

consonant culture An organizational culture that encourages development of a collaborative team environment.

continuing education Formal transmission of a predetermined body of knowledge. Related activities are frequently provided with designated accreditation and generate "credits" for practitioners, necessary for most state licensure and other credentialing processes.

continuous quality improvement (CQI) Measures taken by a healthcare organization to ensure that the best possible care is provided during each patient encounter, that the potential for errors is minimized, and that patient encounters are properly documented to enable later review and improvement.

coordination Organization of care across all elements of the healthcare system.

core measure set Standards relevant to a given field used to objectively assess the efficacy of change efforts.

crew resource management (CRM) A method to support quality care that focuses on leadership, interprofessional communication, and effective decision-making, using all available resources, emphasizing a no-blame culture, and focusing on clear, comprehensive standard operating procedures.

critical reflection The act of questioning clinical practices and assumptions in an effort to improve patient care.

critical thinking Examination of knowledge, intuition, and application of knowledge.

cultural competence A set of congruent behaviors, attitudes, and policies that come together in a system or agency or among professionals, enabling effective work in cross-cultural situations.

culture The prevailing attitudes and beliefs of an organization.

culture of safety An organizational culture in which all members share a sense of accountability in creating a safe, effective care environment.

dashboard A clear visual depiction of data in one view.

data Objective, informative details that are presented without interpretation.

database A method used to organize data so information is easy to store, manage, and access.

decision tree A method of identifying solutions to a problem by treating each potential solution as a "trunk" from which the potential positive and negative outcomes "branch."

deep dive An in-depth brainstorming technique that is used ideally by an interprofessional team.

define and measure-analyze-design-verify (DMADV) A means of assessing care quality by which project goals and outcomes are defined, the process is analyzed, a detailed description of the process is developed, and then performance is verified.

delegation The act of transferring a specific task to another person, or empowering another to act.

delphi technique A problem-solving technique in which staff respond to a questionnaire that focuses on a particular problem, and responses are discussed through multiple rounds until the problem is understood at its most refined level.

diagnostic error Failure to make the appropriate diagnosis given the available evidence.

disclosure The act of informing a patient that an error occurred, assuming the patient does not already know.

discrimination A cause of unequal patient treatment that occurs when healthcare providers view, and consequently treat, patients differently based on their race, ethnicity, sex, or other characteristics not relevant to the health condition at hand.

disease management Use of services to better ensure patient-centered care and improve the quality of care.

disease-specific measure/indicator A quality indicator used by healthcare organizations that focuses on a disease and applies to patients with that disease.

disparity See *healthcare disparity*.

dissonant culture An organizational culture that blocks the development of a collaborative team environment.

diversity Variation in the characteristics of a population, based on gender, religion, ethnicity, and so on.

early warning system A method of measuring patients' physiological status to anticipate and thus prevent catastrophic medical events.

electronic health record (EHR) A digital record that includes the same information as the EMR plus more comprehensive information about the patient's history.

electronic medical record (EMR) A digital record that includes provider medical and clinical data for a patient.

empowerment The act of empowering someone to act.

enterprise data warehouse A data resource that provides a collection of databases that can be accessed and analyzed.

error An unintended and undesired outcome.

error of execution Failure to execute a planned action.

error of planning Failure to anticipate the patient's needs or prepare the correct course of action.

ethical dilemma A situation in which a choice must be made but none of the options are ideal.

ethics An understanding of proper practice behaviors learned through an organized system, such as standardized ethics code developed by a professional group.

evidence-based management (EBM) The use of current research to improve the performance of healthcare organizations.

evidence-based practice (EBP) The use of current research to make clinical decisions.

failure mode and effects analysis (FMEA) An analysis method focused on known or potential problems and errors, with the goal of preventing errors by understanding and addressing all the ways a system could fail.

failure to rescue (FTR) A missed opportunity to provide care that would have prevented complications.

fishbone analysis A problem analysis tool that uses a fishbone graphic to allow a team to identify and address all possible causes of a problem.

flowchart A format used to describe data that enables reviewing or updating of information and that helps keep it current.

fraud Intentional deception for one's own gain; it is a criminal act.

frontline safety Direct care practices in which staff consider patient safety and quality in their daily work.

frontline staff The staff members responsible for providing direct care staff. These staff members often get lost in the big picture but make the biggest difference in quality improvement, regardless of the type or size of the healthcare organization.

GANTT chart A type of chart used to display progress in a project over time.

gap analysis A method for examining current status by focusing on where the organization, department, or unit and the staff want to go. The difference in current status and future vision is referred to as the "gap."

generic measure/indicator A quality indicator used by healthcare organizations to assess factors that are relevant to most patients.

global trigger A signal or a clue that may be used to identify a potential adverse event, not the event itself.

groupthink The tendency of a group member to go along with the group's proposed idea even though the member does not agree with the idea.

handoff The transitioning of a patient from one form of care to another, such as from one clinical site to another.

harm Impaired functioning, whether physical, emotional, or psychological, that causes pain, injury, or distress.

health informatics technology (HIT) The use of technology to study healthcare information and communication systems to improve decision-making and other tasks.

health literacy A person's understanding of his or her own health status and of the variables that lead to good health.

healthcare delivery measure A measure of care delivered to individuals and populations defined by its relationship to clinicians, clinical delivery teams, delivery organizations, or health insurance plans.

healthcare disparity A difference in the quality of health care received by one party versus that received by another party for the same condition. Health disparities in the United States are often based on racial and ethnic differences.

healthcare equity Attainment of the highest level of health for all people.

healthcare inequality The difference in health status or in the distribution of health determinants between different population groups.

high-reliability organization (HRO) A healthcare organization that uses a three-step approach to achieve a high level of reliability: Prevent failure, identify and mitigate failure, and redesign processes.

high-risk A situation in which there is greater chance of near misses and errors occurring.

hospital-acquired condition (HAC) A condition that develops after admission to the hospital that could have been prevented through appropriate care measures.

huddle A short meeting with staff focusing on a specific issue; it can be scheduled or unscheduled.

human error Failure to achieve a desired outcome that can be attributed to skill-, rule-, or knowledge-based performance.

human factors and ergonomics Physical, cognitive, and organizational factors that can have an impact on errors.

human failure A source of error attributed to an individual provider.

incidence An estimate of how frequently new events, cases, etc., develop.

incident report A standardized form created by an organization that addresses specific incidents to ensure that staff provide all relevant details relating to the incident.

incivility Unprofessional conduct such as rude and discourteous behavior, gossiping and spreading rumors, or refusing to help others in the work situation.

indicator An aggregate measure for a specific operation.

interoperability The ability of health systems to easily share electronic health information with one another.

interprofessional education Education for individuals from different professions offered together to promote collaborative working in their professional practice.

just culture An organizational culture in which individuals are not blamed for errors that may be considered organizational shortcomings but are held accountable for negligent or otherwise inappropriate care delivery.

justice The principle that patients should be treated fairly.

lapse Failure to check something that is part of the procedure.

latent conditions Factors that are not readily apparent within an organization that contribute to errors.

latent error See *latent conditions*.

lateral violence Acts of violence occurring between coworkers (e.g., nurse to nurse).

leadership The act of guiding others toward a desired outcome.

lean approach An approach to quality improvement that focuses on value to the customer (i.e., the patient), with efforts made to reduce waste in time, effort, and cost—doing more with less.

learning healthcare system A healthcare system that values and builds upon clinical research and that strives to use population-based data to improve patient interventions and outcomes.

lifelong learning Voluntary and self-motivated pursuit of knowledge for either personal or professional reasons.

linguistic competence The capacity of an organization and its personnel to communicate effectively and convey information in a manner easily understood by diverse audiences, including persons of limited English proficiency, those who have low literacy skills or are not literate, and those with disabilities.

macrosystem The broadest level of the healthcare system, such as the healthcare organization under which several distinct hospitals operate.

macroview The perspective of healthcare quality focused on the broader issues, from a local, state, federal, or even global perspective.

malpractice Failure to provide a level of care appropriate to the provider's professionally licensed capacity.

management The act of ensuring that the structure and resources exist to accomplish a job.

meaningful use Criteria defined by the Centers for Medicare and Medicaid Services that hospitals and providers must meet to be identified as meaningful users of health informatics technology.

measure A standard used as a reference point to compare outcomes.

medication error A preventable event in which medication, while still under the control of the provider, is used in a manner that causes patient harm.

medication reconciliation The act of formulating a list of medications for a patient (e.g., drug name, dosage and frequency, administration method, and purpose of the medication) and reviewing the list to ensure that there are no conflicts in the medications.

mental fatigue Reduced mental performance owing to an overload of mental task demands.

mentoring Use of a role model to assist in career development.

mesosystem A level of the healthcare system beneath the macrosystem in which the departments, clinical centers, or services operate.

metric A means of comparing an aspect of care to a specified criterion.

micromanagement Overinvolvement in the details of subordinates' everyday work functions, thus limiting their views and understanding about processes and outcomes.

microsystem A level of the healthcare system beneath the mesosystem in which the clinical units, the smallest unit of the system, operate; it is here that the patient has the most influence.

microview The perspective of healthcare quality focused on the healthcare provider, which can be a healthcare organization or an individual healthcare provider such as a physician, nurse, or pharmacist.

missed care Nursing care that is delayed, partially completed, or not completed.

mistake A wrong decision, often related to inexperience, inadequate training, or even negligence.

misuse An avoidable event that prevents patients from receiving the full potential benefit of a service.

morbidity Incidence of disease state or condition.

mortality Incidence of death.

near miss An instance in which an error almost happened, but staff caught the problem before it became an error.

negligence Failure to provide a level of care that would be expected of a reasonably prudent person.

nominal group A brainstorming method in which each group member records his or her ideas related to an issue, and the ideas are then shared anonymously and voted on by the group to determine the most important ideas.

nursing regulation Professional oversight intended to ensure nursing services provide for the public's health, safety, and welfare.

omission Failure to provide assessment, planning, or interventions, possibly leading to problems for the patient and affecting expected outcomes.

operational plan A plan relating to the quality improvement program that describes the steps needed to ensure outcomes are met, describes roles and responsibilities, identifies timelines, plans evaluation, and describes the revision process.

organizational culture The values, beliefs, traditions, and communication processes that bring a group of people together and characterize the organization.

organizational failure A source of error attributed to staff orientation and training, policies, procedures, and use of clinical pathways or protocols.

organizational readiness The likelihood that staff and the organization are prepared to handle change.

outcome The result of a patient intervention or treatment, whether acute or long-term.

outcome measure/indicator A means by which an organization evaluates the efficacy of its interventions and practices.

overuse An instance in which the potential for harm from the provision of a service exceeds the possible benefit.

Pareto chart A vertical bar graph with bars ordered from longest to shortest to prioritize the frequency of causes related to one another.

pass the problem A problem-solving method in which participants are divided into two groups and, through a back-and-forth process, develop a list of strategies to address given problems, ending in a group presentation and discussion of all the identified strategies.

patient-centered care Care that respects differences among patients, that seeks to provide optimal patient care that minimizes suffering and ensures continuity of care, and that values the patient's involvement in his or her own care.

patient-centered rounds Clinical rounds that can be configured in a number of ways for different purposes, but the critical element is they focus on the patient and patient needs.

patient safety primer Evidence-based sources of information about patient safety available on the Agency for Healthcare Research and Quality's website.

pay for performance A payment model by which providers and healthcare organizations are financially incentivized to provide care that meets defined care standards.

performance management A forward-looking process used to set goals and regularly check progress toward achieving those goals.

performance measure A measure of the quality of care provided by a healthcare system in which specific measurable elements are used as a quality meter.

performance measurement A forward-looking process used to set goals and regularly check progress toward achieving those goals.

personal health record (PHR) A digital record that includes the same information as the EMR and EHR, but the patient keeps the record and maintains it.

PERT chart A visual or graphic representation describing a project or a process using boxes and arrows to illustrate the sequence of tasks. PERT stands for program evaluation review technique.

physical fatigue Physical discomfort and decreased ability to perform physically due to an overload of physical task demands.

plan-do-study-act Often called the PDSA or Deming cycle, a rapid cycle change method used by healthcare organizations to assist in responding to change and planning.

point of care Direct care experiences when the healthcare provider and patient intersect for care, such as for assessment and intervention.

point-of-care learning A subset of workplace learning that occurs at the time and place (whether virtual such as simulation or actual) of a health professional–patient encounter.

policy A continuous quality improvement measure intended to clarify important communication and consistent processes within a healthcare organization to ensure care quality, consistency, and other objectives.

population health measure A measure that addresses health issues of individuals or populations defined by residence in a geographic area or a relationship to organizations that are not primarily organized to deliver or pay for healthcare services (such as schools or prisons).

power The ability to influence decisions, control situations and resources, and affect others' behavior.

powerlessness The inability to influence decisions or control situations.

presenteeism A potential source of errors in which staff are at work but are not functioning at their fullest, often due to a medical problem, whether physical or psychological.

prevalence The rate of the number of cases at a given time divided by the number in the at-risk population.

primary CQI data Information collected in original sources for the purpose of continuous quality improvement (CQI).

proactive change Change that is planned based on assessment of need.

procedure A step-by-step description of a task or clinical activity.

process The manner in which the parts of the healthcare system function independently and interact.

process measure/indicator A means by which an organization evaluates the processes that it has in place to address specific scenarios.

project plan A plan relating to the quality improvement program that focuses on specific needs, such as a change in the medication administration procedure for the emergency department.

qualitative data Data that provide information about descriptive characteristics, used to make inferences based on observable data, not measurable data.

quality care The competent provision of services with effective communication, involvement of the patient in decision-making, and cultural sensitivity.

quality gap A deficiency in healthcare delivery resulting from a system that is fragmented and poorly organized, confusing, and complex, leading to treatment overuse, underuse, and misuse.

quality improvement plan A detailed, organizational work plan for a healthcare organization's continuous quality improvement activities.

quantitative data Data that focus on numbers and frequencies so that measurable data can be obtained and statistics used to analyze the data.

rapid cycle model An approach to quality improvement that is used to test small changes recommended by frontline staff and actively engage staff in the continuous quality improvement process, recognizing that small changes can impact the healthcare organization with positive outcomes.

rapid response team (RRT) A team formed to identify and quickly respond when patients are experiencing deterioration in their condition.

reactive change Change that occurs in response to a development that requires that an improvement be made.

read-back The act of repeating written or oral information to ensure the message was properly received.

reasonably prudent nurse A nurse who acts in the same manner as would any other nurse who has similar education and experience and average intelligence, judgment, foresight, and skill, given the same care scenario.

red rules Rules that must be followed to ensure continuous quality improvement.

reliability (1) The extent to which repeated measurements yield similar results. (2) The state of being failure-free that develops in an environment over time; *over time* is a critical aspect, as it is not a one-time viewpoint of quality, but rather consistent, effective performance.

report card A summary report of the status of a healthcare organization's quality of care.

responsibility The acceptance of an obligation to do something.

risk management An assessment of a healthcare organization's risk for malpractice claims and thus risk for financial loss.

root cause analysis (RCA) A method used by many healthcare organizations to analyze errors, supporting the recognition that most errors are caused by system issues and not necessarily individual staff issues.

run chart A display of data that illustrates or plots change and patterns over time.

safe zone An atmosphere created to ensure that during certain activities there are no interruptions and distractions so that staff can meet their responsibilities effectively and safely.

safety The assurance patients will not be harmed through the care they receive.

safety walkaround A communication method in which the healthcare organization's leadership directly interacts with direct care staff and patients to receive and provide feedback, thus demonstrating the organization's commitment to quality improvement and helping to reduce adverse events.

science of improvement An approach to quality improvement that emphasizes the use of research, innovative methods, and the rapid cycle method, with focus on three questions: (1) What are we trying to accomplish? (2) How will we know that a change is an improvement? (3) What changes can we make that will result in improvement?

scope of practice The performance expectations relating to tasks common to all registered nurses.

secondary CQI data Information collected in second-hand sources, such as those primarily used in care delivery (e.g., a preoperative checklist), for the purpose of continuous quality improvement (CQI).

self-determination A nurse's assessment of his or her own ability to meet the demands of a given care scenario, taking into account such factors as scope of practice, skills and competencies, and factors relating to the patient and clinical setting.

self-management The patient's ability to meet his or her own health needs, promoted by healthcare providers through patient-centered care.

self-regulation Efforts made by nurses to maintain their competence, often through required continuing education for licensure and/or certification.

sentinel event An unexpected event that happens to patients resulting in major negative outcomes, such as an unexpected death or a critical physical or psychological complication that can lead to major alteration in the patient's health.

sentinel measure A quality indicator used by healthcare organizations to identify outcomes that are intrinsically undesirable and that must always be addressed.

shared governance An approach to decision-making in which staff have substantial input and there is a structure to facilitate this process.

signout The transmission of information about the patient during a patient transfer (i.e., handoff).

situation, background, assessment, recommendation (SBAR) A communication approach designed to ensure structured, clear communication.

six hat method A brainstorming method used by teams to better understand proposals for change. During the process, team members assume one of the roles (hats) and discuss the proposal from that perspective.

Six Sigma An approach to quality improvement that includes three key elements: (1) Measure work output, (2) apply the process throughout all departments in an organization, until it eventually becomes part of the organization's culture, and (3) maintain a goal of no more than 3.4 errors per 1,000,000 operations.

slip An error that occurs due to failure to be clear, such as during documentation.

social determinants of health The everyday factors in a person's life that contribute to his or her overall health. Assessing these factors should take into consideration the equity with which money, power, and resources are distributed within a society.

solution analysis A problem-solving method that considers each of the possible solutions and then ranks them according to how effective the solution might be in meeting the objective, cost, time, and feasibility.

spread Active dissemination of best practice and knowledge gained from the continuous quality improvement process so that individual healthcare organizations can apply them.

stakeholder Any party that has a strong enough interest in an issue to want to give input and engage in actions relating to the issue.

standard A measure, determined by a professional body, of practice, service, or education.

standardization Efforts to make work consistent by regulating procedures, equipment, supplies, and so on.

STEEEP A quality improvement framework that is based on the six aims identified in the *Quality Chasm* series (safety, timeliness, effectiveness, efficiency, equity, patient-centeredness).

strategic plan A plan relating to the quality improvement program that considers long-term goals and outcomes, noting the gaps or what needs to be improved over time.

stress An adverse human experience that occurs when demands exceed the person's resources.

structure The manner in which the parts of the healthcare system's elements are put together and come together to impact quality.

structure measure/indicator A means by which an organization evaluates its resources and how well those resources function as a system.

supervision The act of directing, guiding, and evaluating performance.

surveillance Oversight of patient care intended to prevent adverse outcomes.

swiss cheese model A model for understanding errors that focuses on system failure and recognizes that there is potential for an error in any process.

system thinking Seeing the whole, how its parts interrelate, and how these parts all impact workflow.

systematic review A summary of evidence focused on a specific clinical question that provides critical appraisal of the evidence to determine if bias exists.

tally sheet See *check sheet*.

teach-back The act of asking patients to repeat something they have been told to ensure the message was properly received.

teamSTEPPS A method designed to optimize patient care by using training approaches and relevant materials to improve communication and teamwork skills among healthcare professionals, including frontline staff.

technical failure A source of error attributed to unavailable or malfunctioning physical equipment.

30-day unplanned readmission Unplanned readmission of a patient to an acute care setting within 30 days of discharge.

time-out A method used to stop work or care when staff are concerned there is risk or an error has occurred.

transformational leadership An approach to leadership focused on improving care for patients and also improving the organization's work environment. This approach emphasizes that all staff, whether in formal management positions or not (including staff nurses), need to understand leadership to work effectively in the healthcare environment.

triple aim A quality improvement framework that is designed to (1) improve the patient experience of care, (2) improve the health of populations, and (3) reduce the per capita cost of health care.

underuse Failure to provide a service that would have produced a favorable outcome for the patient.

universal protocol A step-by-step protocol to prevent wrong site, wrong procedure, or wrong person surgery.

utilization review/management An assessment routinely performed by a healthcare organization to collect data about use of services.

validity The degree to which an evaluation method measures the intended variable.

value stream mapping A means of assessing care quality that documents, analyzes, and improves the flow of information or supplies that are needed to complete a process or produce a product.

veracity The principle that patients should be told the truth.

workaround The act of avoiding a work-related problem instead of addressing and resolving it.

workflow The sequencing of tasks involved in a work process.

workplace learning An educational approach that allows individuals or groups to acquire, interpret, reorganize, change, or assimilate a related cluster of information, skills, and feelings, and a means by which individuals construct meaning in their personal and shared organizational lives.

workplace violence A work-related event that is physically and/or psychologically distressing to an employee.

Index

Note: Page numbers followed by *f*, *t* and *b* indicates figures, tables and boxes respectively.